Review Papers in Big Data, Cloud-Based Data Analysis and Learning Systems

Review Papers in Big Data, Cloud-Based Data Analysis and Learning Systems

Editors

Domenico Talia
Fabrizio Marozzo

MDPI • Basel • Beijing • Wuhan • Barcelona • Belgrade • Manchester • Tokyo • Cluj • Tianjin

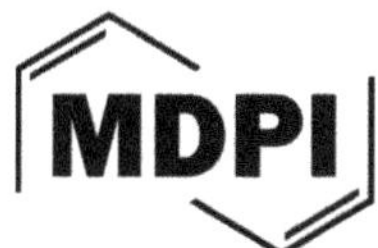

Editors
Domenico Talia
University of Calabria
Rende, Italy

Fabrizio Marozzo
University of Calabria
Rende, Italy

Editorial Office
MDPI
St. Alban-Anlage 66
4052 Basel, Switzerland

This is a reprint of articles from the Special Issue published online in the open access journal *Big Data and Cognitive Computing* (ISSN 2504-2289) (available at: https://www.mdpi.com/journal/BDCC/special_issues/Review_Big_Data).

For citation purposes, cite each article independently as indicated on the article page online and as indicated below:

LastName, A.A.; LastName, B.B.; LastName, C.C. Article Title. *Journal Name* **Year**, *Volume Number*, Page Range.

ISBN 978-3-0365-8000-5 (Hbk)
ISBN 978-3-0365-8001-2 (PDF)

Contents

About the Editors . . . . **vii**

Fabrizio Marozzo and Domenico Talia
Perspectives on Big Data, Cloud-Based Data Analysis and Machine Learning Systems
Reprinted from: *Big Data Cogn. Comput.* **2023**, *7*, 104, doi:10.3390/bdcc7020104 . . . . **1**

Hafiz Suliman Munawar, Fahim Ullah, Siddra Qayyum and Danish Shahzad
Big Data in Construction: Current Applications and Future Opportunities
Reprinted from: *Big Data Cogn. Comput.* **2022**, *6*, 18, doi:10.3390/bdcc6010018 . . . . **5**

Athira Nambiar and Divyansh Mundra
An Overview of Data Warehouse and Data Lake in Modern Enterprise Data Management
Reprinted from: *Big Data Cogn. Comput.* **2022**, *6*, 132, doi:10.3390/bdcc6040132 . . . . **33**

Andrea Ponti, Ilaria Giordani, Matteo Mistri, Antonio Candelieri and Francesco Archetti
The "Unreasonable" Effectiveness of the Wasserstein Distance in Analyzing Key Performance
Indicators of a Network of Stores
Reprinted from: *Big Data Cogn. Comput.* **2022**, *6*, 138, doi:10.3390/bdcc6040138 . . . . **57**

**Zaher Ali Al-Sai, Mohd Heikal Husin, Sharifah Mashita Syed-Mohamad,
Rasha Moh'd Sadeq Abdin, Nour Damer, Laith Abualigah and Amir H. Gandomi**
Explore Big Data Analytics Applications and Opportunities: A Review
Reprinted from: *Big Data Cogn. Comput.* **2022**, *6*, 157, doi:10.3390/bdcc6040157 . . . . **71**

**Krithika Latha Bhaskaran, Richard Sakyi Osei, Evans Kotei, Eric Yaw Agbezuge,
Carlos Ankora and Ernest D. Ganaa**
A Survey on Big Data in Pharmacology, Toxicology and Pharmaceutics
Reprinted from: *Big Data Cogn. Comput.* **2022**, *6*, 161, doi:10.3390/bdcc6040161 . . . . **95**

**Khaled H. Almotairi, Ahmad MohdAziz Hussein, Laith Abualigah, Sohaib K. M. Abujayyab,
Emad Hamdi Mahmoud, Bassam Omar Ghanem and Amir H. Gandomi**
Impact of Artificial Intelligence on COVID-19 Pandemic: A Survey of Image Processing,
Tracking of Disease, Prediction of Outcomes, and Computational Medicine
Reprinted from: *Big Data Cogn. Comput.* **2023**, *7*, 11, doi:10.3390/bdcc7010011 . . . . **115**

Eugenio Cesario, Paolo Lindia and Andrea Vinci
Detecting Multi-Density Urban Hotspots in a Smart City: Approaches, Challenges and
Applications
Reprinted from: *Philosophies* **2023**, *7*, 29, doi:10.3390/bdcc7010029 . . . . **133**

Vincenzo Barbuto, Claudio Savaglio, Min Chen and Giancarlo Fortino
Disclosing Edge Intelligence: A Systematic Meta-Survey
Reprinted from: *Philosophies* **2023**, *7*, 44, doi:10.3390/bdcc7010044 . . . . **151**

Nisrine Berros, Fatna El Mendili, Youness Filaly and Younes El Bouzekri El Idrissi
Enhancing Digital Health Services with Big Data Analytics
Reprinted from: *Big Data Cogn. Comput.* **2023**, *7*, 64, doi:10.3390/bdcc7020064 . . . . **171**

Giuseppe Agapito and Mario Cannataro
An Overview on the Challenges and Limitations Using Cloud Computing in Healthcare
Corporations
Reprinted from: *Philosophies* **2023**, *7*, 68, doi:10.3390/bdcc7020068 . . . . **195**

About the Editors

Domenico Talia

Domenico Talia is a professor of computer engineering at the University of Calabria and an honorary professor at Noida University. He is a member of the editorial boards of Computer, Future Generation Computer Systems, IEEE Transactions on Parallel and Distributed Systems, ACM Computing Surveys, the Journal of Cloud Computing-Advances, Systems and Applications, and the International Journal of Next-Generation Computing. His research interests include parallel and distributed data mining algorithms, cloud computing, machine learning, big data, peer-to-peer systems, and parallel programming models. On these research topics, he has published more than 400 papers and several books. Prof. Talia is a senior member of ACM and IEEE.

Fabrizio Marozzo

Fabrizio Marozzo is an assistant professor of computer engineering at the University of Calabria. He received a Ph.D. in systems and computer engineering at the University of Calabria. In 2011–2012, he visited the Barcelona SuperComputing Center for a research internship with the Grid Computer Research group in the Computer Sciences department. He is a member of the editorial boards of several journals including IEEE Access, IEEE Transactions on Big Data, Journal of Big Data, SN Computer Science, and Big Data and Cognitive Computing. His research focuses on big data analysis, social media analysis, parallel and distributed computing, cloud and edge computing, and machine learning.

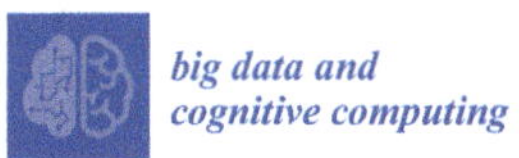

big data and cognitive computing

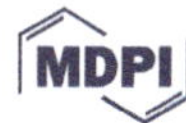

Editorial

Perspectives on Big Data, Cloud-Based Data Analysis and Machine Learning Systems

Fabrizio Marozzo * and Domenico Talia

Department of Informatics, Modeling, Electronics and Systems (DIMES), University of Calabria, 87036 Rende, Italy; talia@dimes.unical.it
* Correspondence: fmarozzo@dimes.unical.it

Citation: Marozzo, F.; Talia, D. Perspectives on Big Data, Cloud-Based Data Analysis and Machine Learning Systems. *Big Data Cogn. Comput.* **2023**, *7*, 104. https://doi.org/10.3390/bdcc7020104

Received: 23 May 2023
Accepted: 24 May 2023
Published: 30 May 2023

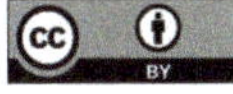

1. Introduction

Huge amounts of digital data are continuously generated and collected from different sources, such as sensors, cameras, in-vehicle infotainment, smart meters, mobile devices, social media platforms, and web applications and services [1]. Those data volumes, commonly referred to as big data, hold immense potential for extracting valuable information and generating useful knowledge in the fields of science, industry, and public services [1,2]. Extracting useful knowledge from huge digital datasets requires smart and scalable analytics algorithms, services, programming tools, and applications. Advanced data analysis techniques and tools are helping to extract patterns, trends, and hidden knowledge from big, complex datasets. Progress in this area is very useful for enabling businesses and research collaborators alike to make informed decisions.

The combination of big data analytics and knowledge discovery techniques with scalable computing systems is an effective strategy for producing new insights in a shorter period of time. Novel technologies, architectures, and algorithms have been developed to manage and analyze big data [3], enabling researchers and data scientists to extract useful information and knowledge to make new discoveries and support decision-making processes [4]. Many researchers have focused on the development of applications for big data analysis in various application fields, including trend discovery, social media analytics, pattern mining, sentiment analysis, and opinion mining. For example, from the analysis of large amounts of user data we can understand human dynamics and behaviors including (i) the main tourist attractions and mobility patterns within a city [5]; (ii) the areas of a city where it is necessary to improve the means of transport [6] or where it is more suitable to open new businesses [7]; (iii) the purchase behavior of users while browsing an ecommerce site [8]; (iv) the behavior of fans following important sporting events [9]; and (v) the political orientation of citizens and estimating the outcome of a political event [10]. To this end, the use of advanced and scalable algorithms, along with parallel programming frameworks and high-performance computers, is commonly used to solve big data problems and obtain valuable information and learning processes in a reasonable time.

From this perspective, this Special Issue aims to contribute to the field by presenting review/survey papers and original research articles in the fields of big data, cloud-based data analysis, and learning systems. Ten papers have been accepted for publication to this Special Issue, which focus on different topics.

The first paper [11] proposes the analysis of urban data to discover multi-density hotspots in metropolitan areas. It examines the limitations of traditional density-based clustering algorithms in handling multi-density data and highlights the need for more suitable techniques. By comparing four approaches (DBSCAN, OPTICS-xi, HDBSCAN, and CHD) for clustering urban data, the study evaluates their performance on state-of-the-art and real-world datasets. The findings demonstrate that multi-density clustering algorithms outperform classic density-based algorithms, providing more accurate results for urban data analysis.

The second paper [12] proposes a novel approach for analyzing customer data in large retail companies. Traditionally, customer behavior is analyzed using simple parameters such as average and variance, which fail to capture the increasing heterogeneity among customers. To address this limitation, the paper suggests representing customer survey samples as discrete probability distributions and assessing their similarities using different models. The study focuses on the Wasserstein distance, a well-defined and interpretable metric for comparing distributions, and on multiple Key Performance Indicators per store. Experimental results using real customer data validate the effectiveness of this approach in providing meaningful global performance measures.

The third paper [13] addresses the challenges and issues associated with the widespread adoption of cloud computing in healthcare corporations for analyzing big data. Technological advancements have facilitated the storage of massive amounts of data, and cloud computing has offered an ideal solution for handling such large datasets by ensuring effective data analysis, sharing, and access; however, the security and privacy of data pose significant concerns, especially when dealing with patients' data. The objective of this study is to highlight the security challenges that hinder the widespread adoption of cloud computing in healthcare corporations.

The fourth paper [14] explores the application of big data in the field of digital health, considering the vast amount of imaging data generated in different medical contexts. The study focuses on recent research efforts in big data analysis within the health domain, along with technical and organizational challenges. Furthermore, a general strategy is proposed for medical organizations seeking to adopt or leverage big data analytics. The study aims to provide healthcare organizations and institutions, both considering and utilizing big data analytics, with a comprehensive understanding of its potential applications, effective targeting, and expected impact.

The fifth paper [15] examines the integration of artificial intelligence technologies to help curb the spread of the COVID-19 pandemic. It assesses various applications and deployments of modern technology, including image processing, disease tracking, outcome prediction, and computational medicine. A comprehensive search of COVID-19-related technology databases was conducted, and the findings were reviewed to explore the potential of technology in addressing the pandemic. While there is existing research on the use of technology for COVID-19, the full extent of its application is still being explored. The study also identifies open research issues and challenges in deploying AI technology to combat the global pandemic.

The sixth paper [16] explores the utilization of big data in healthcare and drug detection sectors. Here the challenge lies in managing and extracting valuable insights from the enormous amount of data generated by patients, hospitals, sensors, and healthcare organizations. Big data has the potential to transform drug development and safety testing in pharmacology, toxicology, and pharmaceutics by providing deeper insights into drug effects on human health; however, challenges include specialized skills and infrastructure requirements. The survey highlights the current applications, challenges, and solutions in using big data in these fields, emphasizing the need for further research.

The seventh paper [17] reviews the literature on big data applications and analytics, highlighting their importance in making strategic decisions, particularly during the COVID-19 pandemic. It compares the use of big data applications in different industry fields (healthcare, education, transportation, and banking) before and during the pandemic. The paper emphasizes the significance of aligning big data applications with relevant analytics models in the COVID-19 era, as they can address the limitations faced by organizations. Additionally, the critical challenges of big data analytics and applications during the pandemic have been investigated.

The eighth paper [18] offers a comprehensive overview of two popular data management platforms in the area of big data analytics: data warehouses and data lakes. It covers the definitions and features of these platforms and existing research related to them, along with architecture and design considerations. The paper concludes by discussing challenges and suggesting promising research directions for the future.

The ninth paper [19] examines the role of big data in the construction industry, exploring trends and identifying opportunities for improvement. Despite the availability of data and digital technologies such as CAD and BIM, the construction industry has been slow in utilizing big data effectively. The paper analyzes the existing literature to highlight gaps and explore ways that big data analysis and storage can be applied in the construction sector, and suggests future opportunities in areas such as construction safety, site management, heritage conservation, and project waste minimization and quality improvements.

Finally, the tenth paper [20] focuses on the emerging paradigm of Edge Intelligence (EI) as a solution to overcome the limitations of cloud computing in the development and provision of IoT services. It conducts a systematic analysis of the state-of-the-art literature on EI, including literature reviews, surveys, and mapping studies, following the PRISMA methodology. The paper provides a comparison framework and identifies research questions to explore the past, present, and future directions of the EI paradigm and its relationship with IoT and cloud computing. The analysis aims to benefit both experts and beginners in understanding and advancing the field of EI.

2. Future Research Directions

Solving problems in science and engineering was the first motivation for inventing computers capable of calculating complex formulas and equations. Today, science and engineering are still the main areas in which innovative solutions and technologies are being developed and applied, although business and industry play a key role in the exploitation of advanced computing solutions. As the data scale increases, we must address new challenges and attack ever-larger problems. New discoveries will be achieved and more accurate investigations can be carried out due to the increasingly widespread availability of large amounts of data and of high-performance computer systems.

Within the scope of this Special Issue, there are several promising research directions that warrant further exploration, particularly in the area of big data and cloud-based data analysis. One significant area is the effective management and extraction of insights from vast-scale data archives. For instance, a pertinent challenge involves designing and optimizing data-intensive computing platforms capable of accommodating an extensive number of CPU cores, such as those of exascale systems [21,22]. These systems demand the management of millions of threads across an extensive array of cores to ensure optimal performance. To achieve this, it becomes imperative for data-intensive applications to minimize synchronization, reduce communication and remote memory usage, and adeptly handle potential software and hardware faults. Presently, no existing programming languages, frameworks, or infrastructures offer comprehensive solutions to tackle exascale complex issues, especially when it comes to data-intensive applications. For these reasons, in the coming years there will be a pressing need to develop new tools and technologies to unlock the full potential of exascale systems and realize their potential in pushing forward the boundaries of scientific research, big data analytics, and computational simulations.

Another significant area of attention lies in the convergence of high-performance computing (HPC), data analytics (DA), and artificial intelligence (AI) [23] for the analysis of large volumes of data. The expansion of traditional HPC applications to encompass DA and AI tasks raises challenges due to the lack of suitable programming models, environments, and deployment tools for seamless integration. To address these new challenges, ongoing efforts are focused on developing new platforms that leverage specialized software stacks capable of effectively managing big data applications and workflows. Embracing these advancements will facilitate the seamless integration of HPC, DA, and AI, resulting in the improved efficiency and scalability of big data application execution in large-scale computing environments.

Conflicts of Interest: The authors declare no conflict of interest.

References

1. Belcastro, L.; Marozzo, F.; Talia, D. Programming Models and Systems for Big Data Analysis. *Int. J. Parallel Emergent Distrib. Syst.* **2019**, *34*, 632–652. [CrossRef]
2. Sagiroglu, S.; Sinanc, D. Big data: A review. In Proceedings of the 2013 International Conference on Collaboration Technologies and Systems (CTS), San Diego, CA, USA, 20–24 May 2013; pp. 42–47.
3. Belcastro, L.; Cantini, R.; Marozzo, F.; Orsino, A.; Talia, D.; Trunfio, P. Programming Big Data Analysis: Principles and Solutions. *J. Big Data* **2022**, *9*, 4. [CrossRef]
4. Talia, D.; Trunfio, P.; Marozzo, F. *Data Analysis in the Cloud: Models, Techniques and Applications*, 1st ed.; Elsevier Science Publishers B.V.: Amsterdam, The Netherlands, 2015.
5. Belcastro, L.; Marozzo, F.; Talia, D.; Trunfio, P. G-RoI: Automatic Region-of-Interest detection driven by geotagged social media data. *ACM Trans. Knowl. Discov. Data* **2018**, *12*, 27. [CrossRef]
6. You, L.; Motta, G.; Sacco, D.; Ma, T. Social data analysis framework in cloud and Mobility Analyzer for Smarter Cities. In Proceedings of the 2014 IEEE International Conference on Service Operations and Logistics, and Informatics, Qingdao, China, 8–10 October 2014; pp. 96–101.
7. Ancillai, C.; Terho, H.; Cardinali, S.; Pascucci, F. Advancing Social Media Driven Sales Research: Establishing Conceptual Foundations for B-to-B Social Selling. *Ind. Mark. Manag.* **2019**, *82*, 293–308. [CrossRef]
8. Branda, F.; Marozzo, F.; Talia, D. Ticket Sales Prediction and Dynamic Pricing Strategies in Public Transport. *Big Data Cogn. Comput.* **2020**, *4*, 36. [CrossRef]
9. Cesario, E.; Marozzo, F.; Talia, D.; Trunfio, P. SMA4TD: A Social Media Analysis Methodology for Trajectory Discovery in Large-Scale Events. *Online Soc. Netw. Media* **2017**, *3–4*, 49–62. [CrossRef]
10. Marozzo, F.; Bessi, A. Analyzing Polarization of Social Media Users and News Sites during Political Campaigns. *Soc. Netw. Anal. Min.* **2018**, *8*, 1–13. [CrossRef]
11. Cesario, E.; Lindia, P.; Vinci, A. Detecting Multi-Density Urban Hotspots in a Smart City: Approaches, Challenges and Applications. *Big Data Cogn. Comput.* **2023**, *7*, 29. [CrossRef]
12. Ponti, A.; Giordani, I.; Mistri, M.; Candelieri, A.; Archetti, F. The "Unreasonable" Effectiveness of the Wasserstein Distance in Analyzing Key Performance Indicators of a Network of Stores. *Big Data Cogn. Comput.* **2022**, *6*, 138. [CrossRef]
13. Agapito, G.; Cannataro, M. An Overview on the Challenges and Limitations Using Cloud Computing in Healthcare Corporations. *Big Data Cogn. Comput.* **2023**, *7*, 68. [CrossRef]
14. Berros, N.; El Mendili, F.; Filaly, Y.; El Bouzekri El Idrissi, Y. Enhancing Digital Health Services with Big Data Analytics. *Big Data Cogn. Comput.* **2023**, *7*, 64. [CrossRef]
15. Almotairi, K.H.; Hussein, A.M.; Abualigah, L.; Abujayyab, S.K.M.; Mahmoud, E.H.; Ghanem, B.O.; Gandomi, A.H. Impact of Artificial Intelligence on COVID-19 Pandemic: A Survey of Image Processing, Tracking of Disease, Prediction of Outcomes, and Computational Medicine. *Big Data Cogn. Comput.* **2023**, *7*, 11. [CrossRef]
16. Latha Bhaskaran, K.; Osei, R.S.; Kotei, E.; Agbezuge, E.Y.; Ankora, C.; Ganaa, E.D. A Survey on Big Data in Pharmacology, Toxicology and Pharmaceutics. *Big Data Cogn. Comput.* **2022**, *6*, 161. [CrossRef]
17. Al-Sai, Z.A.; Husin, M.H.; Syed-Mohamad, S.M.; Abdin, R.M.S.; Damer, N.; Abualigah, L.; Gandomi, A.H. Explore Big Data Analytics Applications and Opportunities: A Review. *Big Data Cogn. Comput.* **2022**, *6*, 157. [CrossRef]
18. Nambiar, A.; Mundra, D. An Overview of Data Warehouse and Data Lake in Modern Enterprise Data Management. *Big Data Cogn. Comput.* **2022**, *6*, 132. [CrossRef]
19. Munawar, H.S.; Ullah, F.; Qayyum, S.; Shahzad, D. Big Data in Construction: Current Applications and Future Opportunities. *Big Data Cogn. Comput.* **2022**, *6*, 18. [CrossRef]
20. Barbuto, V.; Savaglio, C.; Chen, M.; Fortino, G. Disclosing Edge Intelligence: A Systematic Meta-Survey. *Big Data Cogn. Comput.* **2023**, *7*, 44. [CrossRef]
21. Da Costa, G.; Fahringer, T.; Rico-Gallego, J.A.; Grasso, I.; Hristov, A.; Karatza, H.D.; Lastovetsky, A.; Marozzo, F.; Petcu, D.; Stavrinides, G.L.; et al. Exascale machines require new programming paradigms and runtimes. *Supercomput. Front. Innov.* **2015**, *2*, 6–27.
22. Talia, D.; Trunfio, P.; Marozzo, F.; Belcastro, L.; Garcia-Blas, J.; del Rio, D.; Couvée, P.; Goret, G.; Vincent, L.; Fernández-Pena, A.; et al. A Novel Data-Centric Programming Model for Large-Scale Parallel Systems. In Proceedings of the Euro-Par 2019: Parallel Processing Workshops, Göttingen, Germany, 26–30 August 2019; pp. 452–463.
23. Ejarque, J.; Badia, R.M.; Albertin, L.; Aloisio, G.; Baglione, E.; Becerra, Y.; Boschert, S.; Berlin, J.R.; D'Anca, A.; Elia, D.; et al. Enabling dynamic and intelligent workflows for HPC, data analytics, and AI convergence. *Future Gener. Comput. Syst.* **2022**, *134*, 414–429. [CrossRef]

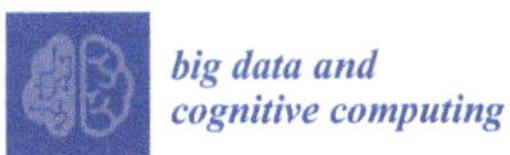
big data and cognitive computing

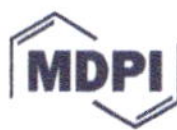

Review

Big Data in Construction: Current Applications and Future Opportunities

Hafiz Suliman Munawar [1], Fahim Ullah [2,*], Siddra Qayyum [1] and Danish Shahzad [3]

[1] School of the Built Environment, University of New South Wales, Sydney, NSW 2052, Australia; h.munawar@unsw.edu.au (H.S.M.); s.qayyum@unsw.edu.au (S.Q.)
[2] School of Surveying and Built Environment, University of Southern Queensland, Springfield Central, QLD 4300, Australia
[3] Department of Visual Computing, University of Saarland, 66123 Saarbrücken, Germany; dani.shahzad87@gmail.com
* Correspondence: fahim.ullah@usq.edu.au

Abstract: Big data have become an integral part of various research fields due to the rapid advancements in the digital technologies available for dealing with data. The construction industry is no exception and has seen a spike in the data being generated due to the introduction of various digital disruptive technologies. However, despite the availability of data and the introduction of such technologies, the construction industry is lagging in harnessing big data. This paper critically explores literature published since 2010 to identify the data trends and how the construction industry can benefit from big data. The presence of tools such as computer-aided drawing (CAD) and building information modelling (BIM) provide a great opportunity for researchers in the construction industry to further improve how infrastructure can be developed, monitored, or improved in the future. The gaps in the existing research data have been explored and a detailed analysis was carried out to identify the different ways in which big data analysis and storage work in relevance to the construction industry. Big data engineering (BDE) and statistics are among the most crucial steps for integrating big data technology in construction. The results of this study suggest that while the existing research studies have set the stage for improving big data research, the integration of the associated digital technologies into the construction industry is not very clear. Among the future opportunities, big data research into construction safety, site management, heritage conservation, and project waste minimization and quality improvements are key areas.

Keywords: big data; big data engineering; construction big data; digital technologies; construction industry

Citation: Munawar, H.S.; Ullah, F.; Qayyum, S.; Shahzad, D. Big Data in Construction: Current Applications and Future Opportunities. *Big Data Cogn. Comput.* **2022**, *6*, 18. https://doi.org/10.3390/bdcc6010018

Academic Editors: Domenico Talia and Fabrizio Marozzo

Received: 6 December 2021
Accepted: 3 February 2022
Published: 6 February 2022

Publisher's Note: MDPI stays neutral with regard to jurisdictional claims in published maps and institutional affiliations.

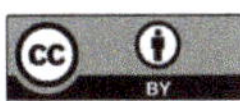

1. Introduction

Big data are increasingly becoming an integral part of almost all fields. The rapidity with which data is generated and piled up in the era of disruptive digital technologies is astounding [1]. Such big data have necessitated the need for efficient data management tools and techniques to deal with the bulk of data. Recently, a great deal of focus has been dedicated to using, storing, and managing big data in various fields [2]. The rise of interest in big data is associated with the easy availability of technology such as smartphones and computers across the globe [3]. The bulk of data generated daily through these technologies has made various researchers interested in using the data for innovative purposes and moving away from traditional time-consuming questionnaire-based approaches for data collection to more digital data management. Algorithm development, machine learning (ML), statistical analysis, and computational model development are among the various techniques that depend on data that can be easily gathered by day-to-day usage gadgets [4,5]. The presence of bulks of data makes it possible for researchers to make informed decisions and conduct relevant analyses for their field of study.

Construction is a data-intensive sector where the bulk of data is generated and not capitalized on adequately due to slow technology adoption [6]. Accordingly, it is not surprising to see the construction sector lagging behind the technology curve by more than five years which is rather slow considering the day-to-day innovations and disruptions brought about by the booming information technology industry [7]. Moreover, big data, a relatively new technology, are not properly adopted by construction. In fact, construction big data management is in its nascency and has a long way to go to mature. However, multiple studies [6,8] show that the potential is enormous if construction big data are fully utilized.

There are various steps involved in using big data, including data acquisition, storage, classification, and refining [8]. These steps are handled through various software programs to refine the associated big data and make it usable for research and practical purposes [9–11]. The biggest challenge in big data management is identifying which data is useful and vice versa through data refinement [12,13]. The immense amounts of data easily available make it hard to identify the datasets used for a particular purpose. Moreover, the available data format may not be ready for use or easily readable for the intended purpose [14,15]. These barriers to accessing, understanding, and utilizing big data make it important to develop systems for extracting key information and analyzing it [16]. In addition, the strategic sorting and analysis of big data have opened up new avenues of research by widening the need to use data appropriately [17]. In the case of construction, some barriers to big data adoption include latency, data privacy, data availability, data governance, poor broadband connectivity at construction sites, and cost implication for long-term use. For instance, big data adoption in construction may have latency issues with lower transfer rate and response time required due to software issues or network problems which may be a hurdle for some time-sensitive construction applications [18].

Furthermore, there is an increase in vulnerability in technology adoption due to the fluidity of security parameters. Storing construction design and financial information in shared resources concerns the construction industry [19]. Afolabi et al. [20] assessed the economies of big data in project delivery and included poor network connect among the threats to adoption by the construction industry.

Sorting big data requires developing database designs that would automate picking the most useful data for a given purpose [21]. Identifying a design that works best for data sorting is an entire research area on its own and has helped expand big data research by a great deal [22]. Currently, the biggest question concerning researchers in the field of big data is to find a way that creates seamless coordination between database systems such that they can hold big data, help process it, and possibly lead to an error-free statistical analysis [23]. Removing the current limitations in understanding big data will enable scientists to utilize the readily available data and make better decisions.

The construction industry is also benefiting from big data in a way that has revolutionized its traditional operational methods to a more automated process. The presence of digital tools and technologies for designing and executing construction projects has made the construction industry take enormous leaps in the last two decades. The possibility of modeling building structures and identifying the functionality of those structures before they are built has led to industrial investments in big data and related technologies [24,25]. Computer-aided design (CAD), such as building information modelling (BIM), is a term now synonymous with the construction industry [26]. The three-dimensional modeling of buildings and other construction infrastructures leads to the generation of digital files which can be stored in various formats, leading to a bulk of data generation [27]. Other digital innovations such as digital twins, 3D laser scanning, and advanced wearable gadgets incorporated in hats, shoes, gloves, and other sensor-based tools have revolutionized the construction industry and helped generate useful big data.

Big data in the construction industry can accumulate quickly and become storage heavy due to the large size of the 3D modeling files and a huge amount of daily data generated by wearable gadgets [28]. Management of such big data is a hectic but essential task as the usefulness of the models lies in ensuring that they are available for viewing and leveraging as and when needed. Apart from providing the ease of modeling infrastructure, big data also provide the opportunity to develop sustainable structures by using test models before actual constructions. These are made possible by using digital twins, geographical information systems (GIS)-based 3D point cloud structures, and other cloud-based scanning systems. Furthermore, the software that enables CAD and BIM further feeds into the databases and contributes to big data. All these variables lead to the possibility of utilizing technology for sustainable construction and associated development in line with the United Nations sustainable development goals and other local development initiatives.

The applications of big data in the construction industry are immense. Identifying how big data can be applied to the construction industry remains the real challenge. Since each construction project leads to more data generation, it is crucial to analyze and sort the data accordingly. Some of the key features within the construction industry that can benefit from big data include construction safety, efficiency, waste minimization, productivity, competitive advantage, and pollution management [29]. The strategic and operational benefits of big data in the construction industry have further been explored by Atuahene et al. [30]. The major benefits of big data were found to be project management, management of claims, and procurement. These aspects of big data application are crucial for managing construction projects. However, many other aspects and applications of big data within the construction industry still need to be explored. While these different aspects of construction projects benefit from big data, it is important to understand how big data can be analyzed and utilized for different projects. Furthermore, the algorithms and frameworks that can integrate big data in the construction industry remain largely unexplored.

Today, studies on construction and its management in relation to big data are scarce, presenting a gap in research. This provides opportunities for further research that can greatly benefit the construction industry in the long run. This gap is targeted in the current study, where the papers published in construction fields focused on big data since 2010 are studied. The key takeaways of these studies are presented here to help the construction researchers build upon these studies and advance the state of research related to big data in construction.

In terms of implications, this study will help both the construction researchers and practitioners, where the former will have the current state of research on big data and can see opportunities for further research. Similarly, the practitioners can ascertain the software and hardware requirements for incorporating big-data-based opportunities in construction and create implementation models and gadgets. This paper is divided into sections exploring big data engineering (BDE), databases, use of big data in construction, the application of big-data-based statistics in construction, and future opportunities for big data in construction.

Research Questions

This study aims to identify ways in which big data can be used for construction and its management based on the review of existing literature. The existing literature on big data does not provide detailed solutions for construction management, which creates a gap in the literature concerning the use of big data in the construction industry. The research questions set for this study are as follows:

- How can we use big data for research in construction engineering and management?
- How is construction big data managed and stored?
- How can big data be used for planning construction projects in a futuristic way?

The rest of the paper is organized as follows. Section 2 presents the method and materials used in the study. Section 3 presents the preliminary analyses conducted in the study. This is followed by Section 4, where the BDE and its subcomponents, including big data processing, big data storage, and big data analytics (BDA), are presented and discussed. Similarly, the 10 vs. of big data and ML techniques are also presented in this section. Section 5 presents the future opportunities for big data in construction. Finally,

Section 6 concludes the study and presents the key takeaways, limitations, and future expansion directions based on the current study.

2. Materials and Methods

This study follows a multi-stepped approach for reviewing the studies on big data in construction. First, a comprehensive literature retrieval mechanism is adopted from published literature and modified accordingly to retrieve pertinent literature on big data in construction. This is followed by analyses of the retrieved articles in the shape of preliminary analyses, BDE, processing, storage, analytics, and statistical and data mining approaches in relation to the construction industry. These steps are subsequently explained.

An extensive literature search was carried out to identify peer-reviewed papers related to big data and construction since 2010, following the approaches adopted in recent studies [31,32]. This was conducted in order to keep a recent focus and study current articles on big data in construction. Some preliminary analyses, as subsequently discussed, highlighted that big data in construction received more attention in 2010 and onwards; hence, the review period of 2010 and onwards makes sense. A number of scholarly research platforms, including Google Scholar, Scopus, Science Direct, Springer, Elsevier, and IEEE Explore, were consulted for literature search based on the high volume of high-quality research papers available on these platforms following recent studies [33–35]. Once the search engines were selected, a combination of different keywords was developed to identify the most useful publications for this study in the next step. The keyword combinations were developed in a tier-based approach, such that terms related to big data, such as "big data", "big data analysis", "big data volume", and "big data analysis tools" fell into category 1 (S1).

Similarly, all keywords pertaining to construction, such as "construction", "construction management", and "construction industry", were classified into category 2 (S2). Different combinations of keywords from both categories were used to retrieve the most relevant publications. Examples of keyword combinations include big data in construction, big data for construction management, construction management, and big data, etc.

Search category was further restricted by including only those papers that were published in 2010 or later years. Since big data technology was used robustly in the last decade, research publications prior to 2010 were left out. Concept papers, editorials, notes, perspectives, closures, discussions, conference papers, and others were also excluded from the search to ensure the inclusion of original research papers only. Other publications dealing with classical definitions were also excluded.

Using different combinations of the keywords to identify papers published from 2010 onwards led to a total of more than 10,000 papers being retrieved from the mentioned search engines. The list of articles was narrowed down using the detailed inclusion criteria set for this study. This included removing duplicates and other exclusions, as previously mentioned, which brought the search results down to around 4000 papers. This was further narrowed down in a stepwise manner to ensure that only those papers were included that fit the scope of the current study. In the final step, the content of the papers was analyzed to determine their suitability for this study, resulting in a total of 156 papers.

Figure 1 shows an overview of the different ways in which research studies have addressed the use of big data in construction. There has been a rise in the interest in big data usage for the construction industry since 2016. However, the interest has been limited in terms of analyses scope as the trends have remained steady. As shown in Figure 1, the publications on this topic have followed similar terms and research themes over the last few years, leading to gradual evolution. For example, in 2016, most papers related to big data and construction focused on the use of cloud computing, while 2017 saw a trend of developing models and frameworks for implementing big data in the construction industry. Similarly, in 2018 and 2019, researchers have mainly explored how different big data models could be implemented within the construction industry. Recently, the research focus has shifted to using big data in real-time construction projects and identifying how these technologies could be harnessed for developing futuristic construction projects.

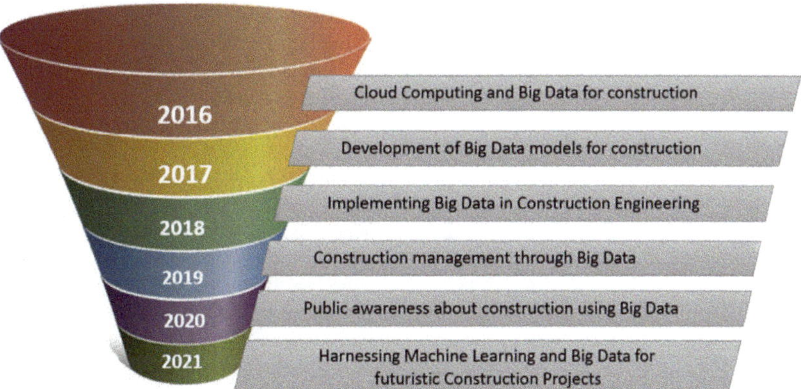

Figure 1. Funnel diagrams showing trends in big data research in construction since 2016.

In addition to big data, some other technologies and methods have been researched in the last couple of years for improving the construction industry. There is a great overlap in the types of technologies studied simultaneously for developing models that could guide future research in the construction industry. Figure 2 shows the overlapping tools and technologies identified from recent literature. It can be observed that big data is not standalone; rather, it depends on other tools and methods, including data analytics, ML, pattern recognition, statistics, deep learning, and artificial intelligence (AI). All these tools and technologies are used in different combinations for developing models that could be used in real time for construction projects. The reliance of all these tools on each other is an important factor to consider when developing construction projects as the computational aspects of the project can only be as good and true and the depth of research is performed for developing and testing the algorithms and frameworks. The construction industry greatly benefits from the overlapping fields of big data technologies. The use of big data requires data mining which generates enormous datasets. The bulk of construction-related data makes the use of statistics inevitable.

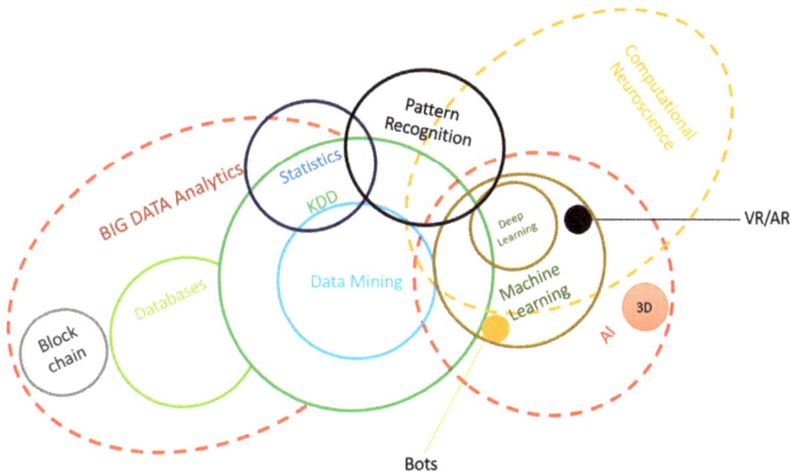

Figure 2. Overlapping fields of research contributing to big data.

Along with data management, statistical analysis, and big data analytics, several different techniques and resources come into use. For example, machine learning tools and artificial intelligence play a crucial role in the construction industry in conjunction with big data. The overlap of all the different fields shown in Figure 2 shows how the field of construction is laden with the use of different technologies, each of which is somehow associated with big data. The use of computational models, databases, deep learning, pattern recognition, virtual reality, bots, and augmented reality contributes to the application of big data in the construction industry. An in-depth analysis of the big data applications and the use of technology in the construction industry results in a much more complex overlap than shown here. However, the core aim of using different technologies is to simplify how datasets can be used to guide future construction projects. Recognizing data patterns and understanding how each dataset fits the needs of a construction project is only possible if the dataset has been analyzed, critically appraised, and classified for its specific usage. The guiding principle here is to use modern technology to upgrade and update the ways in which information could be streamlined for the benefit of different projects. For example, identifying the materials that best suit a particular structure, developing project timelines, and streamlining the resources can become much more straightforward if the construction projects are developed with the help of big data technologies.

As shown in Figure 2, different technologies in the construction industry overlap in different ways. Integrating big data in the construction industry is possible through the combined use of other technologies such as machine learning, AI, VR, AR, pattern recognition, and other such methods.

3. Preliminary Analyses

As mentioned in the method, some preliminary analyses were conducted on the retrieved articles, including the keywords analysis and the countries of origin of the articles following recently published articles [31,35]. Before this, a basic Google Trend (r) search was conducted using trends.google.com (accessed on 20 November 2021). A comparison was made for three iterations of the keywords previously mentioned. These included construction big data (keyword 1), big data in construction (keyword 2), and big data for construction management (keyword 3). As shown in Figure 3, the earliest attention paid to big data in construction was reported in 2010. This was reported for keyword 1, followed by keyword 2 in 2013 and keyword 3 in 2014. Two clusters are clearly visible from Figure 3. The initial interest cluster showed when big data focused on construction and the spike in interest cluster. The first cluster is evident in 2010–2014, whereas the spike in interest cluster started in 2016. This shows the hotness or relevance of the topic under investigation in the current study.

After the Google Trend analyses, the retrieved articles were analyzed using Vos Viewer® tool. The first analysis was that of keywords. The natural distribution of keywords retrieved from the articles shows five distinct clusters: education, city and region, disaster and human interactions, knowledge management, and technology management in relation to construction, as given in Figure 4. The overall top keywords in order of priority retrieved from these articles included big data, information management, AI, data mining, internet of things, ML, advanced analytics, data technologies, students, data handling, digital storage, colleges and universities, smart city, decision making, cloud computing, construction industry, and others. These are based on the appearance of the keywords in the titles, abstract, and keywords of a minimum of 30 papers. These keywords are in line with the natural clusters highlighted in Figure 4.

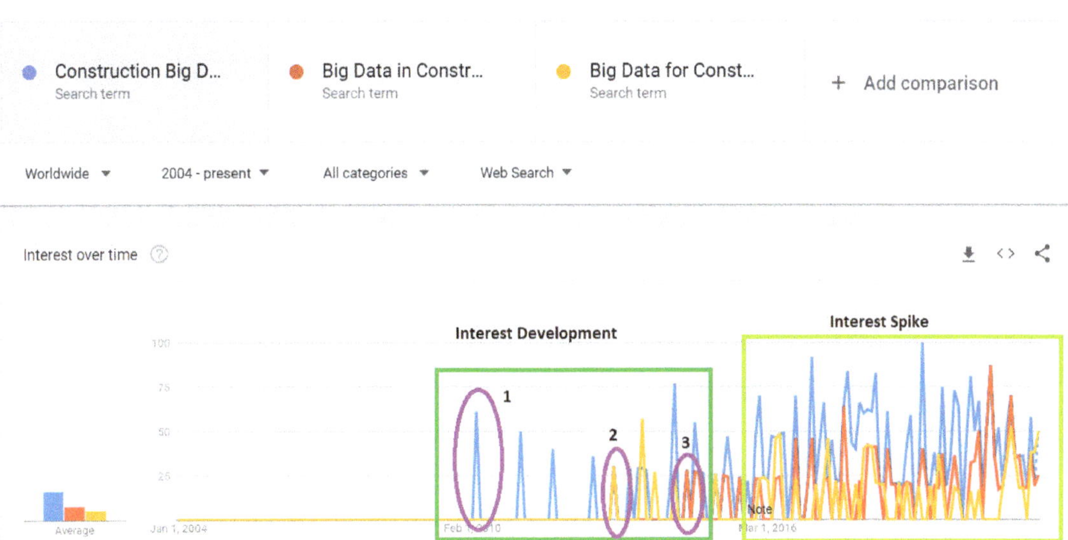

Figure 3. Google Trends analyses for big data in construction, showing interest development and spike in interest.

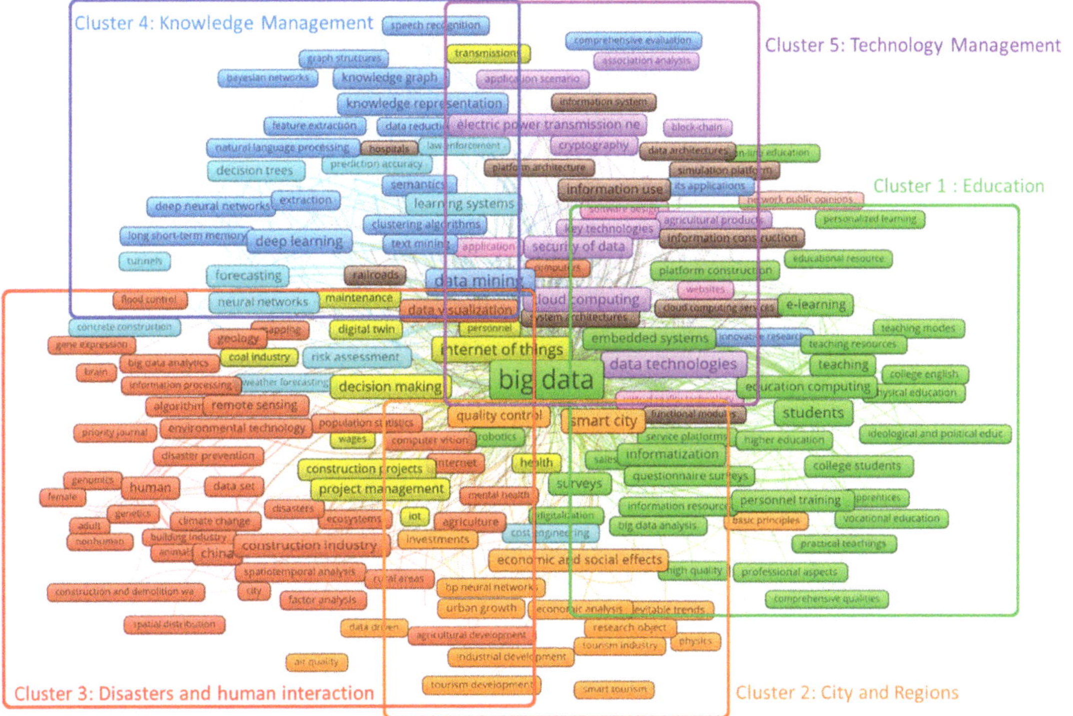

Figure 4. Five key clusters of big data in construction based on keywords reported in the reviewed literature.

In another analysis, the top 10 contributing countries to big data research in construction were investigated. These are China, United States, United Kingdom, Russian Federation, Australia, India, South Korea, Germany, Spain, and Italy in terms of the number of contributions as shown in Figure 5. The colors in the country box show the countries with the strongest collaborations, whereas the size of the box refers to the number of papers. For example, most of the papers authored by Chinese authors are in collaboration with authors from Australia, New Zealand, and Indonesia.

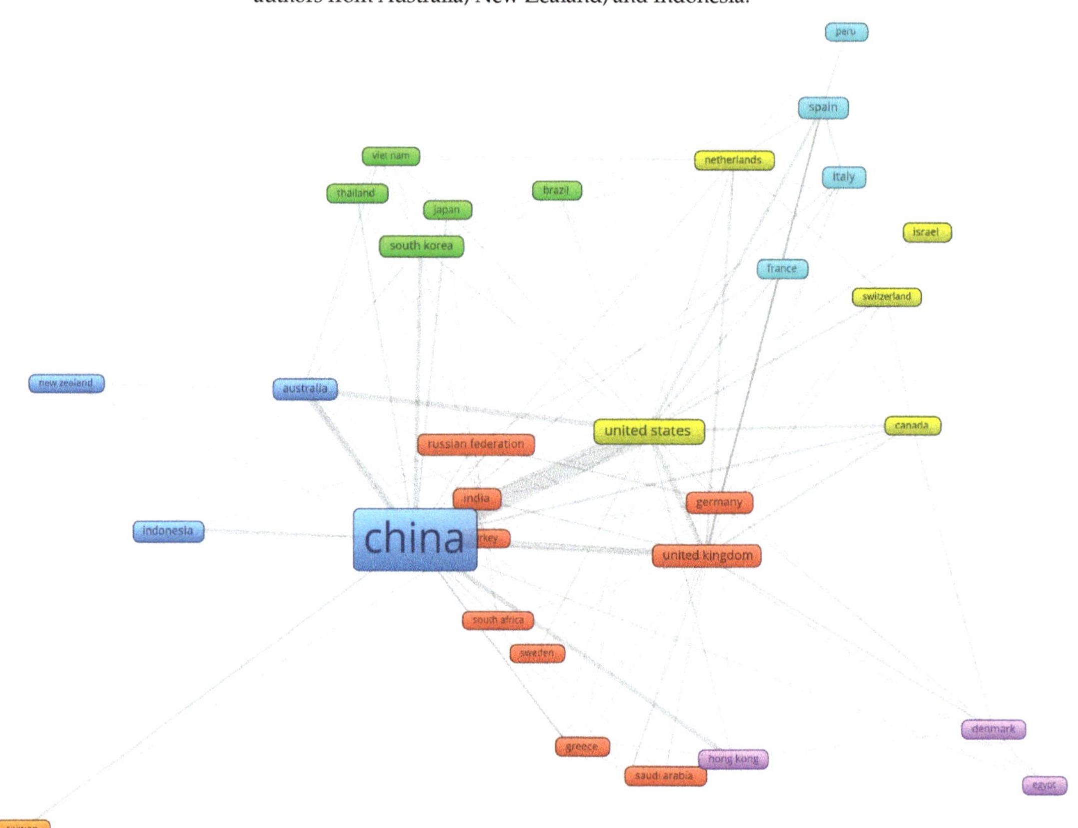

Figure 5. Countries conducting big data research in construction based on reviewed literature.

4. Big Data Engineering (BDE)

Big data analytics (BDA) is supported by BDE that provides a framework to conduct it. BDE has tremendous applications in construction. It has been used for BIM to improve project management [36]. It has also been used to improve building design and for effective performance monitoring [37], project management, safety, energy management, decision-making design frameworks, resource management [38], quality management, waste management, and others [24].

To understand BDE, it is important to discuss big data platforms. These platforms are divided into two groups based on variations in their inherent characteristics. These include horizontal scaling platforms (HSP) and vertical scaling platforms (VSP). HSP utilizes multiple servers by distributing processing across them and bringing new machines into the cluster. VSPs are single-server-based configurations that achieve the scaling by upgrading the hardware of the related server. In construction, HSPs have been used for waste management [25], profitability performance [39], smart road construction, and others [40].

Similarly, VSPs have been reported in one-off construction projects [41], transportation [42], and others. This paper focuses on HSPs, particularly Berkeley Data Analytics Stack (BDAS) and Hadoop.

Recently, BDAS has been in the limelight since it has greater performance gains over Hadoop. However, as it is quite recent, it suffers the drawback of limitation in available supporting tools. On the other side, Hadoop has been widely utilized in big data applications. The tools offered by these platforms are useful in the storage and processing of big data. For instance, Bilal et al. [39] investigated the profitability performance of construction projects using big data and used Hadoop Distributed File System (HDFS) for managing the data within the staging area while employing Resource Description Framework (RDF)-enabled Network Data Model (NDM) for storing the persistent data. Similarly, Jun Ying et al. [43] investigated the development and implementation of BDAS by the relevant building authorities in Singapore, which has enhanced knowledge and expertise in buildability. An overview of big data classification into BDE and BDA is shown in Figure 6 and subsequently explained.

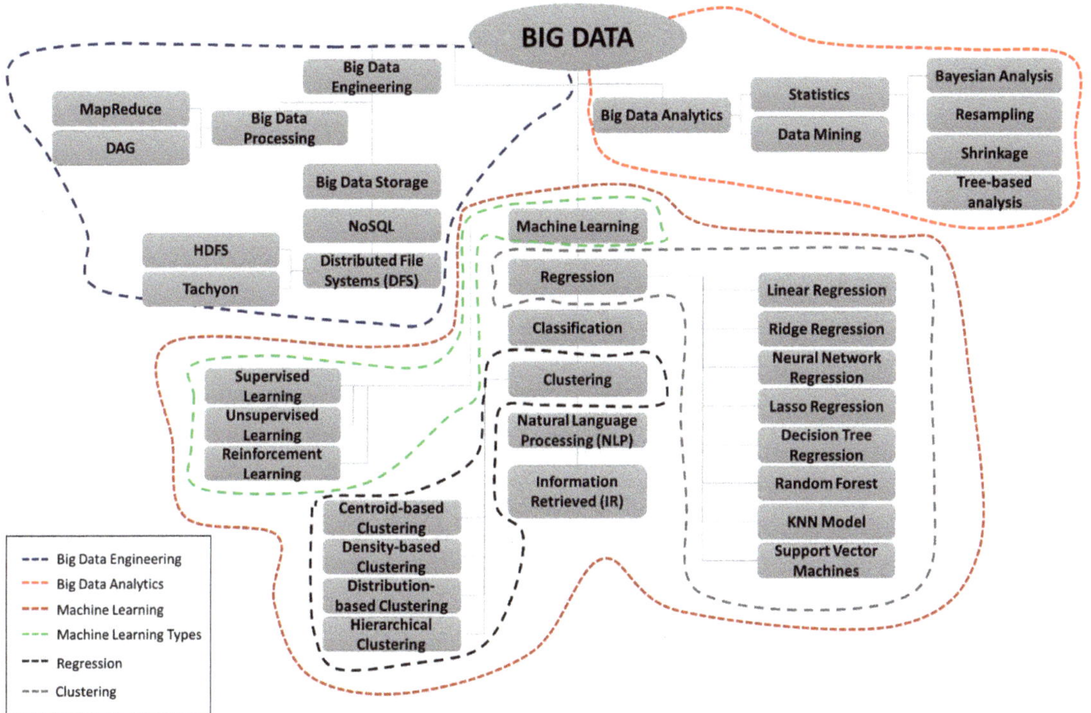

Figure 6. Classification of big data into its key domains.

Big data are classified into two major domains: BDE and BDA. These two main domains are further divided into many classes and subclasses. A third domain that comes under the canopy of big data is ML. The use of ML is inevitable in big data as the data need to be organized, analyzed, and used through ML tools and models such as deep learning and neural networks. Some of the key ML tools and models associated with big data directly or indirectly include regression analysis, clustering, classification, information retrieved (R), and natural language processing (NLP). Some examples of ML in construction include deep-learning-based flood detection and damage assessment [44], projects delay risk prediction [45], construction site safety [46], construction site monitoring [47], neural network models to predict concrete properties [48], and others.

The various algorithms and methods shown in Figure 6 all contribute towards big data in some way. The use of supervised and unsupervised learning approaches is determined depending on the type of datasets available. The major difference between supervised learning and unsupervised learning is that the algorithm for supervised learning utilizes labeled datasets while the unsupervised data do not use labeled data. The supervised and unsupervised algorithms further have different methods and examples. For instance, regression, linear regression, neural network regression, random forest, Naïve Bayes, and lasso regression are examples of supervised learning.

Similarly, clustering, Natural Language Processing (NLP), and KNN are examples of unsupervised learning. The applications of each of these algorithms can differ and hence their integration in the construction industry can vary. The regression models are used in engineering for analyzing trends and correlations between different variables. In the construction industry, these models play a crucial role as the statistical analysis and correlation development between different variables are made easy through linear regression and other similar algorithms. Similarly, machine learning models have made it possible to ensure that construction projects are developed considering safety, time management, and quality.

As shown in Figure 6, the two major big data domains rely on statistics, data processing, and data management. All these features, in turn, are heavily dependent on ML tools and methods. For example, BDE requires data processing and storage, which in turn require regression models, NoSQL, and MapReduce, all of which are different types of computational tools that enable the different applications of big data management. Similarly, BDA heavily depends on ML tools that can use data and statistics to provide organized data solutions. The use of tree-based analysis, Bayesian analysis, and shrinkage are all examples of ML integration in the field of BDA. A wide variety of ML tools have been explored over the years and have been directly or indirectly associated with big data management and analysis. Tools such as linear regression, vector machines, KNN models, clustering, and decision tree regression are among the few examples which enable the use of big data coherently. Furthermore, the classification tree of big data is likely to be further expanded as the ML algorithms are further developed and more analysis methods are added to the list. Therefore, the constant expansion of the big data analysis tools can enable the use of these tools in the construction industry for improving construction projects in the future. Yang and Yu [49] investigated the application of heterogeneous networks oriented to NoSQL database in optimal post-evaluation indexes of construction projects. NoSQL database is scalable with a powerful and flexible data model and a large amount of data and has increasing application potential in the memory field. Sanni-Anibire et al. [50] investigated the increase in delays and abandonment of tall buildings and developed a machine learning model for delay risk assessment. Methods such as K-Nearest Neighbors (KNN), Artificial Neural Networks (ANN), Support Vector Machines (SVM), and Ensemble methods were considered. The model developed for predicting the risk of delay was based on ANN with a classification accuracy of 93.75%. The key components of big data from Figure 6 for its management are discussed below.

4.1. Big Data Processing

Distributed and parallel computation is present in the core of BDE. In construction, big data processing has been utilized for waste management [51], prefabricated construction project management [52], profitability analyses, and other construction management applications [39]. For processing information, a considerable number of models are developed. Some of the key big data models are discussed below.

4.1.1. MapReduce (MR)

MapReduce was developed for the handling of big data. It utilizes a distributed processing model in which two functions, as indicated by the name itself, map and reduce, are employed to write analytical tasks. Mappers and reducers are the processes that collect the data from these functions for further processing. Initially, mappers collect and read the input information to process it for subsequent results generation. The output of mappers is used by reducers which give the results that are ultimately stored in the file system. MR has been used by Jiao et al. [53] to develop an augmented framework for BIM. Similarly, it has also been used in construction knowledge maps [54] and other big data applications [54].

The use of MapReduce in the construction industry is inevitable due to the big data applications within the construction industry. The usability of the MapReduce framework in the construction industry relies on the management of big data in a particular way. Accordingly, the datasets are analyzed and divided into categories to reduce clutter and present an easy-to-understand data output. The basic framework of MapReduce includes data input, data chunks, decomposition mappers, decomposed output, linear mappers, linear reducers, and combined output. The exact series and number of components in the framework can vary depending on the version used. However, the overall features and application of MapReduce remain the same, i.e., reduction of data into manageable chunks. The use of MapReduce not only distributes data into smaller chunks but also helps develop datasets that present a more analytic view of big data. Having organized datasets within the construction industry is of key importance as it can greatly increase the efficiency of data management and decision making based on data analysis.

Hadoop was the popular and first big data platform that introduced and made it easy for people to work on MR by executing its programs successfully. For tasks requiring batch processing, MR proved itself to be an effective tool as a typical cluster contains interlinked mappers and reducers that assist by running MR programs side by side at the same time. Though it has its benefits, these are not devoid of the drawbacks. These drawbacks include running some applications for graph generation and real-time and iterative processing. By dissociating the rest of the ecosystem from the processing of MR, Hadoop's latest versions have tried to sort out the problem. Yet another resource negotiator (YARN) has also been introduced, which functions by providing resource management and scheduling related functions of MR and has made it easy to implement innovative applications by Hadoop.

Hadoop models have been used in construction for smart buildings and disaster management [55], failure prediction of construction firms [56], workers' safe behaviors in a metro construction project [57], and other relevant applications. The overall platform design architecture of Hadoop offers high reliability; adopt cluster technology, multi-copy technology, independent backup technology, and other means to reduce the data failure rate effectively and build a reliable data application service platform. First, the processing of big data into batches and simultaneous reduction and refining of the data are carried out using MR. Next, data are batched into similar items to streamline the analyses. This step further reduces noise or datasets that do not align with a particular batch of data. Finally, a dataset is obtained, which is refined and aligned with the original search purpose.

4.1.2. Directed Acyclic Graph

Big data platforms also use Directed Acyclic Graph (DAG) which is an alternative processing model. In comparison with MR, DAG works by relaxing map-then-reduce, the style of MR, which is supported by Spark. Spark is widely accepted for reactive and iterative applications due to its supremacy over MR in high expressiveness and in-memory computation. Disk-resident and memory-resident tasks are conducted ten and one hundred times faster using Spark than MR. DAGs show relationships among variables, making them easier to understand. DAGs provide major advantages that enable experts and researchers to construct complex causal relationships in which nodes represent stochastic variables, and directed edges (arrows) indicate direct probabilistic dependencies among the relevant variables. DAGs are also able to encode deterministic as well as probabilistic relationships among the variables. The usage of Spark and associated DAGs has been reported for construction profitability analysis [39], waste management [25], energy monitoring service on smart campuses [58], and others.

Spark and Hadoop are among the ML tools with enormous potential in construction engineering and management. Figure 7 compares the two tools that can inform research in construction. The speed of both these systems is better than other algorithms and ML tools currently in use in the construction industry. Moreover, fault tolerance in both these systems is also high and has greater scalability than existing models. The data storage in these systems is slightly different in that Spark uses a memory system while Hadoop utilizes a disk for data storage. The language for both these tools is also different since Spark is written in Scala while Hadoop has been developed using JavaScript. Despite the slight differences, both these tools provide the opportunity to process data in the form of batches and at a higher speed than previously existing models, making them potential tools for futuristic model developments in construction engineering and management. JavaScript has been used in construction to anticipate building material reuse [59], automated progress control coupled with laser scanning [60], shared virtual reality for design and management [61], construction information mining [62], and others. Similarly, Scala has been used for the process information modeling concept for on-site construction management [63].

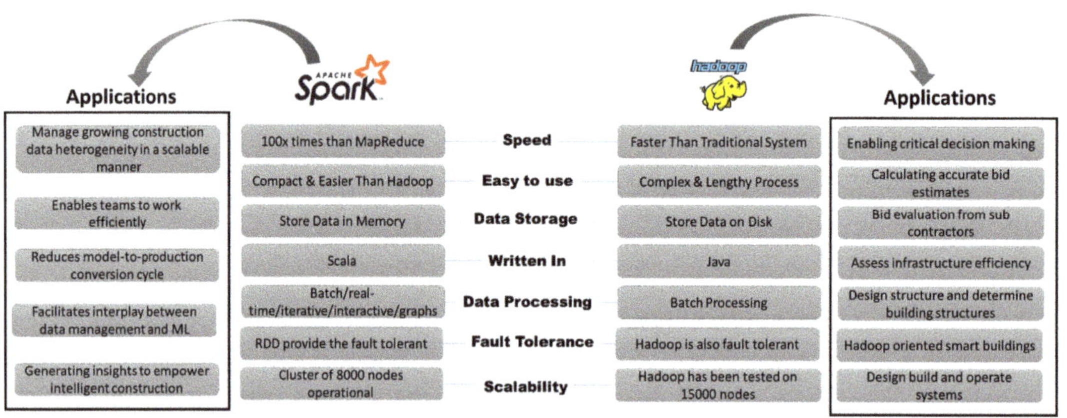

Figure 7. Components of Spark and Hadoop. A side-by-side comparison of Spark and Hadoop provides insights about the usability and applications of each.

4.1.3. Big Data Processing in Construction

Big data processing has been effectively utilized in the construction industry for failure prediction data [56], construction waste analytics [25], profitability data [39], modular and prefabricated construction [52], fire incident management [64], smart campus energy monitoring [58], healthier cities management [28], smart road management [40], and others.

Though MR and Spark have their own significance, these are less frequently employed in the construction industry to process big data such as BIM-associated data. Partial BIM models' retrieval was optimized by MR by Bilal, et al. [65] and Chang and Tsai [66]. The authors found a loop in the Hadoop MR logic of data distribution. For overcoming the query problem, a few steps of prepartitioning and processing are introduced for relevant BIM data parts that are later stored in Hadoop clusters. Node multi-threading during data analysis helped by making the CPU work its maximum. This helped in customizing Hadoop for BIM data while the YARN application implemented querying components. YARN applications are further utilized to develop a BIM system for quantity estimation and clash detection that can execute required tasks with the performance improved many-fold.

Another research group worked for naive and expert BIM users by developing a system for BIM data storage and retrieval [67]. The authors developed a system for cloud BIM to retrieve and represent big data intelligently. This system helped develop an interactive interface to maximize the usability and utility of construction big data. Complex BIM data are retrieved by processing proposed natural languages after reformulating user queries. This data are then visualized by mapping on various visualizations. Before query evaluation, two BIM collections are merged to optimize the process of query execution. Using this technology, a 40% reduction in response time has been witnessed compared to other traditional technologies. Currently, the utilization of BIM is limited across the construction and facilities management stages. The real intent of BIM could only be achieved once applied at each stage of the building lifecycle.

4.2. Big Data Storage

Big data storage is also an important aspect of BDE. In construction, big data storage has been explored for forecasting the success of construction projects [68], smart buildings data storage [69], tender price evaluation [70], and others. Despite the availability of BIM data storage, the current applications in construction still require successful implementation. Social BIM, proposed by Das et al. [71], captures building models and the social interactions among the users. The authors developed BIMCloud based on the distributed BIM framework.

Similarly, a two-tiered hybrid data infrastructure was proposed by Jeong et al. [72] for data management and monitoring of bridges. In this model, the client tier efficiently completes some analytical tasks by storing structured data momentarily using MongoDB, while the central tier stores sensor data permanently using Apache Cassandra. Lin et al. [67] also used MongoDB to store BIM data obtained through building models.

Overall big data storage is provided by either emerging NoSQL databases or distributed file systems, as explained subsequently.

4.2.1. Distributed File Systems

The distributed file systems consist of Hadoop Distributed File System (HDFS) and Tachyon. HDFS is designed to deal with large and complex databases such as those related to BIM, waste, and other construction big data sources. It operates with the commodity servers grouped together in a cluster. As it utilizes several servers, the probability of hardware failure also increases. To overcome this problem, HDFS introduces fault tolerance achieved through the distribution of data and their replication. However, in situations where low-latency data access is required, HDFS is not a suitable option as it shows inferior performance. Moreover, it is also troublesome to save many small files due to issues in managing meta-data. Moreover, it is not useful if modifications must be made concurrently at random locations in the data. Nevertheless, HDFS has been utilized by construction researchers for observing construction workers' behavior [73], improving road performance [39], and investigating profitability performance [39]. Furthermore, based on the distributed input from HDFS, it facilitates building predictive models for conducting building simulations that give output in a predictive model markup language.

Tachyon is a distributed file system designed to extend HDFS benefits by providing access to the distributed data across the cluster at memory speed. It provides better performance through in-memory data caching and backward compatibility allows MR and Spark tasks to run without changing the codes required in those programs. Tachyon has been utilized in construction for handling unstructured documents [65] and file storage [74]. The Tachyon performs better than HDFS, is backward compatible and can handle the MapReduce jobs without any further modifications.

4.2.2. NoSQL Databases

Relational databases have been common for data management in past decades. However, new applications were designed for better performance, scalability, and flexibility as the technology emerged. Relational databases lag because of their special processing and storage needs. As a result, new systems were devised to fill this technology gap. One such system is the "Not only SQL" system that has optimized data management in several ways. For achieving flexibility, it supports schemaless storage rather than schema-oriented storage. NoSQL has been widely used in different industries, including construction, due to its fragmented nature. Some examples of NoSQL in construction include integration of lessons learned knowledge in BIM [75], web service framework for construction supply chain collaboration and management [76], and Social BIMCloud implementation [71]. NoSQL systems store schemaless data in a non-relational model. It does not set too many restrictions on value and allows easy product determination. Generally, when NoSQL databases are set to key values, they carry out only specific tasks without evaluating specific values. The key-value database is mainly tailored to the business accessed through the primary key. These systems have four data models that are briefly discussed below.

- Key-value

This is the simplest data model used for unstructured data storage. However, the data lack self-description. It has been used for knowledge management in construction [77] and integration of lessons learned knowledge in BIM [75]. BIM provides positive outcomes on project success, such as cost and time reduction, communication and coordination improvement, and increased quality. Big data utilization in BIM can be beneficial to discover root causes of poor building performance, perform real-time data queries, improve the decision-making process, improve productivity, and reveal new designs and services in the construction industry, as is the case in every industry.

- Document

This model can store self-describing data. However, this model can lag in terms of efficiency. It has been used for unified lifecycle data management in architecture, engineering, construction, and facilities management through BIM integration [78].

- Columnar

Aggregated columns, grouped sub-columns, and sparse data can be stored by using this model. It has been used for integrating digital construction through the internet of things [79] and smart archiving of energy and petroleum construction projects [80].

- Graph

This model works well for property-graph-based huge datasets in relationship traversal. It has been used for the 4D construction management information model of prefabricated buildings [81] and the development of a BIM-enabled software tool for facility management [82].

Databases concerning big data storage and management are widely used worldwide for research on various topics. The construction industry also relies on big data sources and databases, observed throughout the last five years to a decade. As shown in Figure 8, the search engine is among the most widely searched database in the last five years, followed by relational and graph DBMS. Until the time of analyzing data for this review, i.e., November 2021, other heavily used databases for extracting and using big data for the construction industry include document stores, native XML, key-value stores, and wide column stores. Object-oriented DBMS and multivalued DBMS search are considerably lower than relational DBMS and graph DBMS, whereas the search engines outperform all other DBMS. These different databases provide data sources for BIM and computational sources for developing structures that could guide larger construction projects. The rising trend in using big data sources shows the increasing interest among the construction industries in big data. For example, exchanging and reusing information is critical for engineering and construction project management. The issues pertaining to data exchange have been minimized with the Extensible Markup Language (XML) application. Such an XML-based Distributed Construction Estimating System (XDCES) has been helpful to reduce the overload of cost-estimating information exchange. Similarly, construction-based DBMS enables all construction companies to build and maintain a database easily. It allows supervisors and workers to capture information using a mobile or tablet device, and then all of that information is stored in the cloud and accessible via a desktop version.

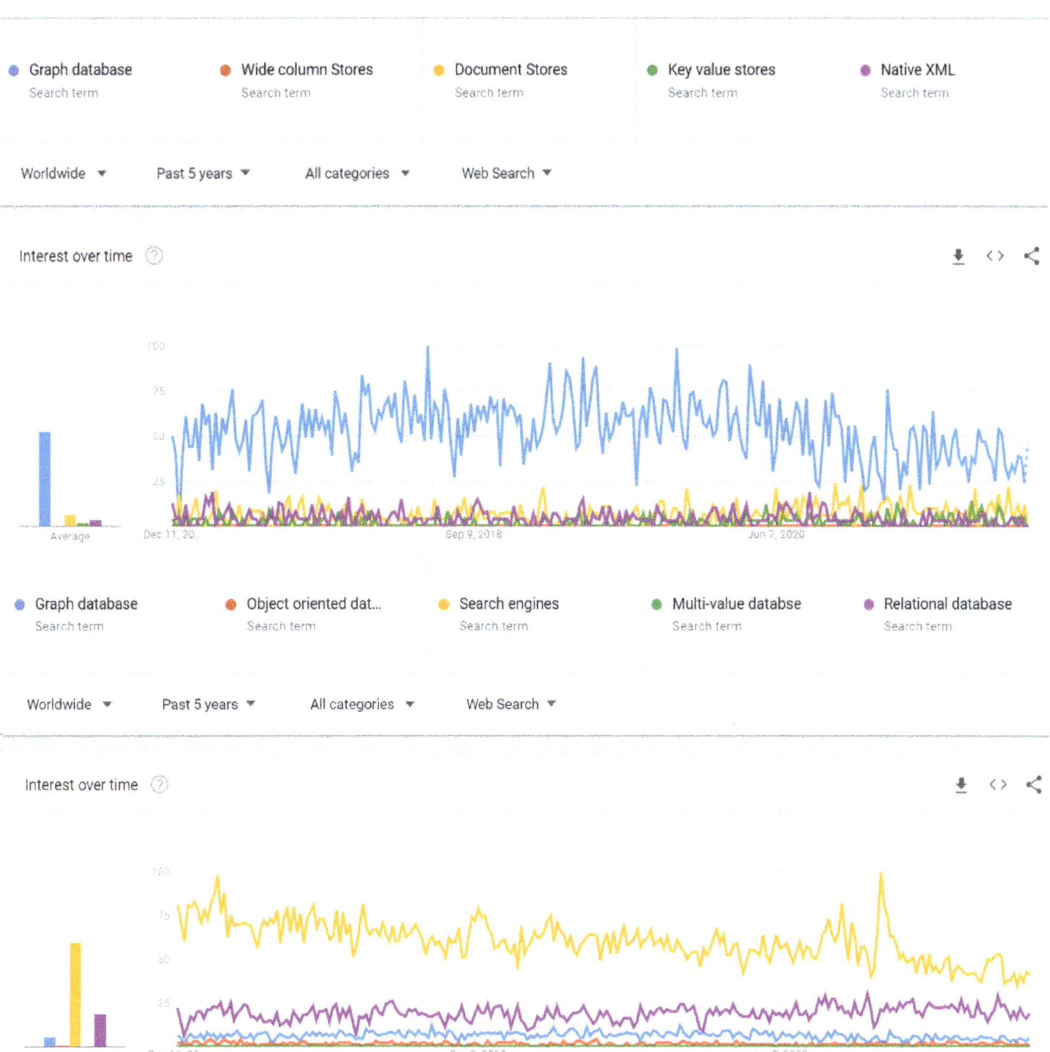

Figure 8. Database popularity in 2016–2021 based on search trends.

4.3. Big Data Analytics (BDA)

BDA gathers information from a variety of disciplines. All these disciplines have one thing in common: to find out data patterns. Some of these related disciplines are data mining, statistics, business analytics, predictive analytics, data analytics, knowledge discovery from data, and the most recent one, big data. Big data use the previous techniques to broaden the field of data analytics. For BDA, some of the ML-based tools are developed. In construction projects, BDA has been used for improving building design and effective performance monitoring [37], project safety, energy, resource, overall management and decision-making frameworks [38], and quality and waste management [24]. Big data analytics has been taken a step further by developing predictive analysis techniques. Ngo et al. [83] used a factor-based big data predictive analytic tool for analyzing the capacity of construction industries to deal with big data. This tool was tested and validated on four different construction organizations to ensure that the predictive analytic method could improve how the construction industry can use big data. The integration of big data in the construction industry remains an avenue that requires further research in terms of big data analytics. The gaps in this area were explored by Atuahene et al. [30] and Atuahene et al. [84]. It was identified that the management and processing of data by firms led to the generation of more data, which made data analysis an uphill task. Developing an integrated framework for managing big data and sorting the useful datasets can greatly increase the usability and application of big data in the construction industry. Overall, data analytics is conducted through statistical, data mining, and regression techniques, as explained below.

4.3.1. Statistics

Statistics has wide applications in the construction industry. Statistical techniques including Monte Carlo simulation, Gaussian distribution, non-Bayesian methods, correlation analysis, factor analysis, decision trees, Naïve Bayes, and others have been reported by various studies in construction [85,86]. Some of the areas that benefitted from statistics include learning from post-project reviews, identifying causes of construction delays, analyzing buildings for structural damages, construction litigation, and identifying and recognizing heavy machinery and workers. Other examples of statistics in construction are those of bidding statistics to predict completed construction cost [87], accidents statistics [88], quality control [89], and six sigma for project success [90,91]. From measuring the bid-to-win ratio to how much a project is over budget or schedule, and KPIs, the more numbers you can put behind your work, the better. Data not only allow for more visibility into the state of a particular project, but relevant industry statistics and facts can provide valuable information needed to make important future decisions regarding preconstruction and planning, productivity tools, risk assessment, and workforce and operational efficiency. Table 1 presents some uses of statistical models in construction.

Table 1. Use of statistical models in construction.

Purpose	Techniques	References
Damage detection in buildings	Monte Carlo simulation Gaussian distribution	[85]
Construction time scheduling	Gaussian distribution	[86]
Predicting project delays	Monte Carlo simulation Non-Bayesian methods Correlation analysis Factor analysis	[92–94]
Decision making	Decision trees Naïve Bayes	[95,96]

4.3.2. Data Mining

Data mining is used to extract meaningful patterns in the data. It has been an integral part of all big data management systems. It employs the techniques used in pattern recognition, ML, and statistics. Several models are assessed, and the ones with the best tolerance and high accuracy are selected and used for obtaining predictive results. In construction, data mining has been reported in waste management [97], BIM-based construction engineering quality management [98], and other relevant areas. Data mining detects useful regularities and information necessary for decision making for construction management projects. A data mining method such as cluster analysis is important for the construction industry, as it combines different construction objects into homogeneous groups and investigates them.

Data mining is supported through data warehousing. Specially structured data is stored in data warehousing for querying and analysis. Extract, transform and load (ETL) is a program that allows the collation of transactional data and operational data. Warehouse data analysis is conducted using Online Analytical Processing (OLAP), which performs better than SQL in computing breakdown and data summaries. OLAP has been used for cost data management in construction cost estimates by Moon et al. [99]. OLAP technology deals with the operational data and data obtained using big data technology. OLAP is presented as a multidimensional cube that rapidly processes datasets.

Similarly, different data mining techniques have been used to identify construction delays. For analyzing construction datasets, Kim et al. [12] presented a framework of knowledge discovery in databases (KDD). In the KDD, the most time-consuming and challenging step is data preprocessing. Nevertheless, KDD is a powerful tool for identifying casual relationships in construction projects and reducing construction variability by identifying and eliminating causes for possible deviations. With the application of KDD, randomness of construction projects and novel patterns can be determined. Other techniques include dimensional matrix analysis, link analysis, and text analysis [100]. Other datasets with information related to delay causes, BIM-based knowledge discovery, intelligent learning, and the prevention of occupational injuries can be easily extended in the domain of data mining.

4.3.3. Regression Techniques

Based on an input variable, regression predicts the value of the target variable. It is a supervised ML method. Regression is categorized into simple linear and multiple linear regression based on explanatory variables. In simple linear regression, the relationship between two variables (an explanatory variable x and a dependent variable y) is modeled using ML. While in multiple linear regression, two or more explanatory variables are used and their relationship with the dependent variable is modeled. The more common regression technique is multiple linear regression.

Regression has been extensively used in construction research. For example, it has been used to predict properties of concrete cured under hot weather [48], predicting final cost for competitive bids on construction projects [101], determining contingency in international construction projects [102], estimating performance time for construction projects [103], and others. Moreover, regression has been used for cost estimation, which is a difficult task in the early stages of the project. Adoption of parametric methods such as regression and multiple regression can be applied as both analytical and predictive techniques to estimate the overall reliability of the cost estimation.

4.4. The 10 vs. of Big Data

The bulk and variety of big data gathering enormously each day make it virtually impossible to deal with the data sources seamlessly. On the other hand, the enormity of big data gives it many characteristics that further expand the potential of big data and its applications in different research fields. Figure 9 provides an overview of some of the crucial characteristics of big data, also known as the vs. of big data. The 10 vs. of big data have been discussed in Figure 9. Understanding these characteristics of big data enables the identification of opportunities and challenges. The most crucial properties of big data include their value, volume, velocity, variety, veracity, volatility, validity, variability, vulnerability, and visualization, also known as the 10 vs. of big data [104]. These characteristics of vs. are used to guide research in different areas and fields.

In terms of the use of big data in the field of construction, analyzing the vs. can help explore how big data can be used for developing better construction models in the future. Firstly, big data provide great value using various databases and sources that inform the research studies and algorithm developments related to computational models of different building structures. In addition to the value of research, big data also provide a bulk of information needed for research simply through the ever-increasing volume of data that becomes available each day. Furthermore, the velocity with which databases expand each day adds variety to the sort of data available for utilization in fields like construction. The variety of data present is not varying just in terms of the data sources but also the types of data. For example, big data can be present in the form of written text, graphs, pictures, and various other formats to help manage construction project schedules and progress reporting. The increasing amounts of data make the visualization process quite complex. Therefore, it is crucial to develop new ways for data visualization and analysis to keep with the volatility of big data.

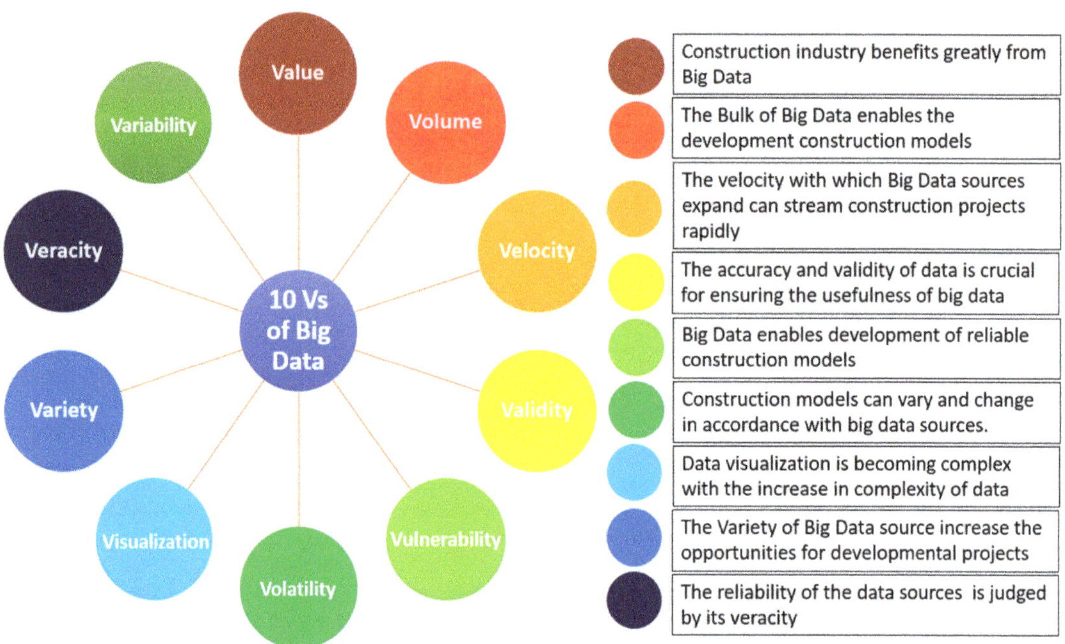

Figure 9. The 10 vs. of big data.

The 10 vs. of big data are among the crucial characteristics representing the true picture of big data as a field of research. The applications of big data in the construction industry are innumerable and they can all be categorized and managed through understanding the characteristic features (or Vs) of big data. The construction industry benefits immensely as a business by integrating big data technologies. The correlation with the business side of the construction industry has been explored in light of the 10 vs. of big data and it has been found that these characteristics provide an immense business growth potential. Starting from the core attributes of volume, variety and velocity, big data have come a long way in terms of their applications and trends. Today, there are 10 characteristics that define big data and are also crucial for implementing big data into different fields. It is crucial to understand that these 10 vs. of big data can be explained in a context-dependent manner considering the field of research. As for the construction industry, the variety and volume of big data are immense, but there is also a great deal of variability in the data present. For example, the choice of building materials and the suitability of the selected materials in different projects depend on several different factors. In this case, analyzing the applicability of big data is possible through data-visualizing techniques that can help deal with the volatility and variability of big data. Similarly, the validity and veracity of big data in construction can be judged only after analyzing the value that the data sources bring and the authenticity that these sources present. Therefore, the increasing velocity of big data is not useful as an independent factor. Instead, the application of big data in the construction industry depends on the 10 different characteristics (Vs) which are associated with big data and are explained in Figure 9.

Similarly, these data types can be refined and unstructured, further adding variety to the type of data present for various reporting and research purposes. Veracity refers to the reliability of big data. This is guided by statistics as the enormity of big data makes it hard to identify reliable data sources. Therefore, validating data sources and ensuring that they can be reliably used to guide construction project developments is crucial for research. The veracity of data sources leads to another important characteristic of big data: variability. It is crucial to understand that big data can be highly variable depending on the sources used for extracting the datasets. Understanding these characteristics of big data and analyzing these characteristics given the use of big data in the construction industry can greatly enhance the potential of future construction projects.

Overall, multiple construction-related studies have reported the usage of vs. of big data. For example, velocity has been reported for high-speed construction data processing [105]. Value has been reported for smarter universities and campuses [106]. Volume has been reported for mass level offsite construction material and component production [107]. Variety has been reported for investigating the profitability performance of construction projects [39]. Veracity has been reported for forecasting the success of construction projects [68]. Similarly, variability has been reported for modeling occupational accidents in construction projects [108].

Big data necessitate cost-effective, innovative information processing forms for enhanced insights and decision making. Construction companies can analyze historical datasets and carry out predictive analytics to forecast future events. Data-driven decision making has the potential to reshape the entire business. Together, the 10 attributes or 10 vs. of big data play a crucial role in the construction industry. The volume of data and the velocity through which data are produced at high speed lead to the possibility of validating information related to construction projects. The ability to visualize big data, keep up with the variety of data, and accept the volatility, vulnerability, and variability that come with the veracity of data helps ensure that big data could be truly applicable in the construction industry. Therefore, the value of big data in the construction industry is high and it helps guide future projects.

4.5. Machine Learning Techniques

One AI subdomain is ML which can be used to learn from the data using computational systems. The tools used for big data ML are presented in Table 2. ML is further categorized into: (i) supervised learning; (ii) unsupervised learning; (iii) association; and (iv) numeric prediction. ML has several applications in the construction industry. It uses different approaches, including rule-based learning approaches, case-based reasoning techniques, artificial neural networks, and hybrid methodologies.

ML has immense potential as a tool in the field of construction. Over the last two decades, several ML algorithms have been proposed to aid and improve the overall process of construction. For example, ML has been used to predict properties of concrete [48], contract management [109], site safety and injury prediction [46], delay risks management [45], BIM integrated on-demand site monitoring [47], and other areas of construction engineering and management.

Various ML tools are integrated at different steps along with the construction management processes. Different ML interfaces such as PyTorch and Keras.io help develop computational models based on existing data for building futuristic construction models. BIM can also be improved by using big data and ML tools, as these technologies allow the opportunity to explore how technology could be applied to the construction industry [110]. Over the last few years, different algorithms have been explored to predict various project phases and guide construction projects from inception to closure [111]. Firstly, decision trees and similar tools are used for developing an overall project timeline to predict or determine construction project performance in various phases. Secondly, statistical analysis tools are used for analyzing previous projects and choosing guiding principles for future projects [112]. Finally, design tools are integrated with ML algorithms to build 3D construction models and graphics for building models. These computational models enable analyzing construction projects by planning through look-up schedules and looking for ways to improve buildings and other structures [113].

The combined use of big data, ML, and AI holds the potential to develop seamless construction projects and enable the development of structures that can withhold severe weather conditions and disasters. For example, one of the key uses of ML tools in futuristic construction projects can be the development of structures that can stand through natural disasters and provide safety nets to communities during floods and other disasters [114]. Similarly, post-disaster evacuation and rescue of individuals can also be carried out more easily if the area contains structures such as roads and buildings built through the use of statistical modeling, thus providing safe routes for people [115]. Although the automation of construction projects remains a future goal, the integration of different ML algorithms is already underway. Managing costs, timelines, and human resources on a construction project are areas guided by various algorithms and computational models [116]. The ML approach can also be applied to develop leading indicators to classify sites according to their safety risk in construction projects.

Table 2. Machine learning tools used for big data.

No.	Tool	Description	Supported Algorithm	Languages	Applications in Construction	Ref.
1	PyTorch	PyTorch is a free tool available for Windows, Mac OS, and Linux for developing ML programs	Regression Classification Clustering Dimensionality reduction Preprocessing	C, C++, Python	Object detection, analyzing buildings and other structures to develop better models	[117]
2	Apache Mahout	An open-source tool that allows high-performing and scalable applications using ML	Distributed Linear Algebra Clustering Regression Preprocessing	Java, Scala	Processing big data for the development of building models and appropriate algorithms	[118,119]
3	Shogun	A diverse ML platform supporting various languages and platforms. Works well with Windows, Linux, and Mac OS	Classification Regression Dimensionality reduction Online learning Support vector machines	C++	Provides a platform for analyzing data and developing strategies for construction projects using available information in the form of big data	[120]
4	SciKit Learn	A free, machine-learning tool that supports Windows, Mac OS, and Linux	Regression Classification Preprocessing Clustering Model selection	C, C++, Cython, Python	Enables statistical analysis for construction projects, particularly using existing data for developing suitable construction models	[121]
5	Keras.io	An ML software that can be used across different platforms	API for neural networks	Python	Provides training models which can be harnessed for improving BIM and creating confident models for construction projects	[122]

5. Future Opportunities of Big Data in Construction

There is immense potential for the use of big data in the construction industry. The use of big data and ML can enable construction automation. These tools can also enhance the overall project by removing various hurdles and roadblocks that tend to slow down different projects. The construction industry is quite dynamic and demanding, with the need for labor strength and human resources to ensure the smooth running of projects. The constant challenge of keeping projects on track and ensuring that new buildings and structures are made up to modern standards puts much strain on the project management teams. These roadblocks can greatly be reduced with the use of big data and ML. The core aim of using big data in the construction industry is to enhance the project planning phases and speed up the overall construction process by predicting the possible timelines for particular projects and identifying what factors can be worked on to improve the overall process [123].

The automation of the construction projects will require the combined use of big data, deep learning, and ML tools. One of the major concerns with such projects is ensuring workers' safety and developing strategies for overcoming potential threats to the overall process. Safety of the workers and the structures is essential for the smoother development of construction projects. The use of big data and related tools can ensure that existing data and information can be used for drafting guiding principles and then building computational models accordingly. For example, using sensor-based wearable personal protective equipment, the big data of near misses, onsite accidents, hazards, and other issues can be generated for developing safety plans and management techniques. Similarly, big data, BIM, and cloud-powered simulations can help minimize project waste and help produce superior quality constructed facilities. Further, big data artifacts generated by 3D scanners for as-built drawing development are another key advantage whereby the rehabilitation plans of ancient heritage sites can be developed.

The future holds great potential for the construction industry through big data integration. Some of the key opportunities for the construction industries lie in using big data for business and environmental sustainability. The current roadblocks faced by the construction industry can be overcome in the future through the integration of information extracted through big data. The use of information gathered from past and present projects can help develop sustainable infrastructure in the long term. It is possible to avoid past mistakes and use better quality products guided by the information found through big data in construction. Future research directions in the field of construction rely heavily on big data as the presence of information sources can help in building better infrastructure and greatly improve building designs and the overall construction business. The construction industry must move towards automation and build upon the integration of technology to make the future use of big data seamless and hassle-free. The use of big data tools, BIM, and CAD can only be possible if the relevant support and integration systems are present [107]. Hence, the future of the construction industry depends on upgrading the present environment gradually.

Overall, the role of big data in enabling the entire process of futuristic construction projects is undeniable. Data play a crucial role in developing training models and smoothly enabling the process of construction. Future developments in this field will also include the generation and use of more algorithms and models that rely on big data, owing to the need to train the models reliably.

6. Conclusions

The construction industry is yet to reap the true benefits of using big data aptly. Over the last two decades, the rapid growth of big data technologies has caused a spike in the number of models and platforms that have been developed for increasing digitalization across different fields. However, the same level of digitalization has not truly been harnessed or integrated by the construction industry. A critical overview of the existing literature points towards the bulk of existing resources and platforms that can easily be applied for construction management. However, the state of implantation of adoption in construction is below par. Therefore, the utilization and commercialization of big data to benefit the construction industry are crucial. An extensive literature review enabled us to identify the potential of big data in construction as the industry generates huge amounts of data daily and can greatly improve using the latest technologies. The development of online tools and software which enable infrastructure modeling and CAD is a crucial step in the right direction for futuristic constructions. Having explored the existing ML tools, we found that these tools, coupled with big data, can be applied in the construction industry. In this paper, we have discussed the existing tools used in big data, the use of statistics, big data storage, and BDE. Overlap between these variables further creates complications in that more data are present and the field of big data is ever-expanding.

The current study contributes to the body of knowledge by providing a state-of-the-art review of relevant articles focused on big data applications in construction published between 2010 and 2021. It further provides various current applications and future opportunities of big data in the construction industry for practitioners and researchers to ponder upon and initiates the necessary debate around practical implementation and adoption of big data applications in construction.

There are currently various gaps and pitfalls that act as barriers to using big data to its full potential. Firstly, data generation is much faster than the tools available for processing it. Moreover, big data integration into the construction industry is quite an uphill task even with the existing data processing tools.

The current study is limited to the literature published in the last decade and may not include all the available papers due to specific selection criteria developed in this study. Similarly, the search terms may not be holistic and thus not exhaustive; a study conducted in the future with slightly different search strings may produce different results. In the future, the researchers can expand upon and explore the five clusters identified in Figure 4. The individual relations and adoption frameworks for big data in these clusters can be explored.

Author Contributions: Conceptualization, H.S.M. and F.U.; methodology, H.S.M., F.U. and S.Q.; software, H.S.M. and F.U.; validation, H.S.M., F.U., S.Q. and D.S.; formal analysis, H.S.M. and F.U.; investigation, H.S.M., F.U. and S.Q.; resources, H.S.M. and F.U.; data curation, H.S.M., F.U., S.Q. and D.S.; writing—original draft preparation, H.S.M. and F.U.; writing—review and editing, H.S.M., F.U., S.Q. and D.S.; visualization, H.S.M. and F.U.; supervision, F.U.; project administration, H.S.M. and F.U.; funding acquisition, H.S.M. and F.U. All authors have read and agreed to the published version of the manuscript.

Funding: This research received no external funding.

Institutional Review Board Statement: Not applicable.

Informed Consent Statement: Not applicable.

Data Availability Statement: Data are available with the first author and can be shared upon reasonable request.

Conflicts of Interest: The authors declare no conflict of interest.

References

1. Villars, R.L.; Olofson, C.W.; Eastwood, M. Big data: What it is and why you should care. *White Pap. IDC* **2011**, *14*, 1–14.
2. Siddiqa, A.; Karim, A.; Gani, A. Big data storage technologies: A survey. *Front. Inf. Technol. Electron. Eng.* **2017**, *18*, 1040–1070. [CrossRef]
3. Phaneendra, S.V.; Reddy, E.M. Big Data-solutions for RDBMS problems-A survey. In Proceedings of the 12th IEEE/IFIP Network Operations & Management Symposium (NOMS 2010), Osaka, Japan, 19–23 April 2013.
4. Henry, R.; Venkatraman, S. Big Data Analytics the Next Big Learning Opportunity. *J. Manag. Inf. Decis. Sci.* **2015**, *18*, 17–29.
5. Xu, W.; Sun, J.; Ma, J.; Du, W. A personalized information recommendation system for R&D project opportunity finding in big data contexts. *J. Netw. Comput. Appl.* **2016**, *59*, 362–369.
6. Sepasgozar, S.M.; Davis, S. Construction technology adoption cube: An investigation on process, factors, barriers, drivers and decision makers using NVivo and AHP analysis. *Buildings* **2018**, *8*, 74. [CrossRef]
7. Ullah, F.; Sepasgozar, S.M.; Wang, C. A systematic review of smart real estate technology: Drivers of, and barriers to, the use of digital disruptive technologies and online platforms. *Sustainability* **2018**, *10*, 3142. [CrossRef]
8. Kwon, O.; Lee, N.; Shin, B. Data quality management, data usage experience and acquisition intention of big data analytics. *Int. J. Inf. Manag.* **2014**, *34*, 387–394. [CrossRef]
9. Cui, L.; Yu, F.R.; Yan, Q. When big data meets software-defined networking: SDN for big data and big data for SDN. *IEEE Netw.* **2016**, *30*, 58–65. [CrossRef]
10. Chaudhary, R.; Aujla, G.S.; Kumar, N.; Rodrigues, J.J. Optimized big data management across multi-cloud data centers: Software-defined-network-based analysis. *IEEE Commun. Mag.* **2018**, *56*, 118–126. [CrossRef]
11. Simmhan, Y.; Aman, S.; Kumbhare, A.; Liu, R.; Stevens, S.; Zhou, Q.; Prasanna, V. Cloud-based software platform for big data analytics in smart grids. *Comput. Sci. Eng.* **2013**, *15*, 38–47. [CrossRef]
12. Kim, K.Y. Business intelligence and marketing insights in an era of big data: The q-sorting approach. *KSII Trans. Internet Inf. Syst. (TIIS)* **2014**, *8*, 567–582.

13. Hu, X. Sorting big data by revealed preference with application to college ranking. *J. Big Data* **2020**, *7*, 1–26. [CrossRef]
14. Custers, B.; Uršič, H. Big data and data reuse: A taxonomy of data reuse for balancing big data benefits and personal data protection. *Int. Data Priv. Law* **2016**, *6*, 4–15. [CrossRef]
15. Majumdar, J.; Naraseeyappa, S.; Ankalaki, S. Analysis of agriculture data using data mining techniques: Application of big data. *J. Big Data* **2017**, *4*, 1–15. [CrossRef]
16. Shadroo, S.; Rahmani, A.M. Systematic survey of big data and data mining in internet of things. *Comput. Netw.* **2018**, *139*, 19–47. [CrossRef]
17. Zhou, R.; Liu, M.; Li, T. Characterizing the efficiency of data deduplication for big data storage management. In Proceedings of the 2013 IEEE international symposium on workload characterization (IISWC), Portland, OR, USA, 22–24 September 2013; pp. 98–108.
18. Petri, I.; Rana, O.; Beach, T.; Rezgui, Y.; Sutton, A. Clouds4Coordination: Managing project collaboration in federated clouds. In Proceedings of the 2015 IEEE/ACM 8th International Conference on Utility and Cloud Computing (UCC), Limassol, Cyprus, 7–10 December 2015; pp. 494–499.
19. Hay, B.; Nance, K.; Bishop, M. Storm clouds rising: Security challenges for IaaS cloud computing. In Proceedings of the 2011 44th Hawaii International Conference on System Sciences, Washington, DC, USA, 4–7 January 2011; pp. 1–7.
20. Afolabi, A.; Ojelabi, R.A.; Fagbenle, O.I.; Mosaku, T. The economics of cloud-based computing technologies in construction project delivery. *Int. J. Civ. Eng. Technol. (IJCIET)* **2017**, *8*, 232–242.
21. Moniruzzaman, A.; Hossain, S.A. Nosql database: New era of databases for big data analytics-classification, characteristics and comparison. *arXiv* **2013**, arXiv:1307.0191.
22. Kouanou, A.T.; Tchiotsop, D.; Kengne, R.; Zephirin, D.T.; Armele, N.M.A.; Tchinda, R. An optimal big data workflow for biomedical image analysis. *Inform. Med. Unlocked* **2018**, *11*, 68–74. [CrossRef]
23. Rodrigues, M.; Santos, M.Y.; Bernardino, J. Big data processing tools: An experimental performance evaluation. *Wiley Interdiscip. Rev. Data Min. Knowl. Discov.* **2019**, *9*, e1297. [CrossRef]
24. Wang, D.; Fan, J.; Fu, H.; Zhang, B. Research on optimization of big data construction engineering quality management based on RNN-LSTM. *Complexity* **2018**, *2018*, 9691868. [CrossRef]
25. Bilal, M.; Oyedele, L.O.; Akinade, O.O.; Ajayi, S.O.; Alaka, H.A.; Owolabi, H.A.; Qadir, J.; Pasha, M.; Bello, S.A. Big data architecture for construction waste analytics (CWA): A conceptual framework. *J. Build. Eng.* **2016**, *6*, 144–156. [CrossRef]
26. Munawar, H.S.; Qayyum, S.; Ullah, F.; Sepasgozar, S. Big data and its applications in smart real estate and the disaster management life cycle: A systematic analysis. *Big Data Cogn. Comput.* **2020**, *4*, 4. [CrossRef]
27. Qadir, Z.; Khan, S.I.; Khalaji, E.; Munawar, H.S.; Al-Turjman, F.; Mahmud, M.P.; Kouzani, A.Z.; Le, K. Predicting the energy output of hybrid PV–wind renewable energy system using feature selection technique for smart grids. *Energy Rep.* **2021**, *7*, 8465–8475. [CrossRef]
28. Miller, H.J.; Tolle, K. Big data for healthy cities: Using location-aware technologies, open data and 3D urban models to design healthier built environments. *Built Environ.* **2016**, *42*, 441–456. [CrossRef]
29. Chen, X.; Lu, W. Scenarios for Applying Big Data in Boosting Construction: A Review. In Proceedings of the 21st International Symposium on Advancement of Construction Management and Real Estate, Guiyang, China, 24–27 August 2018; pp. 1299–1306.
30. Atuahene, B.T.; Kanjanabootra, S.; Gajendran, T. Towards an integrated framework of big data capabilities in the construction industry: A systematic literature review. In Proceedings of the 34th Association of Researchers in Construction Management (ARCOM), Belfast, UK, 3–5 September 2018; p. 547.
31. Ullah, F. A beginner's guide to developing review-based conceptual frameworks in the built environment. *Architecture* **2021**, *1*, 5–24. [CrossRef]
32. Ullah, F.; Al-Turjman, F. A conceptual framework for blockchain smart contract adoption to manage real estate deals in smart cities. *Neural Comput. Appl.* **2021**, 1–22. [CrossRef]
33. Ullah, F. *Developing a Novel Technology Adoption Framework for Real Estate Online Platforms: Users' Perception and Adoption Barriers;* University of New South Wales: Sidney, Australia, 2021.
34. Ullah, F.; Qayyum, S.; Thaheem, M.J.; Al-Turjman, F.; Sepasgozar, S.M. Risk management in sustainable smart cities governance: A TOE framework. *Technol. Forecast. Soc. Change* **2021**, *167*, 120743. [CrossRef]
35. Qayyum, S.; Ullah, F.; Al-Turjman, F.; Mojtahedi, M. Managing smart cities through six sigma DMADICV method: A review-based conceptual framework. *Sustain. Cities Soc.* **2021**, *72*, 103022. [CrossRef]
36. Huang, X. Application of BIM Big Data in Construction Engineering Cost. *J. Phys. Conf. Ser.* **2021**, *1865*, 032016. [CrossRef]
37. Loyola, M. Big data in building design: A review. *J. Inf. Technol. Constr.* **2018**, *23*, 259–284.
38. Ismail, S.A.; Bandi, S.; Maaz, Z.N. An appraisal into the potential application of big data in the construction industry. *Int. J. Built Environ. Sustain.* **2018**, *5*, 145–154. [CrossRef]
39. Bilal, M.; Oyedele, L.O.; Kusimo, H.O.; Owolabi, H.A.; Akanbi, L.A.; Ajayi, A.O.; Akinade, O.O.; Delgado, J.M.D. Investigating profitability performance of construction projects using big data: A project analytics approach. *J. Build. Eng.* **2019**, *26*, 100850. [CrossRef]
40. Sharif, M.; Mercelis, S.; Van Den Bergh, W.; Hellinckx, P. Towards real-time smart road construction: Efficient process management through the implementation of internet of things. In Proceedings of the International Conference on Big Data and Internet of Thing, London, UK, 20–22 December 2017; pp. 174–180.

41. Curtis, C. Architecture at Scale: Reimagining One-Off Projects as Building Platforms. *Archit. Des.* **2020**, *90*, 96–103. [CrossRef]
42. Shtern, M.; Mian, R.; Litoiu, M.; Zareian, S.; Abdelgawad, H.; Tizghadam, A. Towards a multi-cluster analytical engine for transportation data. In Proceedings of the 2014 International Conference on Cloud and Autonomic Computing, London, UK, 8–12 September 2014; pp. 249–257.
43. Ying, L.J.; Pheng, L.S. Enhancing buildability in China's construction industry using Singapore's buildable design appraisal system. *J. Technol. Manag. China* **2007**, *2*, 264–278. [CrossRef]
44. Munawar, H.S.; Ullah, F.; Qayyum, S.; Heravi, A. Application of Deep Learning on UAV-Based Aerial Images for Flood Detection. *Smart Cities* **2021**, *4*, 1220–1242. [CrossRef]
45. Gondia, A.; Siam, A.; El-Dakhakhni, W.; Nassar, A.H. Machine learning algorithms for construction projects delay risk prediction. *J. Constr. Eng. Manag.* **2020**, *146*, 04019085. [CrossRef]
46. Tixier, A.J.-P.; Hallowell, M.R.; Rajagopalan, B.; Bowman, D. Application of machine learning to construction injury prediction. *Autom. Constr.* **2016**, *69*, 102–114. [CrossRef]
47. Rahimian, F.P.; Seyedzadeh, S.; Oliver, S.; Rodriguez, S.; Dawood, N. On-demand monitoring of construction projects through a game-like hybrid application of BIM and machine learning. *Autom. Constr.* **2020**, *110*, 103012. [CrossRef]
48. Maqsoom, A.; Aslam, B.; Gul, M.E.; Ullah, F.; Kouzani, A.Z.; Mahmud, M.; Nawaz, A. Using Multivariate Regression and ANN Models to Predict Properties of Concrete Cured under Hot Weather. *Sustainability* **2021**, *13*, 10164. [CrossRef]
49. Yang, A.; Yu, G. Application of Heterogeneous Network Oriented to NoSQL Database in Optimal Postevaluation Indexes of Construction Projects. *Discret. Dyn. Nat. Soc.* **2022**, *2022*, 4817300. [CrossRef]
50. Sanni-Anibire, M.O.; Zin, R.M.; Olatunji, S.O. Machine learning model for delay risk assessment in tall building projects. *Int. J. Constr. Manag.* **2020**, 1–10. [CrossRef]
51. Lu, W.; Chen, X.; Ho, D.C.; Wang, H. Analysis of the construction waste management performance in Hong Kong: The public and private sectors compared using big data. *J. Clean. Prod.* **2016**, *112*, 521–531. [CrossRef]
52. Han, Z.; Wang, Y. The applied exploration of big data technology in prefabricated construction project management. *ICCREM* **2017**, *2017*, 71–78.
53. Jiao, Y.; Zhang, S.; Li, Y.; Wang, Y.; Yang, B.; Wang, L. An augmented MapReduce framework for building information modeling applications. In Proceedings of the 2014 IEEE 18th International Conference on Computer Supported Cooperative Work in Design (CSCWD), Hsinchu, Taiwan, 21–23 May 2014; pp. 283–288.
54. Yu, T.; Liang, X.; Wang, Y. Factors affecting the utilization of big data in construction projects. *J. Constr. Eng. Manag.* **2020**, *146*, 04020032. [CrossRef]
55. Qadir, Z.; Ullah, F.; Munawar, H.S.; Al-Turjman, F. Addressing disasters in smart cities through UAVs path planning and 5G communications: A systematic review. *Comput. Commun.* **2021**, *168*, 114–135. [CrossRef]
56. Alaka, H.A.; Oyedele, L.O.; Owolabi, H.A.; Bilal, M.; Ajayi, S.O.; Akinade, O.O. A framework for big data analytics approach to failure prediction of construction firms. *Appl. Comput. Inform.* **2018**, *16*, 207–222. [CrossRef]
57. Asadianfam, S.; Shamsi, M.; Kenari, A.R. Hadoop Deep Neural Network for offending drivers. *J. Ambient. Intell. Humaniz. Comput.* **2021**, *13*, 659–671. [CrossRef]
58. Liu, R.-H.; Kuo, C.-F.; Yang, C.-T.; Chen, S.-T.; Liu, J.-C. On construction of an energy monitoring service using big data technology for smart campus. In Proceedings of the 2016 7th International Conference on Cloud Computing and Big Data (CCBD), Macau, China, 16–18 November 2016; pp. 81–86.
59. Song, Y.; Clayton, M.J.; Johnson, R.E. Anticipating reuse: Documenting buildings for operations using web technology. *Autom. Constr.* **2002**, *11*, 185–197. [CrossRef]
60. Zhang, C.; Arditi, D. Automated progress control using laser scanning technology. *Autom. Constr.* **2013**, *36*, 108–116. [CrossRef]
61. Caneparo, L. Shared virtual reality for design and management: The Porta Susa project. *Autom. Constr.* **2001**, *10*, 217–228. [CrossRef]
62. Palaneeswaran, E.; Kumaraswamy, M.M. Knowledge mining of information sources for research in construction management. *J. Constr. Eng. Manag.* **2003**, *129*, 182–191. [CrossRef]
63. Pan, W.; Ilhan, B.; Bock, T. Process information modelling (PIM) concept for on-site construction management: Hong Kong case. *Period. Polytech. Archit.* **2018**, *49*, 165–175. [CrossRef]
64. Kim, J.-S.; Kim, B.-S. Analysis of fire-accident factors using big-data analysis method for construction areas. *KSCE J. Civil Eng.* **2018**, *22*, 1535–1543. [CrossRef]
65. Bilal, M.; Oyedele, L.O.; Qadir, J.; Munir, K.; Ajayi, S.O.; Akinade, O.O.; Owolabi, H.A.; Alaka, H.A.; Pasha, M. Big Data in the construction industry: A review of present status, opportunities, and future trends. *Adv. Eng. Inform.* **2016**, *30*, 500–521. [CrossRef]
66. Chang, C.-Y.; Tsai, M.-D. Knowledge-based navigation system for building health diagnosis. *Adv. Eng. Inform.* **2013**, *27*, 246–260. [CrossRef]
67. Lin, J.R.; Hu, Z.Z.; Zhang, J.P.; Yu, F.Q. A natural-language-based approach to intelligent data retrieval and representation for cloud BIM. *Comput.-Aided Civ. Infrastruct. Eng.* **2016**, *31*, 18–33. [CrossRef]
68. Narayan, S.; Tan, H.C. Adopting big data to forecast success of construction projects: A review. *Malays. Constr. Res. J.* **2019**, *6*, 132–143.

69. Linder, L.; Vionnet, D.; Bacher, J.-P.; Hennebert, J. Big building data—A big data platform for smart buildings. *Energy Procedia* **2017**, *122*, 589–594. [CrossRef]

70. Zhang, Y.; Luo, H.; He, Y. A system for tender price evaluation of construction project based on big data. *Procedia Eng.* **2015**, *123*, 606–614. [CrossRef]

71. Das, M.; Cheng, J.C.; Kumar, S.S. Social BIMCloud: A distributed cloud-based BIM platform for object-based lifecycle information exchange. *Vis. Eng.* **2015**, *3*, 1–20. [CrossRef]

72. Jeong, S.; Byun, J.; Kim, D.; Sohn, H.; Bae, I.H.; Law, K.H. A data management infrastructure for bridge monitoring. In Proceedings of the Sensors and Smart Structures Technologies for Civil, Mechanical, and Aerospace Systems 2015, San Diego, CA, USA, 9–12 March 2015; p. 94350.

73. Guo, S.; Ding, L.; Luo, H.; Jiang, X. A Big-Data-based platform of workers' behavior: Observations from the field. *Accid. Anal. Prev.* **2016**, *93*, 299–309. [CrossRef]

74. Ram, J.; Afridi, N.K.; Khan, K.A. Adoption of Big Data analytics in construction: Development of a conceptual model. *Built Environ. Proj. Asset Manag.* **2019**, *9*, 564–579. [CrossRef]

75. Oti, A.; Tah, J.; Abanda, F. Integration of lessons learned knowledge in building information modeling. *J. Constr. Eng. Manag.* **2018**, *144*, 04018081. [CrossRef]

76. Das, M.; Cheng, J.C.; Law, K.H. An ontology-based web service framework for construction supply chain collaboration and management. *Eng. Constr. Archit. Manag.* **2015**, *22*, 551–572. [CrossRef]

77. Jing, Y.; Wang, Y.-C.; Wang, Z. Knowledge management in construction—The framework of high value density knowledge discovery with graph database. In *Civil, Architecture and Environmental Engineering*; CRC Press: Boca Raton, FL, USA, 2017; pp. 712–715.

78. Jiao, Y.; Wang, Y.; Zhang, S.; Li, Y.; Yang, B.; Yuan, L. A cloud approach to unified lifecycle data management in architecture, engineering, construction and facilities management: Integrating BIMs and SNS. *Adv. Eng. Inform.* **2013**, *27*, 173–188. [CrossRef]

79. Woodhead, R.; Stephenson, P.; Morrey, D. Digital construction: From point solutions to IoT ecosystem. *Autom. Constr.* **2018**, *93*, 35–46. [CrossRef]

80. ElZahed, M.; Marzouk, M. Smart archiving of energy and petroleum projects utilizing big data analytics. *Autom. Constr.* **2022**, *133*, 104005. [CrossRef]

81. Yang, B.; Dong, M.; Wang, C.; Liu, B.; Wang, Z.; Zhang, B. IFC-based 4D construction management information model of prefabricated buildings and its application in graph database. *Appl. Sci.* **2021**, *11*, 7270. [CrossRef]

82. Zibion, D. Development of a BIM-Enabled Software Tool for Facility Management Using Interactive Floor Plans, Graph-Based Data Management and Granular Information Retrieval. Master's Thesis, Aalto University, Espoo, Finland, 2018.

83. Ngo, J.; Hwang, B.-G.; Zhang, C. Factor-based big data and predictive analytics capability assessment tool for the construction industry. *Autom. Constr.* **2020**, *110*, 103042. [CrossRef]

84. Atuahene, B.T.; Kanjanabootra, S.; Gajendra, T. Benefits of Big Data Application Experienced in the Construction Industry: A Case of an Australian Construction Company. In Proceedings of the 36th Annual Association of Researchers in Construction Management (ARCOM) Conference, Virtual Conference, Leeds, UK, 7–8 September 2020.

85. Lam, H.F.; Yang, J.H.; Au, S.K. Markov chain Monte Carlo-based Bayesian method for structural model updating and damage detection. *Struct. Control Health Monit.* **2018**, *25*, e2140. [CrossRef]

86. Ara, J.; Ali, S.; Shah, I. Monitoring schedule time using exponentially modified Gaussian distribution. *Qual. Technol. Quant. Manag.* **2020**, *17*, 448–469. [CrossRef]

87. Wright, M.G.; Williams, T.P. Using bidding statistics to predict completed construction cost. *Eng. Econ.* **2001**, *46*, 114–128. [CrossRef]

88. Abdullah, D.; Wern, G.C.M. An analysis of accidents statistics in Malaysian construction sector. In Proceedings of the International Conference on E-business, Management and Economics, Dubai, United Arab Emirates, 28–30 December 2011; pp. 1–4.

89. Munawar, H.S.; Ullah, F.; Heravi, A.; Thaheem, M.J.; Maqsoom, A. Inspecting Buildings Using Drones and Computer Vision: A Machine Learning Approach to Detect Cracks and Damages. *Drones* **2022**, *6*, 5. [CrossRef]

90. Siddiqui, S.Q.; Ullah, F.; Thaheem, M.J.; Gabriel, H.F. Six Sigma in construction: A review of critical success factors. *Int. J. Lean Six Sigma* **2016**, *7*, 171–186. [CrossRef]

91. Ullah, F.; Thaheem, M.J.; Siddiqui, S.Q.; Khurshid, M.B. Influence of Six Sigma on project success in construction industry of Pakistan. *TQM J.* **2017**, *29*, 276–309. [CrossRef]

92. Shirowzhan, S.; Lim, S. Autocorrelation statistics-based algorithms for automatic ground and non-ground classification of Lidar data. In Proceedings of the ISARC, International Symposium on Automation and Robotics in Construction, Sydney, Australia, 9–11 July 2014; p. 1.

93. Sepasgozar, S.M.; Karimi, R.; Shirowzhan, S.; Mojtahedi, M.; Ebrahimzadeh, S.; McCarthy, D. Delay causes and emerging digital tools: A novel model of delay analysis, including integrated project delivery and PMBOK. *Buildings* **2019**, *9*, 191. [CrossRef]

94. Doloi, H.; Sawhney, A.; Iyer, K. Structural equation model for investigating factors affecting delay in Indian construction projects. *Constr. Manag. Econ.* **2012**, *30*, 869–884. [CrossRef]

95. Baker, H.R.; Smith, S.D.; Masterton, G.; Hewlett, B. Failures in construction: Learning from everyday forensic engineering. In *Forensic Engineering 2018: Forging Forensic Frontiers*; American Society of Civil Engineers: Reston, VA, USA, 2018; pp. 648–658.

96.   Alipour, M.; Harris, D.K.; Barnes, L.E.; Ozbulut, O.E.; Carroll, J. Load-capacity rating of bridge populations through machine learning: Application of decision trees and random forests. *J. Bridge Eng.* **2017**, *22*, 04017076. [CrossRef]

97.   Lu, W.; Chen, X.; Peng, Y.; Shen, L. Benchmarking construction waste management performance using big data. *Resour. Conserv. Recycl.* **2015**, *105*, 49–58. [CrossRef]

98.   Sun, H.; Wang, L.; Yang, Z.; Xie, J. Research on Construction Engineering Quality Management Based on Building Information Model and Computer Big Data Mining. *Arab. J. Sci. Eng.* **2021**, 1–11. [CrossRef]

99.   Moon, S.; Kim, J.; Kwon, K. Effectiveness of OLAP-based cost data management in construction cost estimate. *Autom. Constr.* **2007**, *16*, 336–344. [CrossRef]

100. Carrillo, P.; Harding, J.; Choudhary, A. Knowledge discovery from post-project reviews. *Constr. Manag. Econ.* **2011**, *29*, 713–723. [CrossRef]

101. Williams, T.P. Predicting final cost for competitively bid construction projects using regression models. *Int. J. Proj. Manag.* **2003**, *21*, 593–599. [CrossRef]

102. Polat, G.; Bingol, B.N. A comparison of fuzzy logic and multiple regression analysis models in determining contingency in international construction projects. *Constr. Innov.* **2013**, *13*, 445–462. [CrossRef]

103. Hoffman, G.J.; Thal, A.E., Jr.; Webb, T.S.; Weir, J.D. Estimating performance time for construction projects. *J. Manag. Eng.* **2007**, *23*, 193–199. [CrossRef]

104. Bukowski, L. *Reliable, Secure and Resilient Logistics Networks*; Springer: Cham, Switzerland, 2019.

105. Konikov, A.; Konikov, G. Big Data is a powerful tool for environmental improvements in the construction business. In *IOP Conference Series: Earth and Environmental Science*; IOP Publishing: Bristol, UK, 2017; p. 012184.

106. Williamson, B. The hidden architecture of higher education: Building a big data infrastructure for the 'smarter university'. *Int. J. Educ. Technol. High. Educ.* **2018**, *15*, 1–26. [CrossRef]

107. Gbadamosi, A.-Q.; Oyedele, L.; Mahamadu, A.-M.; Kusimo, H.; Bilal, M.; Delgado, J.M.D.; Muhammed-Yakubu, N. Big data for Design Options Repository: Towards a DFMA approach for offsite construction. *Autom. Constr.* **2020**, *120*, 103388. [CrossRef]

108. Ajayi, A.; Oyedele, L.; Akinade, O.; Bilal, M.; Owolabi, H.; Akanbi, L.; Delgado, J.M.D. Optimised big data analytics for health and safety hazards prediction in power infrastructure operations. *Saf. Sci.* **2020**, *125*, 104656. [CrossRef]

109. Valpeters, M.; Kireev, I.; Ivanov, N. Application of machine learning methods in big data analytics at management of contracts in the construction industry. In Proceedings of the MATEC Web of Conferences, St. Petersburg, Russia, 20–22 December 2017; p. 01106.

110. Braun, A.; Borrmann, A. Combining inverse photogrammetry and BIM for automated labeling of construction site images for machine learning. *Autom. Constr.* **2019**, *106*, 102879. [CrossRef]

111. Huang, M.; Ninić, J.; Zhang, Q. BIM, machine learning and computer vision techniques in underground construction: Current status and future perspectives. *Tunn. Undergr. Space Technol.* **2021**, *108*, 103677. [CrossRef]

112. Cheng, J.C.; Chen, W.; Chen, K.; Wang, Q. Data-driven predictive maintenance planning framework for MEP components based on BIM and IoT using machine learning algorithms. *Autom. Constr.* **2020**, *112*, 103087. [CrossRef]

113. Bloch, T.; Sacks, R. Comparing machine learning and rule-based inferencing for semantic enrichment of BIM models. *Autom. Constr.* **2018**, *91*, 256–272. [CrossRef]

114. Munawar, H.S.; Hammad, A.W.; Waller, S.T. A review on flood management technologies related to image processing and machine learning. *Autom. Constr.* **2021**, *132*, 103916. [CrossRef]

115. Munawar, H.S.; Hammad, A.; Ullah, F.; Ali, T.H. After the flood: A novel application of image processing and machine learning for post-flood disaster management. In Proceedings of the 2nd International Conference on Sustainable Development in Civil Engineering (ICSDC 2019), Jamshoro, Pakistan, 5–7 December 2019; pp. 5–7.

116. Qureshi, A.H.; Alaloul, W.S.; Manzoor, B.; Musarat, M.A.; Saad, S.; Ammad, S. Implications of machine learning integrated technologies for construction progress detection under industry 4.0 (IR 4.0). In Proceedings of the 2020 Second International Sustainability and Resilience Conference: Technology and Innovation in Building Designs (51154), Sakheer, Bahrain, 11–12 November 2020; pp. 1–6.

117. Rozemberczki, B.; Scherer, P.; He, Y.; Panagopoulos, G.; Riedel, A.; Astefanoaei, M.; Kiss, O.; Beres, F.; López, G.; Collignon, N. Pytorch geometric temporal: Spatiotemporal signal processing with neural machine learning models. In Proceedings of the 30th ACM International Conference on Information & Knowledge Management, Gold Coast, Australia, 1–5 November 2021; pp. 4564–4573.

118. Eluri, V.R.; Ramesh, M.; Al-Jabri, A.S.M.; Jane, M. A comparative study of various clustering techniques on big data sets using Apache Mahout. In Proceedings of the 2016 3rd MEC International Conference on Big Data and Smart City (ICBDSC), Muscat, Oman, 15–16 March 2016; pp. 1–4.

119. Solanki, R.; Ravilla, S.H.; Bein, D. Study of distributed framework hadoop and overview of machine learning using apache mahout. In Proceedings of the 2019 IEEE 9th Annual Computing and Communication Workshop and Conference (CCWC), Las Vegas, NV, USA, 7–9 January 2019; pp. 0252–0257.

120. Sonnenburg, S.; Rätsch, G.; Henschel, S.; Widmer, C.; Behr, J.; Zien, A.; Bona, F.d.; Binder, A.; Gehl, C.; Franc, V. The SHOGUN machine learning toolbox. *J. Mach. Learn. Res.* **2010**, *11*, 1799–1802.

121. Jain, A. Scikit-learn: Machine learning in Python. *J. Mach. Learn. Res.* **2011**, *12*, 2825–2830.

122. Majumder, G.; Jain, R. A Comparative Study and Analysis of Classification Methods in Machine Learning. *Think India J.* **2019**, *22*, 709–718.
123. Liu, H.; Lang, B. Machine learning and deep learning methods for intrusion detection systems: A survey. *Appl. Sci.* **2019**, *9*, 4396. [CrossRef]

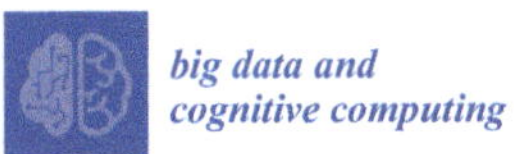

big data and cognitive computing

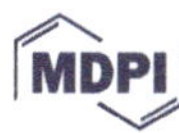

Review

An Overview of Data Warehouse and Data Lake in Modern Enterprise Data Management

Athira Nambiar * and Divyansh Mundra

Department of Computational Intelligence, School of Computing, SRM Institute of Science and Technology, Chennai 603203, India
* Correspondence: athiram@srmist.edu.in

Abstract: Data is the lifeblood of any organization. In today's world, organizations recognize the vital role of data in modern business intelligence systems for making meaningful decisions and staying competitive in the field. Efficient and optimal data analytics provides a competitive edge to its performance and services. Major organizations generate, collect and process vast amounts of data, falling under the category of big data. Managing and analyzing the sheer volume and variety of big data is a cumbersome process. At the same time, proper utilization of the vast collection of an organization's information can generate meaningful insights into business tactics. In this regard, two of the popular data management systems in the area of big data analytics (i.e., data warehouse and data lake) act as platforms to accumulate the big data generated and used by organizations. Although seemingly similar, both of them differ in terms of their characteristics and applications. This article presents a detailed overview of the roles of data warehouses and data lakes in modern enterprise data management. We detail the definitions, characteristics and related works for the respective data management frameworks. Furthermore, we explain the architecture and design considerations of the current state of the art. Finally, we provide a perspective on the challenges and promising research directions for the future.

Keywords: big data; data warehousing; data lake; enterprise data management; OLAP; ETL tools; metadata; cloud computing; Internet of Things

Citation: Nambiar, A.; Mundra, D. An Overview of Data Warehouse and Data Lake in Modern Enterprise Data Management. *Big Data Cogn. Comput.* **2022**, *6*, 132. https://doi.org/10.3390/bdcc6040132

Academic Editors: Domenico Talia and Fabrizio Marozzo

Received: 28 September 2022
Accepted: 2 November 2022
Published: 7 November 2022

Publisher's Note: MDPI stays neutral with regard to jurisdictional claims in published maps and institutional affiliations.

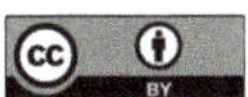

1. Introduction

Big data analytics is one of the buzzwords in today's digital world. It entails examining big data and uncovering the hidden patterns, correlations, etc. available in the data [1]. Big data analytics extracts and analyzes random data sets, forming them into meaningful information. According to statistics, the overall amount of data generated in the world in 2021 was approximately 79 zettabytes, and this is expected to double by 2025 [2]. This unprecedented amount of data was the result of a data explosion that occurred during the last decade, wherein data interactions increased by 5000% [3].

Big data deals with the volume, variety, and velocity of data to process and provides veracity (insightfulness) and value to data. These are known as the 5 Vs of big data [4]. An unprecedented amount of diverse data is acquired, stored, and processed with high data quality for various application domains. These include business transactions, real-time streaming, social media, video analytics, and text mining, creating a huge amount of semi- or unstructured data to be stored in different information silos [5]. The efficient integration and analysis of these multiple data across silos are required to divulge complete insight into the database. This is an open research topic of interest.

Big data and its related emerging technologies have been changing the way e-commerce and e-services operate and have been opening new frontiers in business analytics and related research [6]. Big data analytics systems play a big role in the modern enterprise management domain, from product distribution to sales and marketing, as well as analyzing hidden trends, similarities, and other insights and allowing companies to analyze and optimize their data to find new opportunities [7]. Since organizations with better and more accurate data can make informed business decisions by looking at market trends and customer preferences, they can gain competitive advantages over others. Hence, organizations invest tremendously in artificial intelligence (AI) and big data technologies to strive toward digital transformation and data-driven decision making, which ultimately leads to advanced business intelligence [6]. As per reports, the worldwide big data analytics and business intelligence software applications markets seem as though they will increase by USD 68 billion and 17.6 billion by 2024–2025, respectively [8].

Big data repositories exist in many forms, as per the requirements of corporations [9]. An effective data repository needs to unify, regulate, evaluate, and deploy a huge amount of data resources to enhance the analytics and query performance. Based on the nature and the application scenario, there are many different types of data repositories other than traditional relational databases. Two of the popular data repositories among them are enterprise data warehouses and data lakes [10–12].

A data warehouse (DW) is a data repository which stores structured, filtered, and processed data that has been treated for a specific purpose, whereas a data lake (DL) is a vast pool of data for which the purpose is not defined [9]. In detail, data warehouses store large amounts of data collected by different sources, typically using predefined schemas. Typically, a DW is a purpose-built relational database running on specialized hardware either on the premises or in the cloud [13]. DWs have been used widely for storing enterprise data and fueling business intelligence and analytics applications [14–16].

Data lakes (DLs) have emerged as big data repositories that store raw data and provide a rich list of functionalities with the help of metadata descriptions [10]. Although the DL is also a form of enterprise data storage, it does not inherently include the same analytics features commonly associated with data warehouses. Instead, they are repositories storing raw data in their original formats and providing a common access interface. From the lake, data may flow downstream to a DW to get processed, packaged, and become ready for consumption. As a relatively new concept, there has been very limited research discussing various aspects of data lakes, especially in Internet articles or blogs.

Although data warehouses and data lakes share some overlapping features and use cases, there are fundamental differences in the data management philosophies, design characteristics, and ideal use conditions for each of these technologies. In this context, we provide a detailed overview and differences between both the DW and DL data management schemes in this survey paper. Furthermore, we consolidate the concepts and give a detailed analysis of different design aspects, various tools and utilities, etc., along with recent developments that have come into existence.

The remainder of this paper is organized as follows. In Section 2, the terminology and basic definitions of big data analytics and the data management schemes are analyzed. Furthermore, the related works in the field are also summarized in this section. In Section 3, the architectures of both the data warehouse and data lake are presented. Next, in Section 4, the key design aspects of the DW and DL models along with their practical aspects are presented at length. Section 5 summarizes the various popular tools and services available for enterprise data management. In Sections 6 and 7, the open challenges and promising directions are explained, respectively. In particular, the pros and cons of various methods are critically discussed, and the observations are presented. Finally, Section 8 concludes this survey paper.

2. Definition: Big Data Analytics, Data Warehouses, and Data Lakes

The definitions and fundamental notions of various data management schemes are provided in this section. Furthermore, related works and review papers on this topic are also summarized.

2.1. Big Data Analytics

With significant advancements in technology, unprecedented usage of computer networks, multimedia, the Internet of Things, social media, and cloud computing has occured [17]. As a result, a huge amount of data, known as "big data", has been generated. It is required to collect, manage, and analyze these data efficiently via big data processing. The process of big data processing is aimed at data mining (i.e., extracting knowledge from large amounts of data), leveraging data management, machine learning, high-performance computing, statistics, pattern recognition, etc. The important characteristics of big data (known as the seven Vs of big data) (https://impact.com/marketing-intelligence/7-vs-big-data/, accessed on 25 September 2022) are as follows:

- Volume, or the available amount of data;
- Velocity, or the speed of data processing;
- Variety, or the different types of big data;
- Volatility, or the variability of the data;
- Veracity, or the accuracy of the data;
- Visualization, or the depiction of big data-generated insights through visual representation;
- Value, or the benefits organizations derive from the data.

Typically, there are mainly three kinds of big data processing possible: batch processing, stream processing, and hybrid processing [18]. In batch processing, data stored in the non-volatile memory will be processed, and the probability and temporal characteristics of data conversion processes will be decided by the requirements of the problems. In stream processing, the collected data will be processed without storing them in non-volatile media, and the temporal characteristics of data conversion processes will mainly be determined by the incoming data rate. This is suitable for domains that require low response times. Another kind of big data processing, known as hybrid processing, combines both the batch and stream processing techniques to achieve high accuracy and a low processing time [19]. Some examples of hybrid big data processing are Lambda and Kappa Architecture [20]. The Lambda Architecture processes huge quantities of data, enabling the batch-processing and stream-processing methods with a hybrid approach. The Kappa Architecture is a simpler alternative to the Lambda Architecture, since it leverages the same technology stack to handle both real-time stream processing and historical batch processing. However, it avoids maintaining two different code bases for the batch and speed layers. The major notion is to facilitate real-time data processing using a single stream-processing engine, thus bypassing the multi-layered Lambda Architecture without compromising the standard quality of service.

2.2. Data Warehouses

The concept of data warehouses (DWs) was introduced in the late 1980s by IBM researchers Barry Devlin and Paul Murphy with the aim to deliver an architectural model to solve the flow of data to decision support environments [21]. According to the definition by Inmon, *"a data warehouse is a subject-oriented, nonvolatile, integrated, time-variant collection of data in support of management decisions"* [22]. Formally, a data warehouse (DW) is a large data repository wherein data can be stored and integrated from various sources in a well-structured manner and help in the decision-making process via proper data analytics [23]. The process of compiling information into a data warehouse is known as data warehousing.

In enterprise data management, data warehousing is referred to as a set of decision-making systems targeted toward empowering the information specialist (leader, administrator, or analyst) to improve decision making and make decisions quicker. Hence, DW systems act as an important tool of business intelligence, being used in enterprise data management by most medium and large organizations [24,25]. The past decade has seen unprecedented development both in the number of products and services offered and in the wide-scale adoption of these advancements by the industry. According to a comprehensive research report by Market Research Future (MRFR) titled *"Data Warehouse as a Service Market information by Usage, by Deployment, by Application and Organization Size—forecast to 2028"*, the market size will reach USD 7.69 billion, growing at a compound annual growth rate of 24.5%, by 2028 [26].

In the data warehouse framework, data are periodically extracted from programs that aid in business operations and duplicated onto specialized processing units. They may then be approved, converted, reconstructed, and augmented with input from various options. The developed data warehouse then becomes a primary origin of data for the production, analysis, and presentation of reports via instantaneous reports, e-portals, and digital readouts. It employs "online analytical processing" (OLAP), whose utility and execution needs differ from those of the "online transaction processing" (OLTP) implementations typically backed up by functional databases [27,28]. OLTP programs often computerize the handling of administrative data processes, such as order entry and banking transactions, which are an organization's necessary activities. Data warehouses, on the other hand, are primarily concerned with decision assistance. As shown in Figure 1a, a data warehouse integrates data from various sources and helps with analysis, data mining, and reporting. A detailed description of a DW's architecture is presented in Section 3.1.

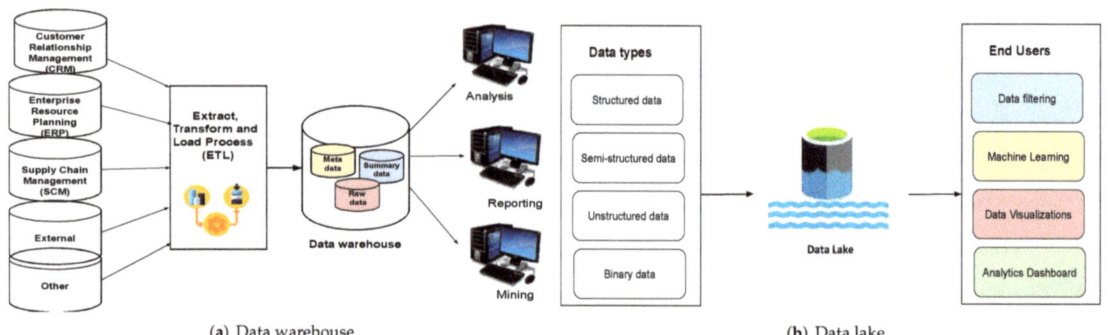

(**a**) Data warehouse   (**b**) Data lake

Figure 1. Data warehouse architecture vs. data lake architecture.

Data warehousing advancements have benefited various sectors, including production (for supply shipment and client assistance), business (for profiling of clients and stock governance), monetary administrations (for claims investigation, risk assessment, billing examination, and detecting fraud), logistics (for vehicle administration), broadcast communications (in order to analyze calls), utility companies (in order to analyze power use), and medical services [29]. The field of data warehousing has seen immense research and developments over the last two decades in various research categories such as data warehouse architecture, data warehouse design, and data warehouse evolution.

2.3. Data Lake

By the beginning of the 21st century, new types of diverse data were emerging in ever-increasing volumes on the Internet and at its interface to the enterprise (e.g., web-based business transactions, real-time streaming, sensor data, and social media). With the huge amount of data around, the need to have better solutions for storing and analyzing large amounts of semi-structured and unstructured data to gain relevant information and valuable insight became apparent. Traditional schema-on-write approaches such as the extract, transform, and load (ETL) process are too inefficient for such data management requirements. This gave rise to another popular modern enterprise data management scheme known as data lakes [30–32].

Data lakes are centralized storage repositories that enable users to store raw, unprocessed data in their original format, including unstructured, semi-structured, or structured data, at scale. These help enterprises to make better business decisions via visualizations or dashboards from big data analysis, machine learning, and real-time analytics. A pictorial representation of a data lake is given in Figure 1b.

According to Dixon, *"whilst a data warehouse seems to be a bottle of water cleaned and ready for consumption, then "Data Lake" is considered as a whole lake of data in a more natural state"* [33]. Another definition for the data lake is provided in [34], and it is as follows: *"a data lake stores disparate information while ignoring almost everything"*. The explanation of data lakes from an architectural viewpoint is given in [35], and it is as follows: *"A data lake uses a flat architecture to store data in its raw format. Each data entity in the lake is associated with a unique, i.e.tifier and a set of extended metadata, and consumers can use purpose-built schemas to query relevant data, which will result in a smaller set of data that can be analyzed to help answer a consumer's question"*. A data lake houses data in its original raw form. The data in data lakes can vary drastically in size and structure, and they lack any specific organizational structure. A data lake can accommodate either very small or huge amounts of data as required. All of these features provide flexibility and scalability to data lakes. At the same time, challenges related to its implementation and data analytics also arise.

Data lakes are becoming increasingly popular for organizations to store their data in a centralized manner. A data lake may contain unstructured or multi-structured data, where most of them may have unrealized value for the enterprise. This allows organizations to store their data from different sources without any overhead related to the transformation of the data [30]. This also allows ad hoc data analyses to be performed on this data, which can then be used by organizations to drive key insights and data-driven decision making. DLs replace the previous way of organizing and processing data from various sources with a centralized, efficient, and flexible repository that allows organizations to maximize their gains from a data-driven ecosystem. Data lakes also allow organizations to scale them to their needs. This is achieved by separating storage from the computational part. Complex transformation and preprocessing of data in the case of data warehouses is eliminated. The upfront financial overhead of data ingestion is also reduced. Once data are collated in the lake or hub, it is available for analysis for the organization.

2.4. The Difference between Data Warehouses and Data Lakes

Although data warehouses and data lakes are used as two interchangeable terms, they are not the same [21]. One of the major differences between them is the different structures (i.e., processed vs. raw data). A data warehouse stores data in processed and filtered form, whereas data lakes store raw or unprocessed data. Specifically, data are processed and organized into a single schema before being put into the warehouse, whereas raw and unstructured data are fed into a data lake. Analysis is performed on the cleansed data in the warehouse. On the contrary, in a data lake, data are selected and organized as and when needed.

As for storing processed data, a data warehouse is economic. On the contrary, data lakes have a comparatively larger capacity than the data warehouse and are ideal for raw and unprocessed data analysis and employing machine learning. Another key difference is the objective or purpose of use. Typically, processed data that flow into data warehouses are used for specific purposes, and hence the storage space will not be wasted, whereas the purpose of usage for the data lake is not defined and can ideally be used for any purpose. To use processed or filtered data, no specialized expertise is required, as merely familiarization with the presentation of data (e.g., charts, sheets, tables, and presentations) will do. Hence, DWs can be used by any business or individual. On the contrary, it is comparatively difficult to analyze DLs without familiarity with unprocessed data, hence requiring data scientists with appropriate skills or tools to comprehend them for specific business use. Accessibility or ease of use of data repositories is yet another aspect that differentiates data warehouses and data lakes. Since the architecture of a data lake has no proper structure, it has flexibility of use. Instead, the structure of a DW makes sure that no foreign particles invade it, and it is very costly to manipulate. This feature makes it very secure, too. A detailed analysis of the differences between data warehouses and data lakes is given in Table 1.

Table 1. Differences between data warehouses and data lakes.

Parameters	Data Warehouse	Data Lake
Data	Data warehouse focuses only on business processes	Data lakes store everything
Processing	Highly processed data	Data are mainly unprocessed
Type of Data	They are mostly in the tabular form and structure	They can be unstructured, semi-structured, or structured
Task	Optimized for data retrieval	Share data stewardship
Agility	Less agile and has fixed configuration compared with data lakes	Highly agile and can configure and reconfigure as needed
Users	Widely used by business professionals and business analysts	Data lakes are used by data scientists, data developers, and business analysts
Storage	Expensive storage that gives fast response times is used	Data lakes are designed for low-cost storage
Security	Allows better control of the data	Offers less control
Schema	Schema on writing (predefined schemas)	Schema on reading (no predefined schemas)
Data Processing	Time-consuming to introduce new content	Helps with fast ingestion of new data
Data Granularity	Data at the summary or aggregated level of detail	Data at a low level of detail or granularity
Tools	Mostly commercial tools	Can use open-source tools such as Hadoop or Map Reduce

2.5. Literature Review

A summary of various research works in the field of data warehouses and data lakes is presented here. A list of various survey articles on data warehouses and data lakes is depicted in Table 2. Mainly, data warehouse review works address architecture modeling and its comparisons [36,37], the evolution of the DW concept [38], real-time data warehousing and ETL [39], etc. Compared with the data warehouse literature reviews, data lake papers are relatively fewer in number. Data lake review works summarize recent approaches and the architecture of DLs [31,32] as well as the design and implementation aspects [30]. To the best of our knowledge, only one work on comparing data warehouses and data lakes was found in the literature [12]. In contrast to that article, our work provides a comprehensive analysis of both data management schemes by addressing various aspects such as, definitions, architecture, practical design considerations, tools and services, challenges, and opportunities in detail. In addition to the survey papers, we also consolidate various works on data warehouses and data lakes in the reported literature and classify them in Table 3 based on their functions and utility.

Table 2. Summary of existing survey articles on data warehouses and data lakes.

Topic	Survey Papers	Contributions
Data warehouse	[28]	Data warehouse concepts, multilingualism issues in data warehouse design and solutions
Data warehouse	[36]	Data warehouse architecture modeling and classifications
Data warehouse and big data	[40]	A comprehensive survey on big data, big data analytics, augmentation, and big data warehouses
Data warehouse	[11]	Data warehouse survey
Data warehouse	[39]	Real-time data warehouse and ETL
Data warehouse	[41]	Architectures of data warehouses (DWs) and their selection

Table 2. *Cont.*

Topic	Survey Papers	Contributions
Data warehouse	[38]	Data warehouse (DW) evolution
Data warehouse	[42]	Data warehouse modeling and design
Data warehouse	[37]	Comparative study on data warehouse architectures
Data lake	[30]	A survey on designing, implementing, and applying data lakes
Data lake	[31]	Recent approaches and architectures using data lakes
Data lake	[32]	Overview of data lake definitions, architectures, and technologies
Data lake vs. data warehouse	[12]	Explores the two architectures of data warehouses and data lakes

Table 3. Related works: classification of data warehouse and data lake solutions.

Systems or Topic Area	Data Warehouse	Data Lake	Function or Work Performed	Reference
OLAP	✓		Online analytical processing (OLAP)	Providing OLAP to User-Analysts: an IT Mandate [28]
GEMMS		✓	Metadata extraction, Metadata modeling	Metadata Extraction and Management in Data Lakes with GEMMS [30]
KAYAK		✓	Dataset preparation and organization	KAYAK: a Framework for Just-in-Time Data Preparation in a Data Lake [43]
DWHA	✓		Modeling and classification of DW	Analysis of Data Warehouse Architectures: Modelling and Classification [36]
DATAMARAN		✓	Metadata extraction	Navigating the Data Lake with DATAMARAN: Automatically Extracting Structure from Log Datasets [44]
Geokettle	✓		Data warehouse architecture, design, and testing	Extraction, Transformation, and Loading (ETL) Module for Hotspot Spatial Data Warehouse Using Geokettle [45]
GOODS		✓	Dataset preparation and organization, metadata enrichment	Managing Google's data lake: an overview of the Goods system [46]
VOLAP	✓		OLAP, query processing, and optimization	VOLAP: a Scalable Distributed System for Real-Time OLAP with High-Velocity Data [47]
Dimension constraints	✓		Multidimensional data modeling, OLAP, query processing, and optimization	Capturing summarizability with integrity constraints in OLAP [48]
CLAMS		✓	Data quality improvement	CLAMS: Bringing Quality to Data Lakes [49]
Juneau		✓	Dataset preparation and organization, discover related data sets, and query-driven data discovery	Juneau: Data Lake Management for Jupyter [50]
JOSIE		✓	Discover related data sets and query-driven data discovery	Josie: Overlap Set Similarity Search for Finding Joinable Tables in Data Lakes [51]
CoreDB		✓	Metadata enrichment and query heterogeneous data	CoreDB: a Data Lake Service [52]
Constance		✓	Unified interface for query processing and data exploration	Constance: An Intelligent Data Lake System [53]
ODS	✓		Operational data store	Combining the Data Warehouse and Operational Data Store [54]

3. Architecture

In this section, the architectures of the data warehouse and data lake schemes are described in detail. Furthermore, the classification of data warehouse and data lake solutions based on function is carried out and summarized as a table.

3.1. Data Warehouse Architecture

The data warehouse architecture contains historical and commutative data from multiple sources. Basically, there are three kinds of architectures [55]:

- *Single-tier architecture*: This kind of single-layer model minimizes the amount of data stored. It helps remove data redundancy. However, its disadvantage is the lack of a component that separates analytical and transactional processing. This kind of architecture is not frequently used in practice.
- *Two-tier architecture*: This model separates physically available sources and the data warehouse by means of a staging area. Such an architecture makes sure that all data loaded into the warehouse are in an appropriate cleansed format. Nevertheless, this architecture is not expandable nor can it support many end users. Additionally, it has connectivity problems due to network limitations.
- *Three-tier architecture*: This is the most widely used architecture for data warehouses [56,57]. It consists of a top, middle, and bottom tier. In the bottom tier, data are cleansed, transformed, and loaded via backend tools. This tier serves as the database of the data warehouse. The middle tier is an OLAP server that presents an abstract view of the database by acting as a mediator between the end user and the database. The top tier, the front-end client layer, consists of the tools and an API that are used to connect and get data out from the data warehouse (e.g., query tools, reporting tools, managed query tools, analysis tools, and data mining tools).

The architecture of a data warehouse is shown in Figure 2. It consists of a central information repository that is surrounded by some key DW components, making the entire environment functional, manageable, and accessible.

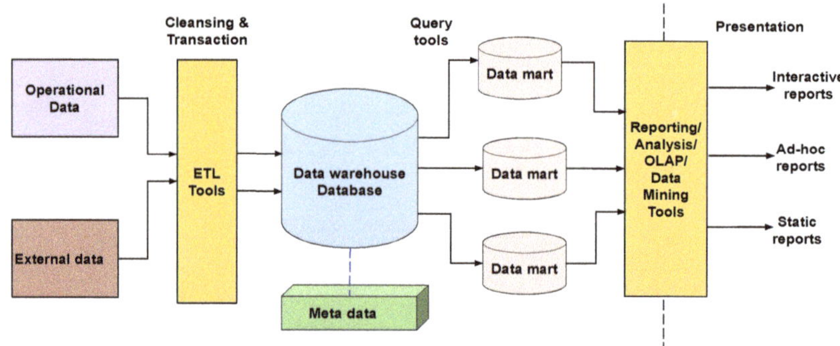

Figure 2. Data warehouse architecture.

- **Data warehouse database**: The core foundation of the data warehouse environment is its central database. This is implemented using RDBMS technology [58]. However, there is a limitation to such implementations, since the traditional RDBMS system is optimized for transactional database processing and not for data warehousing. In this regard, the alternative means are (1) the usage of relational databases in parallel, which enables shared memory on various multiprocessor configurations or parallel processors, (2) new index structures to get rid of relational table scanning and improve the speed, and (3) multidimensional databases (MDDBs) used to circumvent the limitations caused by the relational data warehouse models.
- **Extract, transform, and load (ETL) tools**: All the conversions, summarizations, and changes required to transform data into a unified format in the data warehouse are

carried out via extract, transform, and load (ETL) tools [59]. This ETL process helps the data warehouse achieve enhanced system performance and business intelligence, timely access to data, and a high return on investment:

- *Extraction*: This involves connecting systems and collecting the data needed for analytical processing;
- *Transformation*: The extracted data are converted into a standard format;
- *Loading*: The transformed data are imported into a large data warehouse.

ETL anonymizes data as per regulatory stipulations, thereby anonymizing confidential and sensitive information before loading it into the target data store [60]. ETL eliminates unwanted data in operational databases from loading into DWs. ETL tools carry out amendments to the data arriving from different sources and calculate summaries and derived data. Such ETL tools generate background jobs, Cobol programs, shell scripts, etc. that regularly update the data in the data warehouse. ETL tools also help with maintaining the metadata.

- **Metadata**: Metadata is the data about the data that define the data warehouse [61]. It deals with some high-level technological concepts and helps with building, maintaining, and managing the data warehouse. Metadata plays an important role in transforming data into knowledge, since it defines the source, usage, values, and features of the data warehouse and how to update and process the data in a data warehouse. This is the most difficult tool to choose due to the lack of a clear standard. Efforts are being made among data warehousing tool vendors to unify a metadata model. One category of metadata known as *technical metadata* contains information about the warehouse that is used by its designers and administrators, whereas another category called *business metadata* contains details that enable end users to understand the information stored in the data warehouse.
- **Query Tools**: Query tools allow users to interact with the DW system and collect information relevant to businesses to make strategic decisions. Such tools can be of different types:

  - **Query and reporting tools**: Such tools help organizations generate regular operational reports and support high-volume batch jobs such as printing and calculating. Some popular reporting tools are Brio, Oracle, Powersoft, and SAS Institute. Similarly, query tools help end users to resolve pitfalls in SQL and database structure by inserting a meta-layer between the users and the database.
  - **Application development tools**: In addition to the built-in graphical and analytical tools, application development tools are leveraged to satisfy the analytical needs of an organization.
  - **Data mining tools**: This tool helps in automating the process of discovering meaningful new correlations and structures by mining large amounts of data.
  - **OLAP tools**: Online analytical processing (OLAP) tools exploit the concepts of a multidimensional database and help analyze the data using complex multidimensional views [28,62]. There are two types of OLAP tools: multidimensional OLAP (MOLAP) and relational OLAP (ROLAP) [63]:

    * **MOLAP**: In such an OLAP tool, a cube is aggregated from the relational data source. Based on the user report request, the MOLAP tool generates a prompt result, since all the data are already pre-aggregated within the cube [64].
    * **ROLAP**: The ROLAP engine acts as a smart SQL generator. It comes with a "designer" piece, wherein the administrator specifies the association between the relational tables, attributes, and hierarchy map and the underlying database tables [65].

3.2. Data Lake Architecture

The architecture of a business data lake is depicted in Figure 3. Although it is treated as a single repository, it can be distinguished as separate layers in most cases.

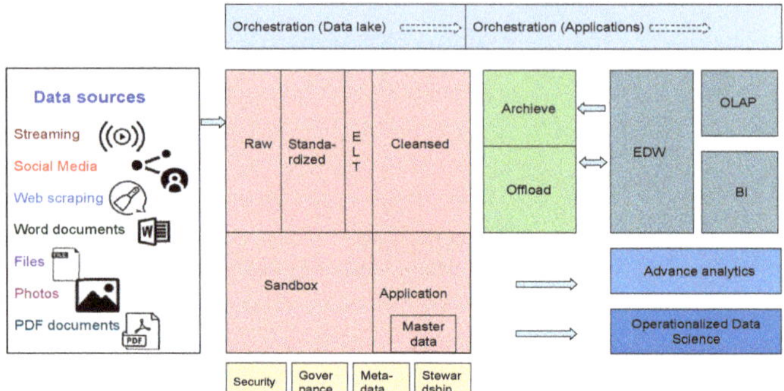

Figure 3. Data lake building blocks.

- **Raw data layer**: This layer is also known as the ingestion layer or landing area because it acts as the sink of the data lake. The prime goal is to ingest raw data as quickly and as efficiently as possible. No transformations are allowed at this stage. With the help of the archive, it is possible to get back to a point in time with raw data. Overriding (i.e., handling duplicate versions of the same data) is not permitted. End users are not granted access to this layer. These are not ready-to-use data, and they need a lot of knowledge in terms of relevant consumption.
- **Standardized data layer**: This is optional in most implementations. If one expects fast growth for his or her data lake architecture, then this is a good option. The prime objective of the standardized layer is to boost the performance of the data transfer from the raw layer to the curated layer. In the raw layer, data are stored in their native format, whereas in the standardized layer, the appropriate format that fits best for cleansing is selected.
- **Cleansed layer or curated layer**: In this layer, data are transformed into consumable data sets and stored in files or tables. This is one of the most complex parts of the whole data lake solution since it requires cleansing, transformation, denormalization, and consolidation of different objects. Furthermore, the data are organized by purpose, type, and file structure. Usually, end users are granted access only to this layer.
- **Application layer**: This is also known as the trusted layer, secure layer, or production layer. This is sourced from the cleansed layer and enforced with requisite business logic. In case the applications use machine learning models on the data lake, they are obtained from here. The structure of the data is the same as in the cleansed layer.
- **Sandbox data layer**: This is also another optional layer that is meant for analysts' and data scientists' work to carry out experiments and search for patterns or correlations. The sandbox data layer is the proper place to enrich the data with any source from the Internet.
- **Security**: While data lakes are not exposed to a broad audience, the security aspects are of great importance, especially during the initial phase and architecture. These are not like relational databases, which have an artillery of security mechanisms.
- **Governance**: Monitoring and logging operations become crucial at some point while performing analysis.
- **Metadata**: This is the data about data. Most of the schemas reload additional details of the purpose of data, with descriptions on how they are meant to be exploited.
- **Stewardship**: Based on the scale that is required, either the creation of a separate role or delegation of this responsibility to the users will be carried out, possibly through some metadata solutions.

- **Master Data**: This is an essential part of serving ready-to-use data. It can be either stored on the data lake or referenced while executing ELT processes.
- **Archive**: Data lakes keep some archive data that come from data warehousing. Otherwise, performance and storage-related problems may occur.
- **Offload**: This area helps to offload some time- and resource-consuming ETL processes to a data lake in case of relational data warehousing solutions.
- **Orchestration and ELT processes**: Once the data are pushed from the raw layer through the cleansed layer and to the sandbox and application layers, a tool is required to orchestrate the flow. Either an orchestration tool or some additional resources to execute them are leveraged in this regard.

Many implementations of a data lakes are originally based on Apache Hadoop. The Highly Available Object Oriented Data Platform (Hadoop) is a widely popular big data tool especially suitable for batch processing workloads of big data [66]. It uses HDFS as its core storage and MapReduce (MR) as the basic computing model. Novel computing models are constantly proposed to cope with the increasing needs for batch processing performance (e.g., Tez, Spark, and Presto) [67,68]. The MR model has also been replaced with the directed acyclic graph (DAG) model, which improves computing models' abstract concurrency. The second phase of data lake evolution has happened with the arrival of the *Lambda Architecture* [69,70], owing to the constant changes in data processing capabilities and processing demand. It presents stream computing engines, such as Storm, Spark Streaming, and Flink [71]. In such a framework, batch processing is combined with stream computing to meet the needs of many emerging applications. Yet another advanced phase is for the *Kappa Architecture* [72]. The two models of batch processing and stream computing are unified by improving the stream computing concurrency and increasing the time window of streaming data. In this regard, stream computing is used that features an inherent and scalable distributed architecture.

4. Design Aspects

The design aspects and practical implementation constraints are to be studied in detail to develop a suitable data management solution. This section presents the design aspects to be considered in data warehouse- and data lake-based enterprise data management.

4.1. Data Warehouse Design Considerations for Business Needs

To design a successful data warehouse, one should also realize the requirements of an organization and develop a framework for them. Some of the key criteria to keep in mind when choosing a data warehouse are as follows:

- **User needs and appropriate data model**: The very first design consideration in a data warehouse is the business and user needs. Hence, during the designing phase, the integration of the data warehouse with existing business processes and compatibility checks with long-term strategies have to be ensured. Enterprises have to clearly comprehend the purpose of their data warehouse, any technical requirements, benefits of end users from the system, improved means of reporting for business intelligence (BI), and analytics. In this regard, finding the notion of what information is important to the business is quintessential to the success of the data warehouse. To facilitate this, creating an appropriate data model of the business is a key aspect when designing DWs (e.g., SQL Developer Data Modeler (SDDM)). Furthermore, a data flow diagram can also help in depicting the data flow within the company in diagram format.
- **Adopting a standard data warehouse architecture and methodology**: While designing a DW, yet another important practical consideration is to leverage a recognized DW modeling standard (e.g., 3NF, star schema (dimensional), and Data Vault) [73]. Selecting such a standard architecture and sticking to the same one can augment the efficiency within a data warehouse development approach. Similarly, an agile data warehouse methodology is also an important practical aspect. With proper planning,

DW projects can be compartmentalized to smaller pieces capable of delivering faster. This design trick helps to prioritize the DW as a business's needs change.

- **Cloud vs. on-premise storage**: Enterprises can opt for either on-premises architecture or a cloud data warehouse [13]. The former category requires setting up the physical environment, including all the servers necessary to power ETL processes, storage, and analytic operations, whereas the latter can skip this step. However, a few circumstances exist where it still makes sense to consider an on-premises approach. For example, if most of the critical databases are on-premises and are old enough, they will not work well with cloud-based data warehouses. Furthermore, if the organization has to deal with strict regulatory requirements, which might include no offshore data storage, an on-premise setting might be the better choice. Nevertheless, cloud-based services provide the most flexible data warehousing service in the market in terms of storage and the pay-as-you-go nature.

- **Data tool ecosystem and data modeling**: The organization's ecosystem plays a key role. Adopting a DW automation tool ensures the efficient usage of IT resources, faster implementation through projects, and better support by enforcing coding standards (Wherescape (https://www.wherescape.com, accessed on 25 September 2022), AnalytixDS, Ajilius (https://tracxn.com/d/companies/ajilius.com, accessed on 25 September 2022), etc.).The data modeling planning step imparts detailed, reusable documentation of a data warehouse's implementation. Specifically, it assesses the data structures, investigates how to efficiently represent these sources in the data warehouse, specifies OLAP requirements, etc.

- **ETL or ELT design**: Selection of the appropriate ETL or ELT solution is yet another design concern [39]. When businesses use expensive in-house analytics systems, much prep work including transformations can be conducted, as in the ETL scheme. However, ELT is a better approach when the destination is a cloud data warehouse. Once data are colocated, the power of a single cloud engine can be leveraged to perform integrations and transformations efficiently. Organizations can transform their raw data at any time according to their use case, rather than a step in the data pipeline.

- **Semantic and reporting layers**: Based on previously documented data models, the OLAP server is implemented to facilitate the analytical queries of the users and to empower BI systems. In this regard, data engineers should carefully consider time-to-analysis and latency requirements to assess the analytical processing capabilities of the data warehouse. Similarly, while designing the reporting layer, the implementation of reporting interfaces or delivery methods as well as permissible access have to be set by the administrator.

- **Ease of scalability**: Understanding current business needs is critical to business intelligence and decision making. This includes how much data the organization currently has and how quickly its needs are likely to grow. Staffing and vendor costs need to be taken into consideration while deciding the scale of growth.

4.2. Data Lake Design Aspects for Enterprise Data Management

At a high level, the concept of a data lake seems to be simple. Irrespective of the format, it stores data from multiple sources in one place, leverages big data technologies, and deploys on a commodity infrastructure. However, many a time, reality may fail due to various practical constraints. Hence, it is quite important to consider several key criteria while designing an enterprise data lake:

- **Focus on business objectives rather than technology**: By anchoring the business objectives, a data lake can prioritize the efforts and outcomes accordingly. For instance, for a particular business objective, there may be some data that are more valuable than others. This kind of comprehension and analysis is the key to an enterprise's data lake success. With such an oriented goal, data lakes can start small and then accordingly learn, adapt, and produce accelerated outcomes for a business. In particular, some key factors in this regard are (1) whether it solves an actual business problem, (2) if it imparts new capabilities, and (3) the access or ownership of data, among others.

- **Scalability and durability** are two more major criteria [74]. Scalability enables scaling to any size of data while importing them in real time. This is an essential criterion for a data lake since it is a centralized data repository for an entire organization. Another important aspect (i.e., durability) deals with providing consistent uptime while ensuring no loss or corruption of data.

- Another key design aspect in a data lake is its **capability to store unstructured, semi-structured, and structured data**, which helps organizations to transfer anything from raw, unprocessed data to fully aggregated analytical outcomes [75]. In particular, the data lake has to deliver business-ready data. Practically speaking, data by themselves have no meaning. Although file formats and schemas can parse the data (e.g., JSON and XML), they fail at delivering insight into their meaning. To circumvent such a limitation, a critical component of any data lake technical design is the incorporation of a knowledge catalog. Such a catalog helps in finding and understanding information assets. The knowledge catalog's contents include the semantic meaning of the data, format and ownership of data, and data policies, among other elements.

- **Security** considerations are also of prime importance in a data lake in the cloud. The three domains of security are encryption, network-level security, and access control. Network-level security imparts a robust defense strategy by denying inappropriate access at the network level, whereas encryption ensures security at least for those types of data that are not publicly available. Security should be part of data lake design from the beginning. Compliance standards that regulate data protection and privacy are incorporated in many industries, such as the Payment Card Industry Data Security Standard (PCI DSS) for financial services and Health Insurance Portability and Accountability Act (HIPAA) for healthcare [76]. Furthermore, two of the biggest regulations regarding consumer privacy (i.e., California's Consumer Privacy Act (CCPA) and the European Union's General Data Protection Regulation (GDPR)) restrict the ownership, use, and management of personal and private data.

- A data lake design must include **metadata storage functionality** to help users to search and learn about the data sets in the lake [77]. A data lake allows the storage of all data that are **independent of the fixed schema**. Instead, data are read at the time of processing, should they be parsed and adapted into a schema, only as necessary. This feature saves plenty of time for enterprises.

- **Architecture in motion** is another interesting concept (i.e., the architecture will likely include more than one data lake and must be adaptable to address changing requirements). For instance, on-premises work with Hadoop could be moved to the cloud or a hybrid platform in the future. By facilitating the innovation of multi-cloud storage, a data lake can be easily upgraded to be used across data centers, on premises, and in private clouds. In addition, machine learning and automation can augment the data flow capabilities of an enterprise's data lake design.

5. Tools and Utilities

In this section, we categorize and detail the popular data warehouse and data lake tools and services in Sections 5.1 and 5.2, respectively.

5.1. Popular Data Warehouse Tools and Services

An enterprise data warehouse is one of the primary components of business intelligence [14,16]. It stores data from one or more heterogeneous sources and then analyzes and extracts insights from them to support decision making. Some of the popular top data warehousing tools are explained below:

- **Amazon Web Services (AWS) data warehouse tools**: AWS is one of the major leaders in data warehousing solutions [78] (https://aws.amazon.com/training/classroom/data-warehousing-on-aws/, accessed on 25 September 2022). AWS has many services, such as AWS Redshift, AWS S3, and Amazon RDS, making it a very cost-effective and highly scalable platform. **AWS Redshift** is a suitable platform for businesses that require very advanced capabilities that exploit high-end tools [79]. It consists of an in-house team that organizes AWS's extensive menu of services. **Amazon Simple Storage Service (AWS S3)** is a low-cost storage solution with industry-leading scalability, performance, and security features. **Amazon Relational Database Service (Amazon RDS)** is an AWS cloud data storage service that runs and scales a relational database. It has resizable and cost-effective technology that facilitates an industry-standard relational database and manages all database management activities.

- **Google data warehouse tools**: Google is highly acclaimed for its data management skills along with its dominance as a search engine (https://cloud.google.com, accessed on 25 September 2022). Google's data warehouse tools (https://research.google/research-areas/data-management/, accessed on 25 September 2022) excel in cutting-edge data management and analytics by incorporating machine intelligence. **Google BigQuery** is a business-level cloud-based data warehousing solution platform specially designed to save time by storing and querying large data sets through using super-fast SQL searches against multi-terabyte data sets in seconds, offering customers real-time data insights. **Google Cloud Data Fusion** is a cloud ETL solution which is entirely managed and allows data integration at any size with a visual point-and-click interface. **Dataflow** is another cloud-based data-processing service that can be used to stream data in batches or in real time. **Google Data Studio** enables turning the data into entirely customizable, easy-to-read reports and dashboards.
- **Microsoft Azure Data Warehouse tools**: Microsoft Azure is a recent cloud computing platform that provides Infrastructure as a Service (IaaS), Platform as a Service (PaaS), and Software as a Service (SaaS) as well as 200+ products and cloud services [80] (https://azure.microsoft.com/en-in/, accessed on 25 September 2022). **Azure SQL Database** is suitable for data warehousing applications with up to 8 TB of data volume and a large number of active users, facilitating advanced query processing. **Azure Synapse Analytics** consists of data integration, big data analytics, and enterprise data warehousing capabilities by also integrating machine learning technologies.
- **Oracle Autonomous Data Warehouse**: Oracle Autonomous Data Warehouse [81] is a cloud-based data warehouse service that manages the complexities associated with data warehouse development, data protection, data application development, etc. The setting, safeguarding, regulating, and backing up of data are all automated using this technology. This cloud computing solution is easy to use, secure, quick to respond, as well as scalable.
- **Snowflake**: Snowflake [82] is a cloud-based data warehouse tool offering a quick, easy-to-use, and adaptable data warehouse platform (https://www.snowflake.com, accessed on 25 September 2022). It has a comprehensive Software as a Service (SaaS) architecture since it runs entirely in the cloud. This makes data processing easier by permitting users to work with a single language, SQL for data blending, analysis, and transformations on a variety of data types. Snowflake's multi-tenant design enables real-time data exchange throughout the enterprise without relocating data.
- **IBM Data Warehouse tools**: IBM is a preferred choice for large business clients due to its huge install base, vertical data models, various data management solutions, and real-time analytics (https://www.ibm.com/in-en/analytics, accessed on 25 September 2022). One DW tool (i.e., **IBM DB2 Warehouse**) is a cloud DW that enables self-scaling data storage and processing and deployment flexibility. Another tool is **IBM Datastage**, which can take data from a source system, transform it, and feed it into a target system. This enables the users to merge data from several corporate systems using either an on-premises or cloud-based parallel architecture.

5.2. Popular Data Lake Tools and Services

A data lake stores structured data from relational databases, where semi-structured data, unstructured data, and binary data and can be set up "on the premises" or in the "cloud" [83,84]. Some of the most popular data lake tools and services are analyzed below:

- **Azure Data Lake**: Azure Data Lake makes it easy for developers and data scientists to store data of any size, shape, and speed and conduct all types of processing and analytics across platforms and languages (https://azure.microsoft.com/en-in/solutions/data-lake/, accessed on 25 September 2022). It removes the complexities associated with ingesting and storing the data and makes it faster to bring up and execute with batch, streaming, and interactive analytics [85]. Some of the key features of Azure Data Lake include unlimited scale and data durability, on-par performance even with demanding workloads, high security with flexible mechanisms, and cost optimization through independent scaling of storage.

- **AWS**: Amazon Web Services claims to provide "the most secure, scalable, comprehensive, and cost-effective portfolio of services for customers to build their data lake in the cloud" (https://aws.amazon.com/lake-formation/?whats-new-cards.sort-by=item.additionalFields.postDateTime&whats-new-cards.sort-order=desc, accessed on 25 September 2022). AWS Lake Formation helps to set up a secure data lake that can collect and catalog data from databases and object storage, move the data into the new Amazon Simple Storage Service (S3) data lake, and clean and classify the data using ML algorithms. It offers various aspects of scalability, agility, and flexibility that are required by the companies to fuse data and analytics approaches. AWS customers include NETFLIX, Zillow, NASDAQ, Yelp, and iRobot.

- **Google BigLake**: BigLake is a storage engine that unifies data warehouses and lakes (https://cloud.google.com/biglake, accessed on 25 September 2022). It removes the need to duplicate or move data, thus making the system efficient and cost-effective. BigLake provides detailed access controls and performance acceleration across BigQuery and multi-cloud data lakes, with open formats to ensure a unified, flexible, and cost-effective lakehouse architecture. The top features of BigLake include (1) users being able to enforce consistent access controls across most analytics engines with a single copy of data and (2) unified governance and management at scale. Users can extend BigQuery to multi-cloud data lakes and open formats with fine-grained security controls without setting up a new infrastructure.

- **Cloudera**: Cloudera SDX is a data lake service for creating safe, secure, and governed data lakes with protective rings around the data wherever they stored, from object stores to the Hadoop Distributed File System (HDFS) (https://www.cloudera.com, accessed on 25 September 2022). It provides the capabilities needed for (1) data schema and metadata information, (2) metadata governance and management, (3) data access authorization and authentication, and (4) compliance-ready access auditing.

- **Snowflake**: Snowflake's cross-cloud platform breaks down silos and enables a data lake strategy (https://www.snowflake.com/workloads/data-lake/, accessed on 25 September 2022). Data scientists, analysts, and developers can seamlessly leverage governed data self-service for a variety of workloads. The key features of Snowflake include (1) all data on one platform that combines structured, semi-structured, and unstructured data of any format across clouds and regions, (2) fast, reliable processing and querying, simplifying the architecture with an elastic engine to power many workloads, and (3) secure collaboration via easy integration of external data without ETL.

6. Challenges

This section addresses some of the key challenges in big data analytics problems. In addition, the implementation challenges encountered in data warehouses and data lake paradigms are also critically analyzed.

6.1. Challenges in Big Data Analytics

In the past few years, big data have been accumulated in every walk of human life, including healthcare, retail, public administration, and research. Web-based applications have to deal with big data frequently, such as Internet text and documents (corpus, etc.), social network analysis, prediction markets, and Internet search indexing [86]. Although we can clearly observe the potential and current advantages of big data, there are some inherent challenges also present that have to be tackled to achieve the full potential of big data analytics [87].

The first hurdle for big data analytics is the **storage mediums and higher I/O speed** [88]. Storage of big data causes a financial overhead which is not affordable or profitable for many enterprises. Furthermore, this also results in slower processes [89]. In decades gone by, analysts made use of hard disk drives for data storage purposes, but this is slower in terms of random I/O performance compared with sequential I/O. To overcome this limitation, the concept of solid-state drives (SSDs) and phase change memory were introduced. However, the currently available storage tech simply does not possess the required performance for processing big data and delivering insights in a timely fashion. Companies opt for various modern techniques to handle large data sets, such as compression (reducing the number of bits within the data), data tiering (storing data in several storage tiers), and deduplication (the process of removing duplicates and unwanted data).

Anther challenge is **the lack of proper understanding of big data and the lack of knowledge professionals**. Due to insufficient understanding, organizations may fail in big data initiatives. This may be due to the absence of skilled data professionals, the lack of a transparent picture for employees, or improper usage of data repositories, among other reasons. It is highly encouraged to conduct big data workshops and seminars at companies to enable every level of the organization to inculcate a basic understanding of knowledge concepts. Furthermore, companies should invest in recruiting skilled professionals, supplying training programs to the staff, as well as purchasing knowledge analytics solutions powered by advanced artificial intelligence or machine learning tools.

Yet another challenge in big data analytics is the **confusion with suitable tool selection**. For instance, many a time, it is not so clear whether Hadoop or Spark is a better option for data analytics and storage. Sometimes, the wrong selection may result in poor decisions and the selection of inappropriate technology. Hence, money, time, effort, and work hours are wasted. The best solution would be to make use of experienced professionals or data consulting to obtain a recommendation for the tools that can support a company based on its scenario.

Data in a corporation come from various sources, such as customer logs, financial reports, social media platforms, e-mails, and reports created by employees. **Integrating data from such a huge spread of sources** is another challenging task [90]. This consolidation task, known as data integration, is crucial for business intelligence. Hence, enterprises purchase proper tools for data integration purposes. Talend Data Integration, IBM InfoSphere Xplenty, Informatica PowerCenter, and Microsoft SQL QlikView are some of the popular data integration tools [91].

Security of huge sets of knowledge, especially ones that involve many confidential details of customers, is one of the, inevitable challenges in big data analytics [92,93]. The careless treatment of data repositories may invite malicious hackers, which can cost millions for a stolen record or a knowledge breach. The remedy would be to foster a cybersecurity division of a company to guard their data and to implement various security actions such as data encryption, data segregation, identity and access control, implementation of endpoint security, real-time security monitoring, and using big data security tools (e.g., IBM Guardian).

6.2. Data Warehouse Implementation Challenges

Implementation of a data warehouse requires proper planning and execution based on proper methods. Some of the major challenging considerations that arise with data warehousing are design, construction, and implementation [94,95].

The efficiency and working of a warehouse are **dependent on the data** that support its operations. With incorrect or redundant data, warehouse managers cannot accurately measure the exact costs. A key solution is to automate the system to improve the lead data quality and make sure that the sales team receives complete, correct, and consistent lead information. Another major concern in a data warehouse is the **quality control of data (i.e., quality and consistency of data)** [96]. The business intelligence process can be fine-tuned by incorporating flexibility to accept and integrate analytics as well as update the warehouse's schema to handle evolutions.

Another major challenge is **differences in naming, domain definitions, and identification numbers from heterogeneous sources**. The data warehouse has to be designed in such a way that it can accommodate the addition and attrition of data sources and the evolution of the sources and source data, thus avoiding major redesign. Yet another challenge is **customizing the available source data into the data model of the warehouse** because the capabilities of a DW may change over time based on the change in technology [97]. Further, **broader skills** are required for the administration of data warehouses in traditional database administration. Hence, managing the data warehouse in a large organization, the design of the management function, and selecting the management team for a database warehouse are some of the important aspects of a data warehouse.

Data security is another critical requirement in DWs, given that business data are extremely sensitive and can be easily obtained [98]. Unfortunately, the typical security paradigm—based on tables, lines, and characteristics—is incompatible with DWs. Following that, the model should be changed to one that is firmly integrated with the applicable model and is focused on the key notions of multidimensional display, such as facts, aspects, and measures. Furthermore, as is frequently advised in computer programming, **information security** should be considered at all stages of the improvement process, from prerequisite analysis to execution and upkeep. In addition, **data warehouse governance** is yet another important consideration, which includes approval of the data modeling standards and metadata standards, the design of a data access policy, and a data backup strategy [99].

6.3. Data Lake Implementation Challenges

The data lake is relatively novel technology and has not matured yet. Hence, there are many challenges in its implementation, including many of the same challenges that early data warehouses confronted [75,100]. The first challenge is the **high cost of data lakes**. They are expensive to implement and maintain. Data lake platforms that exploit the cloud may be easier to deploy, but they may also come with high fees. Some of the platforms such as Hadoop are open source and hence free of cost. Nevertheless, the implementation and management may take more time and more expert staff. **Management difficulty** is another issue [75]. The management of the DL involves various complex tasks, such as ensuring the capacity of the host infrastructure to cope with the growth of the DL and dealing with data redundancy and data security. This puts forth challenges even to skilled engineers. Furthermore, it is required to have more domain experts and engineers with real expertise in setting up and managing data lakes. In the current scenario, there is a shortage of both data scientists and data engineers in the field. This **lack of skills** is yet another challenge.

Another aspect for consideration is the **long time to value** (i.e., it takes years to become full-fledged and to be integrated well with the workflow and analytics tools to impart real value to the enterprise) [101]. As mentioned in the case of data warehouses, in the case of DLs, **data security** is also a major concern. It requires special security measures to be considered to enforce data governance rules and to secure the data in the DL with the help of cyber security specialists and security tools. Another critical challenge is the **computation resources and increase in computing power**. This is due to the fact that data are growing unprecedentedly faster than computing power. At the same rate, the existing computers are not well equipped to host and manage them at the same rate due to a lack of power. Similarly, open-source data platforms also find many core problems surrounding data lakes which are too costly to manage. This also requires massive computing power to overcome such serious skill gaps.

To build a better data lake, it is required to modernize the way businesses build and manage data lakes. One key takeaway is to take full **advantage of the cloud**, as opposed to building cumbersome data lakes on a tailor-made infrastructure [102]. It helps to get rid of data silos and to build data lakes that are applicable to various use cases, rather than only fitting them to a certain range of needs.

7. Opportunities and Future Directions

Based on our survey, we discuss novel trends in modern enterprise data management and point out some promising directions for future research in this section.

7.1. Data Warehouses: Opportunities and Future Directions

The business management landscape has witnessed a massive change with the emergence of the data warehouse. The **advancements in cloud technology, the Internet of Things, and big data analytics** have brought effective data solutions in modern data warehouses [77,103]. With the rapid evolution of technology, many enterprises have migrated their data to the cloud to expand their networks and markets. **Cloud data warehouses** help to overcome the huge costs of purchasing, infrastructure, installation, etc. [104]. Hence, in the coming years, more sophisticated technology in cloud DWs is envisaged to enhance intense, easy-to-use, and economical data clouds as well. The long-term gains for the adoption of cloud warehousing are mainly data availability and scalability. The flexibility to store a variety of data formats—not just relational—combined with the intrinsic flexibility of cloud-based services enables a very broad distribution of cloud services.

Another massive change is in the means of **data analytics**. In contrast to the older times, wherein data analytics and business intelligence occurred in two different divisions, which delayed the overall efficiency of the system, the modern data warehouse provides an advanced structure for storage and faster data flow, thus making them easily accessible for business users. Such an agility model is powered by data fragmentation, allowing access to and the analysis of data across the enterprise in real time.

Another big advancement is in the **Internet of Things (IoT)** platforms for sharing and storing data. This has changed the face of data streaming by enabling users to store and access data across multiple devices. The concept of the IoT is more pertinent to the real world due to the increasing popularity of mobile devices, embedded and ubiquitous communication technologies, cloud computing, and data analytics. In a broader sense, as with the Internet, the IoT enables devices to exist in many places and facilitates applications from trivial to the most crucial. Several technologies such as computational intelligence and big data can be incorporated together with the IoT to improve data management and knowledge discovery on a large scale. Much research in this sense has been carried out by Mishra et al. [105].

In summary, the future of data warehouses comprises features that enable the following:

- All the data are accessible from a single location;
- The capability to outsource the task of maintaining that service's high availability to all customers;
- Governance based on policies;
- Platforms with high user experience (UX) discoverability;
- Platforms that cater to all customers.

7.2. Data Lakes: Opportunities and Future Directions

One of the core capabilities of a data lake architecture is its ability to quickly and easily ingest multiple types of data (e.g., real-time streaming data from on-premises storage platforms, structured data generated and processed by mainframes and data warehouses, and unstructured or semi-structured data). The ingestion process makes use of a high degree of parallelism and low latency since it requires interfacing with external data sources with limited bandwidth. Hence, ingestion will not carry out any deep analysis of the downloaded data. However, there are possibilities for **applying shallow data sketches**

on the downloaded contents and their metadata to maintain a basic organization of the ingested data sets.

In another phase of data lake management (i.e., **the data extraction stage**), the raw data are transformed into a predetermined data model. Although various studies have been conducted on this topic, there still remains room for improvement. Rather than conducting extraction on one file at a time, one can take advantage of the knowledge from the history of extractions. Similarly, in the cleaning phase of the data lake, not much work has not been performed in the literature other than some approaches such as CLAMS [49]. One opportunity in this regard will be to make use of the lake's wisdom and perform collective data cleaning. In addition, it is important to investigate the possible means of errors in the lake and to get rid of them efficiently to obtain a clean data lake.

The common methods to retrieve the data from the data lake are query-based retrieval (a user starts a search with a query for data retrieval) and data-based retrieval (a user navigates a data lake as a linkage graph or a hierarchical structure to find data of interest) [75]. A new direction may be to incorporate **analysis-driven or context-driven** approaches (i.e., augmenting a data set with relevant data and some contextual information to facilitate learning tasks).

Another direction of research is related to the exploration of **machine learning in data lakes**. Specifically, many studies are underway focusing on ML application toward data set organization and discovery. The data set discovery task is often associated with finding "similar" attributes extracted from the data, metadata, etc. which could be further coupled with classification or clustering tasks. Some recent works have leveraged ML techniques, such as the KNN classifier [106] and a logistic regression model for optimizing feature coefficients [107]. More advanced deep learning and similar sophisticated ML techniques are envisaged to augment the data set discovery process in the coming years.

Metadata management is an important task in a data lake, since a DL does not come with descriptive data catalogs [75,77]. Due to the lack of such explicit metadata of data sets, especially during the discovery and cleaning of data, there is a chance for a data lake to become a data swamp. Hence, it is quite necessary to extract meaningful metadata from data sources and to support efficient storage and query answering of metadata. In this field of metadata management, there remain more topics to explore further in extracting knowledge from lake data and incorporating them into existing knowledge bases. Yet another key aspect is **data versioning**, wherein new versions of the already existing files enter into a dynamic data lake [77]. Since versioning-related operations can affect all stages of a data lake, it is a very crucial aspect to address. There are some large-scale data set version control tools, such as DataHub (https://datahubproject.io, accessed on 25 September 2022), that provide a git-like interface to handle version creation, branching, and merging operations. Nevertheless, more research and development may be carried out further to deal with schema evolution.

As a final note, there is an emerging data management architecture trend called the *data lakehouse* that couples the flexibility of a data lake with the data management capabilities of a data warehouse. Specifically, it is considered a unique data storage solution for all data—unstructured, semi-structured, and structured—while providing the data quality and data governance standards of a data warehouse [108]. Such a data lakehouse would be capable of imparting better data governance, reduced data movement and redundancy, efficient use time, etc., even with a simplified schema. This topic of the *data lakehouse* is envisaged to be an excellent research area of data management in the future.

8. Conclusions

Enterprises and business organizations exploit a huge volume of data to understand their customers and to make informed business decisions to stay competitive in the field. However, big data come in a variety of formats and types (e.g., structured, semi-structured and unstructured data), making it difficult for businesses to manage and use them effectively. Based on the structure of the data, typically, two types of data storage are utilized in enterprise data management: the data warehouse (DW) and data lake (DL). Although being used as interchangeable terms, they are two distinct storage forms with unique characteristics that serve different purposes.

In this review, a comparative analysis of data warehouses and data lakes by highlighting the key differences between the two data management approaches was envisaged. In particular, the definitions of the data warehouse and data lake, highlighting their characteristics and key differences, were detailed. Furthermore, the architecture and design aspects of both DWs and DLs are clearly discussed. In addition, a detailed overview of the popular DW and DL tools and services was also provided. The key challenges of big data analytics in general, as well as the challenges of implementation of DWs and DLs, were also critically analyzed in this survey. Finally, the opportunities and future research directions were contemplated. We hope that the thorough comparison of existing data warehouses vs. data lakes and the discussion of open research challenges in this survey will motivate the future development of enterprise data management and benefit the research community significantly.

Author Contributions: Conceptualization, A.N. and D.M.; methodology, A.N. and D.M.; validation, A.N.; formal analysis, D.M.; investigation, A.N.; data curation, A.N. and D.M.; writing—original draft preparation, A.N. and D.M.; writing—review and editing, A.N. and D.M.; visualization, A.N.; supervision, A.N.; project administration, A.N. All authors have read and agreed to the published version of the manuscript.

Funding: This research received no external funding.

Institutional Review Board Statement: Not applicable.

Informed Consent Statement: Not applicable.

Data Availability Statement: Not applicable.

Conflicts of Interest: The authors declare no conflict of interest.

References

1. Tsai, C.W.; Lai, C.F.; Chao, H.C.; Vasilakos, A.V. Big data analytics: A survey. *J. Big Data* **2015**, *2*, 21. [CrossRef]
2. Big Data—Statistics & Facts. Available online: https://www.statista.com/topics/1464/big-data/ (accessed on 27 October 2022).
3. Wise, J. Big Data Statistics 2022: Facts, Market Size & Industry Growth. Available online: https://earthweb.com/big-data-statistics/ (accessed on 27 October 2022).
4. Jain, A. The 5 V's of Big Data. 2016. Available online: https://www.ibm.com/blogs/watson-health/the-5-vs-of-big-data/ (accessed on 27 October 2022).
5. Gandomi, A.; Haider, M. Beyond the hype: Big data concepts, methods, and analytics. *Int. J. Inf. Manag.* **2015**, *35*, 137–144. [CrossRef]
6. Sun, Z.; Zou, H.; Strang, K. Big Data Analytics as a Service for Business Intelligence. In *Open and Big Data Management and Innovation*; Springer International Publishing: Cham, Switzerland, 2015; Volume 9373, pp. 200–211. [CrossRef]
7. Big Data and Analytics Services Global Market Report. Available online: https://www.reportlinker.com/p06246484/Big-Data-and-Analytics-Services-Global-Market-Report.html (accessed on 27 October 2022).
8. BI & Analytics Software Market Value Worldwide 2019–2025. Available online: https://www.statista.com/statistics/590054/worldwide-business-analytics-software-vendor-market/ (accessed on 27 October 2022).
9. Kumar, S. What Is a Data Repository and What Is it Used for? 2019. Available online: https://stealthbits.com/blog/what-is-a-data-repository-and-what-is-it-used-for/ (accessed on 27 October 2022).
10. Khine, P.P.; Wang, Z.S. Data lake: A new, ideology in big data era. *ITM Web Conf.* **2018**, *17*, 03025. [CrossRef]
11. Arif, M.; Mujtaba, G. A Survey: Data Warehouse Architecture. *Int. J. Hybrid Inf. Technol.* **2015**, *8*, 349–356. [CrossRef]
12. El Aissi, M.E.M.; Benjelloun, S.; Loukili, Y.; Lakhrissi, Y.; Boushaki, A.E.; Chougrad, H.; Elhaj Ben Ali, S. Data Lake Versus Data Warehouse Architecture: A Comparative Study. In *WITS 2020*; Bennani, S., Lakhrissi, Y., Khaissidi, G., Mansouri, A., Khamlichi, Y., Eds.; Springer: Singapore, 2022; Volume 745, pp. 201–210. [CrossRef]
13. Rehman, K.U.u.; Ahmad, U.; Mahmood, S. A Comparative Analysis of Traditional and Cloud Data Warehouse. *VAWKUM Trans. Comput. Sci.* **2018**, *6*, 34–40. [CrossRef]
14. Devlin, B.A.; Murphy, P.T. An architecture for a business and information system. *IBM Syst. J.* **1988**, *27*, 60–80. [CrossRef]
15. Garani, G.; Chernov, A.; Savvas, I.; Butakova, M. A Data Warehouse Approach for Business Intelligence. In Proceedings of the 2019 IEEE 28th International Conference on Enabling Technologies: Infrastructure for Collaborative Enterprises (WETICE), Napoli, Italy, 12–14 June 2019; pp. 70–75. [CrossRef]

16. Gupta, V.; Singh, J. A Review of Data Warehousing and Business Intelligence in different perspective. *Int. J. Comput. Sci. Inf. Technol.* **2014**, *5*, 8263–8268.

17. Sagiroglu, S.; Sinanc, D. Big data: A review. In Proceedings of the 2013 International Conference on Collaboration Technologies and Systems (CTS), San Diego, CA, USA, 20–24 May 2013; pp. 42–47. [CrossRef]

18. Miloslavskaya, N.; Tolstoy, A. Application of Big Data, Fast Data, and Data Lake Concepts to Information Security Issues. In Proceedings of the 2016 IEEE 4th International Conference on Future Internet of Things and Cloud Workshops (FiCloudW), Vienna, Austria, 22–24 August 2016; pp. 148–153. [CrossRef]

19. Giebler, C.; Stach, C.; Schwarz, H.; Mitschang, B. BRAID—A Hybrid Processing Architecture for Big Data. In Proceedings of the 7th International Conference on Data Science, Technology and Applications, Porto, Portugal, 26–28 July 2018; pp. 294–301. [CrossRef]

20. Lin, J. The Lambda and the Kappa. *IEEE Internet Comput.* **2017**, *21*, 60–66. [CrossRef]

21. Devlin, B. Thirty Years of Data Warehousing—Part 1. 2020. Available online: https://www.irmconnects.com/thirty-years-of-data-warehousing-part-1/ (accessed on 27 October 2022).

22. Inmon, W.H. *Building the Data Warehouse*, 4th ed.; Wiley Publishing: Indianapolis, IN, USA, 2005.

23. Chandra, P.; Gupta, M.K. Comprehensive survey on data warehousing research. *Int. J. Inf. Technol.* **2018**, *10*, 217–224. [CrossRef]

24. Simões, D.M. Enterprise Data Warehouses: A conceptual framework for a successful implementation. In Proceedings of the Canadian Council for Small Business & Entrepreneurship Annual Conference, Calgary, AL, Canada, 28–30 October 2010.

25. Al-Debei, M.M. Data Warehouse as a Backbone for Business Intelligence: Issues and Challenges. *Eur. J. Econ. Financ. Adm. Sci.* **2011**, *33*, 153–166.

26. Report by Market Research Future (MRFR). Available online: https://finance.yahoo.com/news/data-warehouse-dwaas-market-predicted-153000649.html (accessed on 27 October 2022).

27. Chaudhuri, S.; Dayal, U. An overview of data warehousing and OLAP technology. *ACM Sigmod Rec.* **1997**, *26*, 65–74. [CrossRef]

28. Codd, E.F.; Codd, S.B.; Salley, C.T. In *Providing OLAP to User-Analysts: An IT Mandate*; Codd & Associates: Ladera Ranch, CA, USA, 1993; pp. 1–26.

29. The Best Applications of Data Warehousing. 2020. Available online: https://datachannel.co/blogs/best-applications-of-data-warehousing/ (accessed on 27 October 2022).

30. Hai, R.; Quix, C.; Jarke, M. Data lake concept and systems: A survey. *arXiv* **2021**, arXiv:2106.09592.

31. Zagan, E.; Danubianu, M. Data Lake Approaches: A Survey. In Proceedings of the 2020 International Conference on Development and Application Systems (DAS), Suceava, Romania, 21–23 May 2020; pp. 189–193. [CrossRef]

32. Cherradi, M.; El Haddadi, A. Data Lakes: A Survey Paper. In *Innovations in Smart Cities Applications*; Ben Ahmed, M., Boudhir, A.A., Karaş, R., Jain, V., Mellouli, S., Eds.; Lecture Notes in Networks and Systems; Springer International Publishing: Cham, Switzerland, 2022; Volume 5, pp. 823–835. [CrossRef]

33. Dixon, J. Pentaho, Hadoop, and Data Lakes. 2010. Available online: https://jamesdixon.wordpress.com/2010/10/14/pentaho-hadoop-and-data-lakes/ (accessed on 27 October 2022).

34. King, T. The Emergence of Data Lake: Pros and Cons. 2016. Available online: https://solutionsreview.com/data-integration/the-emergence-of-data-lake-pros-and-cons/ (accessed on 27 October 2022).

35. Alrehamy, H.; Walker, C. Personal Data Lake with Data Gravity Pull. In Proceedings of the IEEE Fifth International Conference on Big Data and Cloud Computing 2015, Beijing, China, 26–28 August 2015. [CrossRef]

36. Yang, Q.; Ge, M.; Helfert, M. Analysis of Data Warehouse Architectures: Modeling and Classification. In Proceedings of the 21st International Conference on Enterprise Information Systems, Heraklion, Greece, 3–5 May 2019; pp. 604–611.

37. Yessad, L.; Labiod, A. Comparative study of data warehouses modeling approaches: Inmon, Kimball and Data Vault. In Proceedings of the 2016 International Conference on System Reliability and Science (ICSRS), Paris, France, 15–18 November 2016; pp. 95–99. [CrossRef]

38. Oueslati, W.; Akaichi, J. A Survey on Data Warehouse Evolution. *Int. J. Database Manag. Syst.* **2010**, *2*, 11–24. [CrossRef]

39. Ali, F.S.E. A Survey of Real-Time Data Warehouse and ETL. *Int. J. Sci. Eng. Res.* **2014**, *5*, 3–9.

40. Aftab, U.; Siddiqui, G.F. Big Data Augmentation with Data Warehouse: A Survey. In Proceedings of the 2018 IEEE International Conference on Big Data (Big Data), Seattle, WA, USA, 10–13 December 2018; pp. 2785–2794. [CrossRef]

41. Alsqour, M.; Matouk, K.; Owoc, M. A survey of data warehouse architectures—Preliminary results. In Proceedings of the Federated Conference on Computer Science and Information Systems, Wroclaw, Poland, 9–12 September 2012; pp. 1121–1126.

42. Rizzi, S.; Abelló, A.; Lechtenbörger, J.; Trujillo, J. Research in data warehouse modeling and design: Dead or alive? In Proceedings of the 9th ACM international workshop on Data warehousing and OLAP, DOLAP '06, Arlington, VA, USA, 10 November 2006; Association for Computing Machinery: New York, NY, USA, 2006; pp. 3–10. [CrossRef]

43. Maccioni, A.; Torlone, R. KAYAK: A Framework for Just-in-Time Data Preparation in a Data Lake. In *Advanced Information Systems Engineering*; Krogstie, J., Reijers, H.A., Eds.; Lecture Notes in Computer Science; Springer International Publishing: Cham, Switzerland, 2018; pp. 474–489. [CrossRef]

44. Gao, Y.; Huang, S.; Parameswaran, A. Navigating the Data Lake with DATAMARAN: Automatically Extracting Structure from Log Datasets. In Proceedings of the 2018 International Conference on Management of Data, Houston, TX, USA, 10–15 June 2018; ACM: Houston, TX, USA, 2018; pp. 943–958. [CrossRef]

45. Astriani, W.; Trisminingsih, R. Extraction, Transformation, and Loading (ETL) Module for Hotspot Spatial Data Warehouse Using Geokettle. *Procedia Environ. Sci.* **2016**, *33*, 626–634. [CrossRef]
46. Halevy, A.V.; Korn, F.; Noy, N.F.; Olston, C.; Polyzotis, N.; Roy, S.; Whang, S.E. Managing Google's data lake: An overview of the Goods system. *IEEE Data Eng. Bull.* **2016**, *39*, 5–14.
47. Dehne, F.; Robillard, D.; Rau-Chaplin, A.; Burke, N. VOLAP: A Scalable Distributed System for Real-Time OLAP with High Velocity Data. In Proceedings of the 2016 IEEE International Conference on Cluster Computing (CLUSTER), Taipei, Taiwan, 13–15 September 2016; pp. 354–363. [CrossRef]
48. Hurtado, C.A.; Gutierrez, C.; Mendelzon, A.O. Capturing summarizability with integrity constraints in OLAP. *ACM Trans. Database Syst.* **2005**, *30*, 854–886. [CrossRef]
49. Farid, M.; Roatis, A.; Ilyas, I.F.; Hoffmann, H.F.; Chu, X. CLAMS: Bringing Quality to Data Lakes. In Proceedings of the 2016 International Conference on Management of Data, SIGMOD '16, San Francisco, CA, USA, 26 June–1 July 2016; Association for Computing Machinery: New York, NY, USA, 2016; pp. 2089–2092. [CrossRef]
50. Zhang, Y.; Ives, Z.G. Juneau: Data lake management for Jupyter. *Proc. VLDB Endow.* **2019**, *12*, 1902–1905. [CrossRef]
51. Zhu, E.; Deng, D.; Nargesian, F.; Miller, R.J. JOSIE: Overlap Set Similarity Search for Finding Joinable Tables in Data Lakes. In Proceedings of the 2019 International Conference on Management of Data, SIGMOD '19, Amsterdam, The Netherlands, 30 June–5 July 2019; Association for Computing Machinery: New York, NY, USA, 2019; pp. 847–864. [CrossRef]
52. Beheshti, A.; Benatallah, B.; Nouri, R.; Chhieng, V.M.; Xiong, H.; Zhao, X. CoreDB: A Data Lake Service. In Proceedings of the 2017 ACM on Conference on Information and Knowledge Management, CIKM '17, Singapore, 6–10 November 2017; Association for Computing Machinery: New York, NY, USA, 2017; pp. 2451–2454. [CrossRef]
53. Hai, R.; Geisler, S.; Quix, C. Constance: An Intelligent Data Lake System. In Proceedings of the 2016 International Conference on Management of Data, SIGMOD '16, San Francisco, CA, USA, 26 June–1 July 2016; Association for Computing Machinery: New York, NY, USA, 2016; pp. 2097–2100. [CrossRef]
54. Ahmed, A.S.; Salem, A.M.; Alhabibi, Y.A. Combining the Data Warehouse and Operational Data Store. In Proceedings of the Eighth International Conference on Enterprise Information Systems, Paphos, Cyprus, 23–27 May 2006; pp. 282–288. [CrossRef]
55. Software Architecture: N Tier, 3 Tier, 1 Tier, 2 Tier Architecture. Available online: https://www.appsierra.com/blog/url (accessed on 27 October 2022).
56. Han, S.W. Three-Tier Architecture for Sentinel Applications and Tools: Separating Presentation from Functionality. Ph.D. Thesis, University of Florida, Gainesville, FL, USA, 1997.
57. What Is Three-Tier Architecture. Available online: https://www.ibm.com/in-en/cloud/learn/three-tier-architecture (accessed on 27 October 2022).
58. Phaneendra, S.V.; Reddy, E.M. Big Data—Solutions for RDBMS Problems—A Survey. *Int. J. Adv. Res. Comput. Commun. Eng.* **2013**, *2*, 3686–3691.
59. Simitsis, A.; Vassiliadis, P.; Sellis, T. Optimizing ETL processes in data warehouses. In Proceedings of the 21st International Conference on Data Engineering (ICDE'05), Tokyo, Japan, 5–8 April 2005; pp. 564–575. [CrossRef]
60. Prasser, F.; Spengler, H.; Bild, R.; Eicher, J.; Kuhn, K.A. Privacy-enhancing ETL-processes for biomedical data. *Int. J. Med. Inform.* **2019**, *126*, 72–81. [CrossRef]
61. Rousidis, D.; Garoufallou, E.; Balatsoukas, P.; Sicilia, M.A. Metadata for Big Data: A preliminary investigation of metadata quality issues in research data repositories. *Inf. Serv. Use* **2014**, *34*, 279–286. [CrossRef]
62. Mailvaganam, H. Introduction to OLAP—Slice, Dice and Drill! 2007. Data Warehousing Review. Retrieved on 18 March 2008. Available online: https://web.archive.org/web/20180928201202/http://dwreview.com/OLAP/Introduction_OLAP.html (accessed on 25 September 2022).
63. Pendse, N. What is OLAP? Available online: https://dssresources.com/papers/features/pendse04072002.htm (accessed on 27 October 2022).
64. Xu, J.; Luo, Y.Q.; Zhou, X.X. Solution for Data Growth Problem of MOLAP. *Appl. Mech. Mater.* **2013**, *321–324*, 2551–2556. [CrossRef]
65. Dehne, F.; Eavis, T.; Rau-Chaplin, A. Parallel multi-dimensional ROLAP indexing. In Proceedings of the CCGrid 2003. 3rd IEEE/ACM International Symposium on Cluster Computing and the Grid, Tokyo, Japan, 12–15 May 2003; pp. 86–93. [CrossRef]
66. Shvachko, K.; Kuang, H.; Radia, S.; Chansler, R. The Hadoop Distributed File System. In Proceedings of the 2010 IEEE 26th Symposium on Mass Storage Systems and Technologies (MSST), Incline Village, NV, USA, 3–7 May 2010; pp. 1–10. [CrossRef]

67. Luo, Z.; Niu, L.; Korukanti, V.; Sun, Y.; Basmanova, M.; He, Y.; Wang, B.; Agrawal, D.; Luo, H.; Tang, C.; et al. From Batch Processing to Real Time Analytics: Running Presto® at Scale. In Proceedings of the 2022 IEEE 38th International Conference on Data Engineering (ICDE), Kuala Lumpur, Malaysia, 9–12 May 2022; pp. 1598–1609. [CrossRef]
68. Sethi, R.; Traverso, M.; Sundstrom, D.; Phillips, D.; Xie, W.; Sun, Y.; Yegitbasi, N.; Jin, H.; Hwang, E.; Shingte, N.; et al. Presto: SQL on Everything. In Proceedings of the 2019 IEEE 35th International Conference on Data Engineering (ICDE), Macao, China, 8–1 April 2019; pp. 1802–1813. [CrossRef]
69. Kinley, J. The Lambda Architecture: Principles for Architecting Realtime Big Data Systems. 2013. Available online: http://jameskinley.tumblr.1084com/post/37398560534/thelambda-architecture-principles-for (accessed on 27 October 2022).
70. Ferrera Bertran, P. Lambda Architecture: A state-of-the-Art. Datasalt. 17 January 2014. Available online: https://github.com/pereferrera/trident-lambda-splout (accessed on 25 September 2022).
71. Carbone, P.; Katsifodimos, A.; Ewen, S.; Markl, V.; Haridi, S.; Tzoumas, K. Apache Flink™: Stream and Batch Processing in a Single Engine. *Bull. IEEE Comput. Soc. Tech. Comm. Data Eng.* **2015**, *36*, 28–38.
72. Kreps, J. Questioning the Lambda Architecture. 2014. Available online: https://www.oreilly.com/radar/questioning-the-lambda-architecture/ (accessed on 27 October 2022).
73. Data Vault vs Star Schema vs Third Normal Form: Which Data Model to Use? Available online: https://www.matillion.com/resources/blog/data-vault-vs-star-schema-vs-third-normal-form-which-data-model-to-use (accessed on 27 October 2022).
74. Patranabish, D. Data Lakes: The New Enabler of Scalability in Cross Channel Analytics—Tech-Talk by Durjoy Patranabish | ET CIO. Available online: http://cio.economictimes.indiatimes.com/tech-talk/data-lakes-the-new-enabler-of-scalability-in-cross-channel-analytics/585 (accessed on 27 October 2022).
75. Nargesian, F.; Zhu, E.; Miller, R.J.; Pu, K.Q.; Arocena, P.C. Data lake management: Challenges and opportunities. *Proc. VLDB Endow.* **2019**, *12*, 1986–1989. [CrossRef]
76. A Brief Look at 4 Major Data Compliance Standards: GDPR, HIPAA, PCI DSS, CCPA. Available online: https://www.pentasecurity.com/blog/4-data-compliance-standards-gdpr-hipaa-pci-dss-ccpa/ (accessed on 27 October 2022).
77. Sawadogo, P.; Darmont, J. On data lake architectures and metadata management. *J. Intell. Inf. Syst.* **2021**, *56*, 97–120. [CrossRef]
78. Overview of Amazon Web Services: AWS Whitepaper. 2022. Available online: https://d1.awsstatic.com/whitepapers/aws-overview.pdf (accessed on 27 October 2022).
79. Pandis, I. The evolution of Amazon redshift. *Proc. VLDB Endow.* **2021**, *14*, 3162–3174. [CrossRef]
80. Microsoft Azure Documentation. Available online: http://azure.microsoft.com/en-us/documentation/ (accessed on 27 October 2022).
81. Automate Your Data Warehouse. Available online: https://www.oracle.com/autonomous-database/autonomous-data-warehouse/ (accessed on 27 October 2022).
82. Dageville, B.; Cruanes, T.; Zukowski, M.; Antonov, V.; Avanes, A.; Bock, J.; Claybaugh, J.; Engovatov, D.; Hentschel, M.; Huang, J.; et al. The Snowflake Elastic Data Warehouse. In Proceedings of the 2016 International Conference on Management of Data, San Francisco, CA, USA, 26 June–1 July 2016; ACM: San Francisco, CA, USA, 2016; pp. 215–226. [CrossRef]
83. Mathis, C. Data Lakes. *Datenbank-Spektrum* **2017**, *17*, 289–293. [CrossRef]
84. Zagan, E.; Danubianu, M. Cloud DATA LAKE: The new trend of data storage. In Proceedings of the 2021 3rd International Congress on Human-Computer Interaction, Optimization and Robotic Applications (HORA), Online, 11–13 June 2021; IEEE: Ankara, Turkey, 2021; pp. 1–4. [CrossRef]
85. Ramakrishnan, R.; Sridharan, B.; Douceur, J.R.; Kasturi, P.; Krishnamachari-Sampath, B.; Krishnamoorthy, K.; Li, P.; Manu, M.; Michaylov, S.; Ramos, R.; et al. Azure Data Lake Store: A Hyperscale Distributed File Service for Big Data Analytics. In Proceedings of the 2017 ACM International Conference on Management of Data, SIGMOD '17, Chicago, IL, USA, 14–19 May 2017; Association for Computing Machinery: New York, NY, USA, 2017; pp. 51–63. [CrossRef]
86. Elgendy, N.; Elragal, A. Big Data Analytics: A Literature Review Paper. In *Advances in Data Mining. Applications and Theoretical Aspects*; Perner, P., Ed.; Lecture Notes in Computer Science; Springer International Publishing: Cham, Switzerland, 2014; pp. 214–227. [CrossRef]
87. Jin, X.; Wah, B.W.; Cheng, X.; Wang, Y. Significance and Challenges of Big Data Research. *Big Data Res.* **2015**, *2*, 59–64. [CrossRef]
88. Agrawal, R.; Nyamful, C. Challenges of big data storage and management. *Glob. J. Inf. Technol. Emerg. Technol.* **2016**, *6*, 1–10. [CrossRef]
89. Padgavankar, M.H.; Gupta, S.R. Big Data Storage and Challenges. *Int. J. Comput. Sci. Inf. Technol.* **2014**, *5*, 2218–2223.
90. Kadadi, A.; Agrawal, R.; Nyamful, C.; Atiq, R. Challenges of data integration and interoperability in big data. In Proceedings of the 2014 IEEE International Conference on Big Data (Big Data), Washington, DC, USA, 27–30 October 2014; IEEE: Washington, DC, USA, 2014; pp. 38–40. [CrossRef]
91. Best Data Integration Tools. Available online: https://www.peerspot.com/categories/data-integration-tools (accessed on 27 October 2022).
92. Toshniwal, R.; Dastidar, K.G.; Nath, A. Big Data Security Issues and Challenges. *Int. J. Innov. Res. Adv. Eng.* **2014**, *2*, 15–20.
93. Demchenko, Y.; Ngo, C.; de Laat, C.; Membrey, P.; Gordijenko, D. Big Security for Big Data: Addressing Security Challenges for the Big Data Infrastructure. In *Secure Data Management*; Jonker, W., Petković, M., Eds.; Lecture Notes in Computer Science; Springer International Publishing: Cham, Switzerland, 2014; pp. 76–94. [CrossRef]
94. Chen, E.T. Implementation issues of enterprise data warehousing and business intelligence in the healthcare industry. *Commun. IIMA* **2012**, *12*, 3.

95. Cuzzocrea, A.; Bellatreche, L.; Song, I.Y. Data warehousing and OLAP over big data: Current challenges and future research directions. In Proceedings of the Sixteenth International Workshop on Data Warehousing and OLAP, DOLAP '13, San Francisco, CA, USA, 28 October 2013; Association for Computing Machinery: New York, NY, USA, 2013; pp. 67–70. [CrossRef]
96. Singh, R.; Singh, K. A Descriptive Classification of Causes of Data Quality Problems in Data Warehousing. *Int. J. Comput. Sci. Issues* **2010**, *7*, 41.
97. Longbottom, C.; Bamforth, R. Optimising the Data Warehouse. 2013. Available online: https://www.it-daily.net/downloads/WP_Optimising-the-data-warehouse.pdf (accessed on 27 October 2022).
98. Santos, R.J.; Bernardino, J.; Vieira, M. A survey on data security in data warehousing: Issues, challenges and opportunities. In Proceedings of the 2011 IEEE EUROCON—International Conference on Computer as a Tool, Lisbon, Portugal, 27–29 April 2011, pp. 1–4. [CrossRef]
99. Responsibilities of a Data Warehouse Governance Committee. Available online: https://docs.oracle.com/cd/E29633_01/CDMOG/GUID-7E43F311-4510-4F1E-A17E-693F94BD0EC7.htm (accessed on 28 October 2022).
100. Gupta, S.; Giri, V. *Practical Enterprise Data Lake Insights: Handle Data-Driven Challenges in an Enterprise Big Data Lake*, 1st ed.; Apress: Berkeley, CA, USA, 2018.
101. Giebler, C.; Gröger, C.; Hoos, E.; Schwarz, H.; Mitschang, B. Leveraging the Data Lake: Current State and Challenges. In *Big Data Analytics and Knowledge Discovery*; Ordonez, C., Song, I.Y., Anderst-Kotsis, G., Tjoa, A.M., Khalil, I., Eds.; Lecture Notes in Computer Science; Springer International Publishing: Cham, Switzerland, 2019; pp. 179–188. [CrossRef]
102. Lock, M. Maximizing Your Data Lake with a Cloud or Hybrid Approach. 2016. Available online: https://technology-signals.com/wp-content/uploads/download-manager-files/maximizingyourdatalake.pdf (accessed on 27 October 2022).
103. Kumar, N. Cloud Data Warehouse Is the Future of Data Storage. 2020. Available online: https://www.sigmoid.com/blogs/cloud-data-warehouse-is-the-future-of-data-storage/ (accessed on 27 October 2022).
104. Kahn, M.G.; Mui, J.Y.; Ames, M.J.; Yamsani, A.K.; Pozdeyev, N.; Rafaels, N.; Brooks, I.M. Migrating a research data warehouse to a public cloud: Challenges and opportunities. *J. Am. Med. Inform. Assoc.* **2022**, *29*, 592–600. [CrossRef]
105. Mishra, N.; Lin, C.C.; Chang, H.T. A Cognitive Adopted Framework for IoT Big-Data Management and Knowledge Discovery Prospective. *Int. J. Distrib. Sens. Netw.* **2015**, *2015*, 1–12. [CrossRef]
106. Alserafi, A.; Abelló, A.; Romero, O.; Calders, T. Keeping the Data Lake in Form: DS-kNN Datasets Categorization Using Proximity Mining. In *Model and Data Engineering*; Schewe, K.D., Singh, N.K., Eds.; Lecture Notes in Computer Science; Springer International Publishing: Cham, Switzerland, 2019; pp. 35–49. [CrossRef]
107. Bogatu, A.; Fernandes, A.A.A.; Paton, N.W.; Konstantinou, N. Dataset Discovery in Data Lakes. In Proceedings of the 2020 IEEE 36th International Conference on Data Engineering (ICDE), Dallas, TX, USA, 20–24 April 2020; IEEE: Dallas, TX, USA, 2020; pp. 709–720. [CrossRef]
108. Armbrust, M.; Ghodsi, A.; Xin, R.; Zaharia, M. Lakehouse: A New Generation of Open Platforms that Unify Data Warehousing and Advanced Analytics. In Proceedings of the Conference on Innovative Data Systems Research, Virtual Event, 11–15 January 2021.

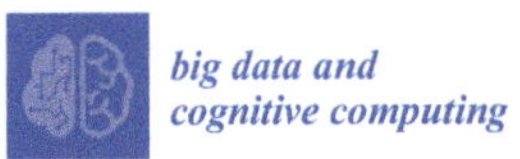

big data and cognitive computing

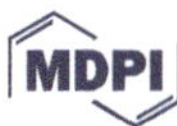

Article

The "Unreasonable" Effectiveness of the Wasserstein Distance in Analyzing Key Performance Indicators of a Network of Stores

Andrea Ponti [1,2,*], Ilaria Giordani [1,3], Matteo Mistri [1], Antonio Candelieri [2] and Francesco Archetti [3]

[1] Oaks S.R.L., 20125 Milan, Italy
[2] Department of Economics, Management and Statistics, University of Milano-Bicocca, 20126 Bicocca, Italy
[3] Department of Computer Science, Systems and Communication, University of Milano-Bicocca, 20126 Bicocca, Italy
* Correspondence: andrea.ponti@unimib.it

Abstract: Large retail companies routinely gather huge amounts of customer data, which are to be analyzed at a low granularity. To enable this analysis, several Key Performance Indicators (KPIs), acquired for each customer through different channels are associated to the main drivers of the customer experience. Analyzing the samples of customer behavior only through parameters such as average and variance does not cope with the growing heterogeneity of customers. In this paper, we propose a different approach in which the samples from customer surveys are represented as discrete probability distributions whose similarities can be assessed by different models. The focus is on the Wasserstein distance, which is generally well defined, even when other distributional distances are not, and it provides an interpretable distance metric between distributions. The support of the distributions can be both one- and multi-dimensional, allowing for the joint consideration of several KPIs for each store, leading to a multi-variate histogram. Moreover, the Wasserstein barycenter offers a useful synthesis of a set of distributions and can be used as a reference distribution to characterize and classify behavioral patterns. Experimental results of real data show the effectiveness of the Wasserstein distance in providing global performance measures.

Keywords: Wasserstein distance; customer experience; key performance indicators

Citation: Ponti, A.; Giordani, I.; Mistri, M.; Candelieri, A.; Archetti, F. The "Unreasonable" Effectiveness of the Wasserstein Distance in Analyzing Key Performance Indicators of a Network of Stores. *Big Data Cogn. Comput.* **2022**, *6*, 138. https://doi.org/10.3390/bdcc6040138

Academic Editors: Domenico Talia, Fabrizio Marozzo and Min Chen

Received: 7 October 2022
Accepted: 11 November 2022
Published: 15 November 2022

Publisher's Note: MDPI stays neutral with regard to jurisdictional claims in published maps and institutional affiliations.

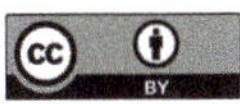

1. Introduction

1.1. Motivations

Among the many facets of omni-channel retailing, this paper refers to a set of analytics and decision processes that support the seamless focus of a brand across many channels (in-store, online, mobile, call center or social). Retailers have come to recognize the importance of integrating information and services from multiple available channels to reduce data mismatch in order to create a seamless Customer eXperience (CX) and to obtain data-supported insight into the management of a network of stores. However, it is important to identify, promote and provide customers with various experiential benefits to enhance both shopping intentions and satisfaction. Although price and convenience are still primary considerations, customers are putting more emphasis on competence in specific categories and the overall customer experience. This aspect is particularly strong for categories that are highly fragmented or in which advice to customer plays a large role in sales, such as furniture, do-it-yourself products, apparel and consumer electronics. Personalization, meaning the quality of individual attention and tailored service, is largely regarded as the top criterion in evaluating CX. The analysis of customer data, from questionnaires and the analyses of online behavior, is instrumental in providing personalized services such as customized purchase recommendations, sending promotion information based on individual preferences and providing location-based services. The focus of this paper is on the analysis of CX while considering a multinational retail company operating through a network of stores. To enable this analysis, a number of key performance indicators (KPI), acquired for each customer through different channels, are associated to the main drivers of the customer experience. It is important to remark that this analysis must be performed from a granular perspective on what a consumer really wants, today and in the future, in order to understand which services/products to offer on which channel. Developing this detailed understanding of consumers requires harnessing consumer data, which should be combined with consumer behavior insight from interviews and observations. It also requires analytics, which can work at the required granular level, gain a clear understanding of consumer expectations and derive a global picture of the strengths and weaknesses of each store. Capturing the full potential of omni-channel retailing requires a cross-channel perspective and transparency to measure and manage channel interplay, obtaining at the same time measures for the entire network of stores and improvement actions. More recently, the use of machine learning methods has been gaining more importance to leverage the wealth of customer data into a richer representation of the CX. It is the opinion of the authors of this paper that, given the growing number of channels and heterogeneity of customers, the standard statistical approach, which analyzes samples of the customer behavior only on parameters such as average and variance, might capture only a part of the hidden value of the data.

This paper proposes a different approach in which the samples from customer surveys are represented as discrete probability distributions, in particular as histograms or cloud points. In this distributional context, the variation in performance between two stores, considering one KPI, is the distance between two univariate histograms. The method can be naturally extended to jointly consider several KPIs, leading, for each store, to a multivariate histogram. The statistical and, more recently, the machine learning communities have developed many alternative models to measure the distance between distributions. A general class of distances, known as f-divergences, is based on the expected value of a convex function of the ratio of two distributions. Some examples are Kullback–Leibler (and its symmetrized version Jensen–Shannon), Hellinger, Total Variation and χ-square divergence. In this paper, the focus is on the Wasserstein (WST) distance. Although other distances measure pointwise differences in densities (or weights), the WST distance (also known as the optimal transport distance) is a cross-binning distance; this distinction can be summed up by saying that the optimal transport distance is horizontal, whereas other distances are based on vertical displacement. Two important elements of the WST theory are the barycenter and WST clustering. The WST barycenter offers a useful synthesis of a set of distributions. A standard clustering method such as k-means can be generalized to WST spaces, enabling the WST barycenters and k-mean WST clustering, which is used to characterize and classify behavioral patterns. In general, WST enables the synthetization of a comparison between two multi-dimensional distributions through a single metric by using all information in the distributions. Moreover, the WST distance is generally well defined and provides an interpretable distance metric between distributions.

This study was motivated by the emerging need for a multination retailer to revise the performance measurement system—currently based on NPS—which has been adopted to rank the 50 stores of its commercial network. The limitations of NPS and the desire to design a new performance measurement system able to deal with multiple KPIs coming from omni-channel customer surveys lead us to propose a completely new analytical framework based on multi-variate discrete distributions and the Wasserstein distance. Indeed, using a more comprehensive system to evaluate the relative performance of each store with respect to the others is a critical decision for the company as a basis for the distribution of a performance-related bonus (on a quarterly basis), which is subject to negotiation with trade unions. Although multi-channel surveys are available, this study focuses on only one specific channel to better evaluate the benefits and limitations of the new framework.

1.2. Related Works

The cornerstone of the implementation of a CX strategy is the metric used to measure the performance of a company. A widely used such metric is the Net Promoter Score [1], which is associated with customer loyalty and is considered a reliable indicator of the future of a company's performance.

The author of [2] offered a view about a complete system of performance measurements for an enterprise based on over twenty years of research and development activities. The system was designed to provide key persons at different units/levels with useful quantitative information, such as board members to exercise due diligence, leaders to decide where to focus attention next and people to carry out their work well. Later, the author of [3] provided a review of various methods for tackling performance measurement problems. Although technical statistical issues are buried somewhat below the surface, statistical thinking is very much part of the main line of the argument, meaning that performance measurements should be an area attracting serious attention from statisticians. More recently, the authors of [4] re-visited the use of NPS (Net Promoter Score) as a predictor of sales growth by analyzing data from seven brands operating in the U.S. sportswear industry measured over five years. Interestingly, the results confirmed that, although the original premises are reasonable, methodological concerns arise when NPS is used as a metric for tracking overall brand health. Only the more recently developed brand health measure of NPS (using an all-potential customer samples) is effective at predicting future sales growth.

An interesting approach leveraging machine learning to analyze Customer Experience (CX) was proposed in [5,6]. The authors of these works considered beyond the NPS and the Customer SATisfaction score (CSAT) to measure the CX, and they performed a wide comparative evaluation of several machine learning approaches, analyzing the specific case of a telecommunication company and applying a wide set of classification methods to categorize the survey results.

In this paper we propose a distributional approach to performance evaluation; the performance is measured through KPIs represented as discrete probability distributions whose similarities are computed through the Wasserstein distance. The Wasserstein distance can be traced back to the works of Gaspard Monge [7] and Lev Kantorovich [8]. Recently, also under the name of the Earth Mover Distance (EMD), it has been gaining increasing importance in several fields, such as Imaging [9], Natural Language Processing [10] and a generation of adversarial networks [11]. Important references include [12], which gave a complete mathematical characterization, and [13], which also gave an up-to-date survey of numerical methods. The authors of [14] provided an overview of the Wasserstein space. A specific analysis of its geometry and geodesic Principal Components Analysis was given in [15]. Specific computational results related to barycenters and clustering were given in [16]. A novel Wasserstein distance and fast clustering method were proposed in [17]. One should note that the computational cost of the WST distance is amplified in computations of the barycenters of multi-variate distributions for computational as well as theoretical reasons [13].

The Wasserstein distance has also been receiving attention in economic theory, where the key reference is [18], in which it was shown that a number of seemingly unrelated problems can be modelled and solved as optimal transport problems. For the term "unreasonable effectiveness" in the title of this paper, we are indebted to [19]. Some key problems in finance have been also dealt with using optimal transport as the pricing of financial derivatives [18] and the analysis of robustness in risk management [20]. Other contributions to finance are [21], which provided a Wasserstein-based analysis of stability in finance, and [22], which proposed Wasserstein k-means clustering to classify market regimes. An important application domain of the Wasserstein distance is the analysis of distributional robustness. In [23], the authors analyzed Wasserstein-based distributionally robust optimization and its application in machine learning using the Wasserstein metric [24,25]. Two contributions, along the line of stochastic programming, were given in [26], which proposed an approximation of data-driven chance-constrained programs over Wasserstein balls, and in [27], which proposed a distributionally robust two-stage Wasserstein model with recourse. We are not aware of significant applications of the Wasserstein distance in management science. A management topic where the Wasserstein distance enables significant contributions is the design of recommender systems using metric learning [28,29], which has shown to enable the measurement of uncertainty and the embedding of user/item representations in a low-dimensional space.

1.3. Contributions

The main contribution of this paper is the representation of performance metrics as measured through KPIs as discrete probability distributions. Embedding these distributions in the "Wasserstein space" enables the comparison and ranking of different stores. In addition, through the definition of Wasserstein barycenters, it is possible to perform clustering in the Wasserstein space with the aim of finding groups of similar stores. Moreover, since some KPIs are correlated with each other, in this paper, a subset of the most "informative" ones are chosen using feature selection and information gain. To further motivate the usage of the Wasserstein distance, a barycenter-based measure of how KPI data are not Euclidean is proposed; the computational results show that the discrepancy between the analysis in the Euclidean space and the WST space grows with the size of the subset.

2. Key Performance Indicators and the Formulation of the Problem

The focus of this paper is on a multinational retailer company which operates through a network of stores. The performance of each store is characterized in terms of service to the customer and is evaluated by the customers themselves through a number of Key Performance Indicators. Each store receives its evaluation through a survey composed of a number of questions. For each question, a customer can answer with a number on a scale from -100 to 100, which represents the satisfaction of a specific service. Each KPI_i, with $i = 1, \ldots, K$, is computed as the average of a set of questions and captures one feature of the customer experience. Figure 1 shows an example considering the experience of a customer inside a store. This aspect of the CX can be evaluated through seven different KPIs, each of which is obtained from the answers to a set of different questions.

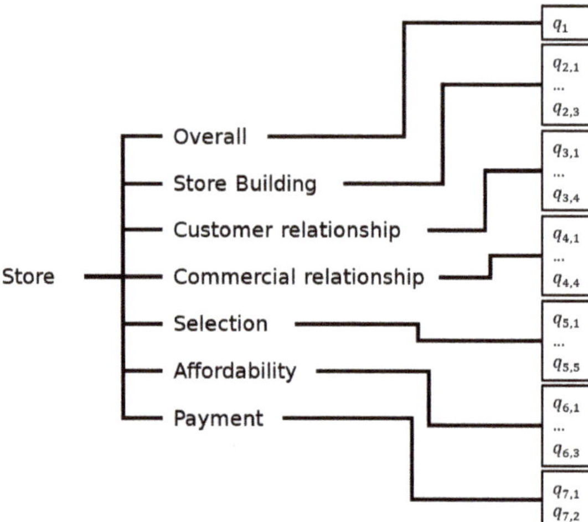

Figure 1. An example of the KPI tree related to the experience inside a store.

The objective of this study is to propose a system to assess stores' performances while simultaneously considering different KPIs. As a case study, a network of 50 stores owned and operated by a multinational retailer is considered. In this paper, the seven KPIs related to the customer experience inside the store are considered. The following list of KPIs provides an idea of the scope of this study:

- Overall: Measures the overall sentiment of the customer for the whole process.
- Store Building: Features of the store, such as parking spaces and cleanliness.
- Customer Relationship: Measures sentiment about the vendors.
- Commercial Relationship: Aggregates scores given by customers in the customer relation before conversion.
- Selection: Aggregates scores from features such as the availability of products and clarity of presentation.
- Affordability: Aggregates scores from customers related to prices and discounts.
- Payment: Aggregates scores such as the length of the queue and easy payment.

Usually, the mean of each KPI for each store is analyzed to build a ranking or to evaluate different aspects of the stores. A very effective way to visualize these means is by using the parallel coordinates plot, as shown in Figure 2. This chart enables the easy and clear visualization of a set of points (stores) in a multi-dimensional space (KPIs).

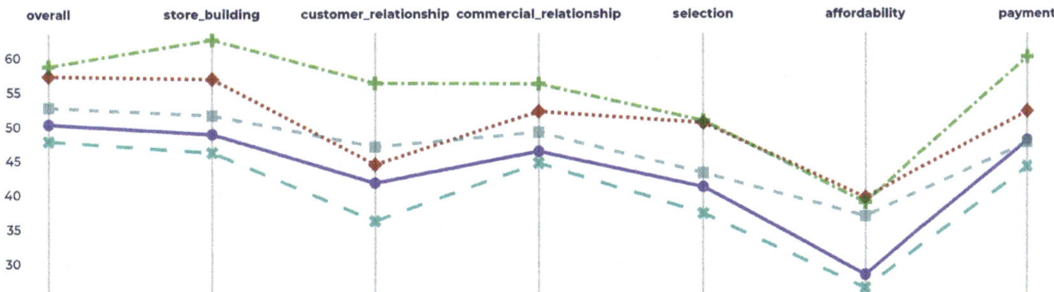

Figure 2. Parallel coordinates plot showing the seven KPIs of five stores (each line represents a store).

3. Space of Data and Distributional Representation

3.1. Distributional Representation

All the data of a store s_i can be stored in a matrix $L^{(s_i)} \in \mathbb{R}^{m \times K}$, in which the columns represent the K KPIs, and the rows represent the m users that completed the survey for a specific store s_i (Table 1). Then, each cell contains the value of a KPI for a customer.

Table 1. Matrix representing store s_i. Each column refers to a KPI, and each row refers to a customer.

$L^{(s_i)}$	KPI_1	KPI_2	...	KPI_K
1				
2				
...				
m				

Each column of $L^{(s_i)}$ can be considered to be a sample of the data related to a KPI. A column k can then be represented as a one-dimensional histogram $h_k^{(s_i)}$, whose support space $[z_k, u_k]$ can be divided into η bins. The weight of each bin is given by the number of customers of the sample, whose score for the specific KPI falls into that bin. Figure 3 shows an example of the histograms associated with three different stores regarding a KPI.

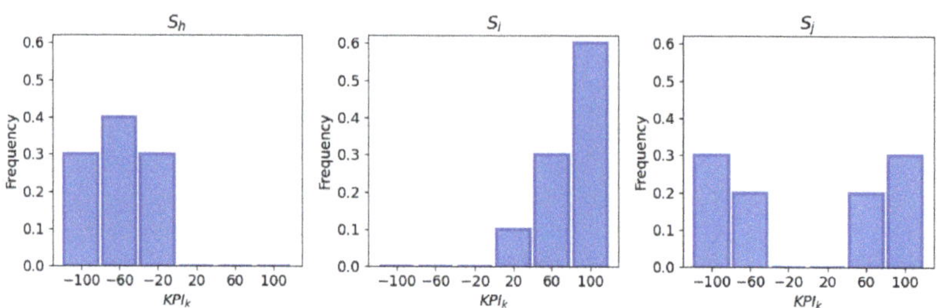

Figure 3. Three different stores represented as univariate histograms. KPI values are on the x-axis, and their relative frequencies are on the y-axis.

As each histogram represents a single KPI, it is possible to compute the distance between two stores as the distance between the two histograms given by the same KPI. This representation naturally extends to multi-dimensional histograms. Characterizing a store using all KPIs, each store is represented as a K-dimensional histogram. For instance, considering two KPIs, the supports of the two-dimensional bins are squares, and the weights of the bins are the number of customers whose KPI_i and KPI_j scores fall into that bin. The natural representation is a heatmap, as shown in Figure 4.

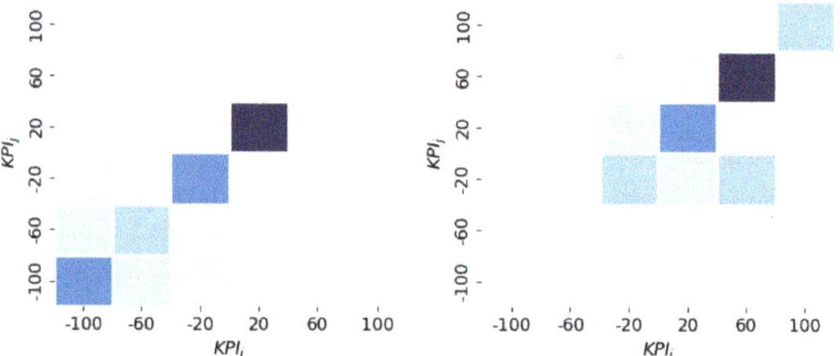

Figure 4. Two different stores represented as bivariate histograms. KPI values related to KPI_i and KPI_j are on the x-axis and y-axis, respectively, and each bin is colored by their relative frequencies.

Since histograms are instances of discrete probability distributions, the stores become elements in a probabilistic space. Another characterization of stores in this probabilistic space can be obtained by representing the matrices $L^{(s_i)}$ as point clouds. Figure 5 displays an example of point cloud representation. On the left, one KPI for two stores is shown, and on the right, a plot of the same two stores for two KPIs is shown.

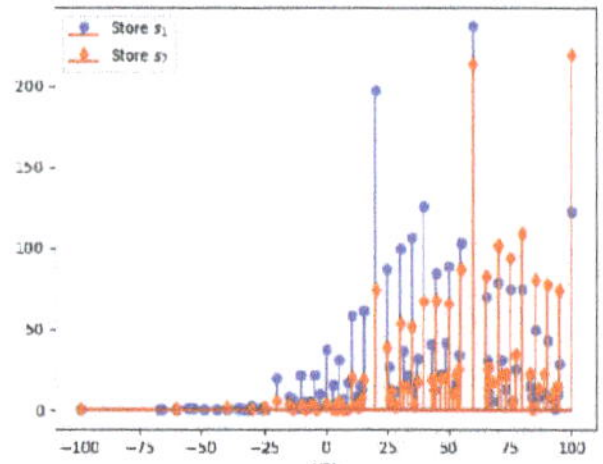
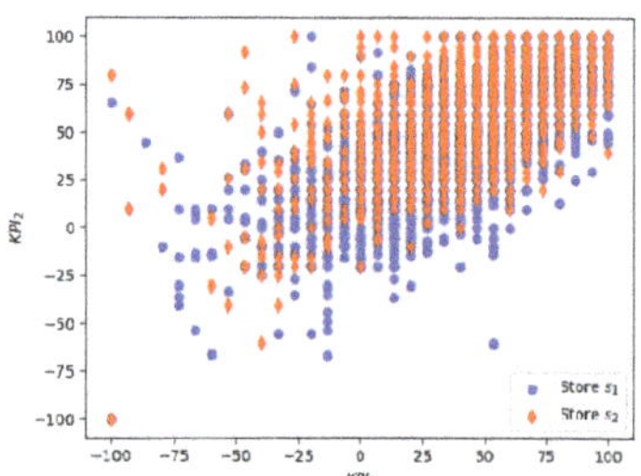

Figure 5. Point cloud representations of two stores. The **left** plot considers one KPI: KPI values are on the x-axis, and the absolute frequency is on the y-axis. The **right** plot considers two KPIs: KPI values are on the x-axis and y-axis, and each point represents a user.

The set of all KPIs is denoted as S. The power set of S is the set of all subsets, including the empty one and S itself. If S has cardinality K, then the number of subsets is 2^K. All subsets but the empty one can be regarded as a description of a store. Therefore, the analysis can be performed on each element (except the empty one) of the power set of S.

A subset of cardinality $k = 1, \ldots, K$ is associated with store k's KPIs, which can be analyzed as k one-dimensional histograms or one k-dimensional histogram. The informational value of the two approaches is different, and the computational cost is also very different, as it increases with k. To mitigate this cost, one can choose the most significant KPIs using feature selection methods, as outlined in Section 5.1.

The histogram is a convenient representation of the $m \times K$ matrix $L^{(s_i)}$ in a space $\mathbb{R}^d$, where $d = \eta^K$, with η representing the number of bins. It is important to remark that d does not depend on the number of users m and can be reduced by considering an element of the power set S of cardinality $k < K$ or a smaller number of bins.

3.2. Graph Representation

An effective way to visualize all the stores and their similarities is by building a graph $G = (V, E)$, where the vertices V represent the stores that are connected with an edge if their similarities are above a given threshold. As previously mentioned, each store can be represented as a k-dimensional histogram $H^{(s_i)}$. Therefore, the set of edges can be given by $E = \left\{ (s_i, s_j) : D\left(H^{(s_i)}, H^{(s_j)}\right) < \tau \right\}$. Any distance between histograms can be used, and in this case, the Wasserstein distance (whose basic definition and properties are provided in Section 3) is considered. Figure 6 shows an example of the graph resulting from 4 KPIs and 50 stores. In this case, only the stores whose distances are below the first decile are connected.

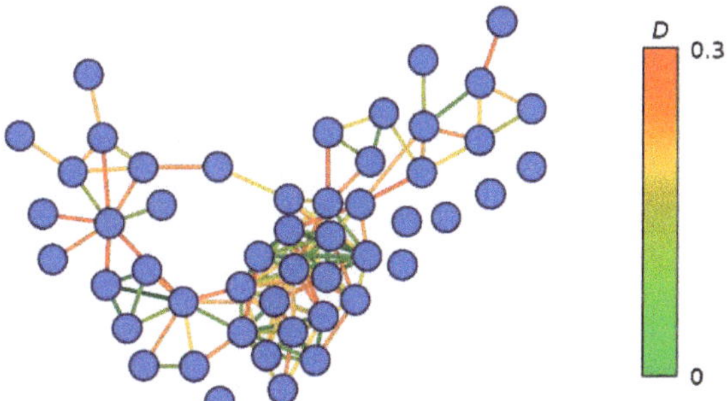

Figure 6. Graph representation of 50 stores. Edges are colored from green to red based on the distance from each other.

4. Wasserstein Distance

4.1. Basic Definitions

Consider the case of a discrete distribution P specified by a set of support points x_i with $i = 1, \ldots, m$ and their associated probabilities w_i, such that $\sum_{i=1}^{m} w_i = 1$ with $w_i \geq 0$ and $x_i \in M$ for $i = 1, \ldots, m$. Usually, $M = \mathbb{R}^d$ is the d-dimensional Euclidean space where x_i are the support vectors. M can also be a symbolic set provided with a symbol-to-symbol similarity. Therefore, P can be written as follows in Equation (1):

$$P(x) = \sum_{i=1}^{m} w_i \delta(x - x_i) \tag{1}$$

where $\delta(\cdot)$ is the Kronecker delta.

The WST distance between two distributions $P^{(1)} = \left\{w_i^{(1)}, x_i^{(1)}\right\}$ with $i = 1,\dots,m_1$ and $P^{(2)} = \left\{w_i^{(2)}, x_i^{(2)}\right\}$ with $i = 1,\dots,m_2$ is obtained by solving the following linear program (2):

$$W\left(P^{(1)}, P^{(2)}\right) = \min_{\gamma_{ij} \in \mathbb{R}^+} \sum_{i \in I_1,\, j \in I_2} \gamma_{ij}\, d\left(x_i^{(1)}, x_j^{(2)}\right) \tag{2}$$

The cost of transport between $x_i^{(1)}$ and $x_j^{(2)}$, $d\left(x_i^{(1)}, x_j^{(2)}\right)$ is defined by the p-th power of the norm $\|x_i^{(1)},\ x_j^{(2)}\|$, which is usually the Euclidean distance.

Two index sets can be defined as $I_1 = \{1,\dots,m_1\}$ and I_2 likewise, such that

$$\sum_{i \in I_1} \gamma_{ij} = w_j^{(2)},\ \forall j \in I_2 \tag{3}$$

$$\sum_{j \in I_2} \gamma_{ij} = w_i^{(1)},\ \forall i \in I_1 \tag{4}$$

Equations (3) and (4) represent the in-flow and out-flow constraints, respectively. The terms γ_{ij} are called matching weights between support points $x_i^{(1)}$ and $x_j^{(2)}$ or the optimal coupling for $P^{(1)}$ and $P^{(2)}$. The basic computation of OT between two discrete distributions involves solving a network flow problem whose computation typically scales cubically in the sizes of the measure. In the case of a one-dimensional histograms, the computation of the Wasserstein distance can be performed by a simple sorting algorithm and with the application of Equation (5).

$$W_p\left(P^{(1)}, P^{(2)}\right) = \left(\frac{1}{n}\sum_i^n \left|x_i^{(1)*} - x_i^{(2)*}\right|^p\right)^{\frac{1}{p}} \tag{5}$$

where $x_i^{(1)*}$ and $x_i^{(2)*}$ are the sorted samples. The discrete version of the WST distance is usually called the Earth Mover Distance (EMD). For instance, when measuring the distance between grey scale images, the histogram weights are given by the pixel values and the coordinates by the pixel positions.

Consider now the three univariate histograms in Figure 3, which represent three different stores. Support x_i is the range of values of the KPI, and the weights w_i are the number of users whose KPI score falls into that interval. Table 2 shows the differences between the Wasserstein distance and the Manhattan and Euclidean distances.

Table 2. The difference between Manhattan, Euclidean and Wasserstein distances.

Distance	Order	$D(S_h,S_i)$	$D(S_h,S_j)$	$D(S_i,S_j)$
Manhattan	1	2.000	1.000	1.000
Euclidean	2	0.894	0.510	0.490
Wasserstein	1	0.583	0.250	0.333
	2	0.677	0.324	0.374

The Wasserstein distance agrees with the intuition that S_h is closer to S_j than S_i. Instead, the Manhattan distance does not discriminate because it assigns the same value to the pairs (S_h, S_j) and (S_i, S_j). In [30], it was remarked that the information reflected in histograms lies more in the relative value of their coordinates rather than on their absolute value.

The computational cost of optimal transport can quickly become prohibitive. The method of entropic regularization [13] enables scalable computations, but large values of the regularization parameter can induce an undesirable smoothing effect, whereas low values not only reduce the scalability but might induce several numerical instabilities.

4.2. Barycenter and Clustering

Under the optimal transport metric, it is possible to compute the mean of a set of empirical probability measures. This mean is known as the Wasserstein barycenter and is the measure that minimizes the sum of its Wasserstein distances to each element in that set. Consider a set of N discrete distributions, $\mathbf{P} = \left\{ P^{(1)}, \ldots, P^{(N)} \right\}$, with $P^{(k)} = \left\{ \left(w_i^{(k)}, x_i^{(k)} \right) : i = 1, \ldots, m_k \right\}$ and $k = 1, \ldots, N$. Therefore, the associated barycenter, denoted with $\overline{P} = \left\{ (\overline{w}_1, x_1), \ldots, (\overline{w}_m, x_m) \right\}$, is computed as follows in Equation (6):

$$\overline{P} = \underset{P}{\arg\min} \frac{1}{N} \sum_{k=1}^{N} \lambda_k W\left(P, P^{(k)} \right) \tag{6}$$

where the values λ_k are used to weigh the different contributions of each distribution in the computation. Without the loss of generality, they can be set to $\lambda_k = \frac{1}{N} \ \forall \ k = 1, \ldots, N$.

The concept of the barycenter enables clustering among distributions in a space whose metric is the Wasserstein distance. More simply, the barycenter in a space of distributions is the analog of the centroid in a Euclidean space. The most common and well-known algorithm for clustering data in the Euclidean space is k-means. Since it is an iterative distance-based (also known as representative-based) algorithm, it is easy to propose variants of k-means by simply changing the distance adopted to create clusters, such as the Manhattan distance (leading to k-medoids) or any kernel allowing for non-spherical clusters (i.e., kernel k-means). The crucial point is that only the distance is changed, and the overall iterative two-step algorithm is maintained. This is also valid in the case of the Wasserstein k-means, where the Euclidean distance is replaced by the Wasserstein distance and where centroids are replaced by barycenters.

5. Results

5.1. Feature Selection

The computational complexity of the Wasserstein distance can quickly become intractable in the case of multi-variate histograms, as already mentioned. The computation of the barycenter and performing the clustering procedure using the WST distance add substantially to the computational cost. It is therefore important to reduce the number of variables to consider, and for this reason, a feature selection strategy based on the Information Gain (IG) is used to select the most relevant KPIs. In turn, each KPI is considered as a target variable in a classification problem, and the IGs of all the others KPIs are computed. Since seven KPIs are considered, for each of them, six different values of IG are obtained, each of which represents the importance for the specific KPI in predicting the other six. Therefore, for each KPI, the average of these six represents its IG. Table 3 reports these results. In the following analysis, the four most relevant KPIs are considered.

Table 3. Information Gain of the seven KPIs.

KPI	Information Gain
Selection	0.37
Customer Relationship	0.34
Commercial Relationship	0.33
Store Building	0.32
Affordability	0.30
Overall	0.29
Payment	0.26

5.2. Wasserstein Analysis

The distributional representation of the stores enables the definition of an ideal store that can be used to build a Wasserstein-based ranking. The histogram associated with the ideal store has the entire mass concentrated on the bin of the most favorable assessment.

For instance, Figure 7 shows the ideal univariate and bivariate histograms. This definition can be naturally extended to multi-dimensional histograms.

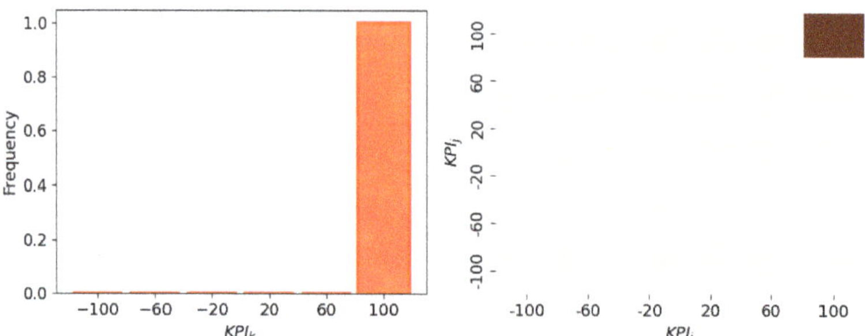

Figure 7. Univariate histogram associated with the ideal store (**left**): KPI values are on the x-axis, and their relative frequencies are on the y-axis. Bivariate histogram associated with the ideal store (**right**): KPI values related to KPI_i and KPI_j are on the x-axis and y-axis, respectively, and each bin is colored by their relative frequencies.

Given such a histogram, it is now possible to build a ranking computing the Wasserstein distance between the histograms associated with each store and the ideal one. In this way, the ranking is built upon the entire distributions of the KPIs' values and not only considering their means. To highlight the advantages of this framework, Figure 8 shows the correlation between the distances of the stores for the ideal and different statistics of the KPIs' distributions while considering histograms in one to four dimensions.

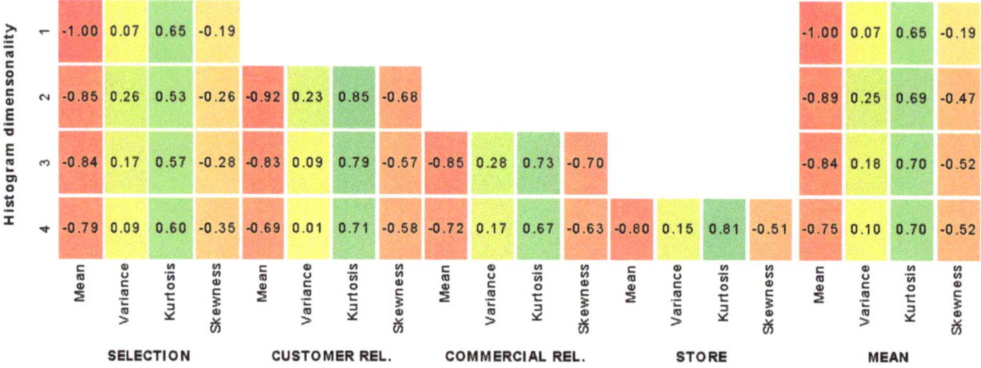

Histogram dimensionality	SELECTION				CUSTOMER REL.				COMMERCIAL REL.				STORE				MEAN			
	Mean	Variance	Kurtosis	Skewness	Mean	Variance	Kurtosis	Skewness	Mean	Variance	Kurtosis	Skewness	Mean	Variance	Kurtosis	Skewness	Mean	Variance	Kurtosis	Skewness
1	-1.00	0.07	0.65	-0.19													-1.00	0.07	0.65	-0.19
2	-0.85	0.26	0.53	-0.26	-0.92	0.23	0.85	-0.68									-0.89	0.25	0.69	-0.47
3	-0.84	0.17	0.57	-0.28	-0.83	0.09	0.79	-0.57	-0.85	0.28	0.73	-0.70					-0.84	0.18	0.70	-0.52
4	-0.79	0.09	0.60	-0.35	-0.69	0.01	0.71	-0.58	-0.72	0.17	0.67	-0.63	-0.80	0.15	0.81	-0.51	-0.75	0.10	0.70	-0.52

Figure 8. Pearson correlation between the distances of stores from the ideal and four statistics (mean, variance, kurtosis and skewness).

In the case of univariate histograms related to the KPI "selection", the correlation between the distance from the ideal and the mean is at a maximum; therefore, the rankings built upon the mean and the distance from being ideal are the same. By increasing the dimensionality of the data, the correlation of the Wasserstein distance with the mean tends to decrease, but the correlation with other statistics, such as kurtosis and skewness, tends to increase. The Wasserstein distance is able to capture other aspects or statistics of a distribution rather than just the mean, resulting in a more robust ranking.

5.3. Clustering Analysis

The barycenters enable the clustering of a set of distributions using the Wasserstein distance in a framework similar to k-means, as explained in Section 3.2. Two different clustering approaches are considered and compared with the standard k-means.

Consider a network of n stores and a set of k KPIs. Each store can be represented as k univariate histograms (one for each KPI) or one k-dimensional histogram. Clustering can be performed to divide the stores into two different groups. In the first case, each clustering iteration requires the computation of $2k$ different univariate barycenter and $2kS$ Wasserstein distances between univariate histograms. In the second case, each clustering iteration requires the computation of two different k-dimensional barycenter and $2S$ Wasserstein distances between k-dimensional histograms. The first approach considers just the marginals of the entire distribution of KPIs, losing the correlations between them and resulting in a more efficient but less effective algorithm. The second approach can instead quickly become too computationally expensive as the number of KPIs k grows.

These two approaches are compared with the k-means algorithm performed on the mean of KPIs. Each store is represented as a k-dimensional vector, where each component contains the mean of a KPI. To enable the visualization of the clustering, the results of the three algorithms are mapped on the network representation of the stores, as shown in Figure 9.

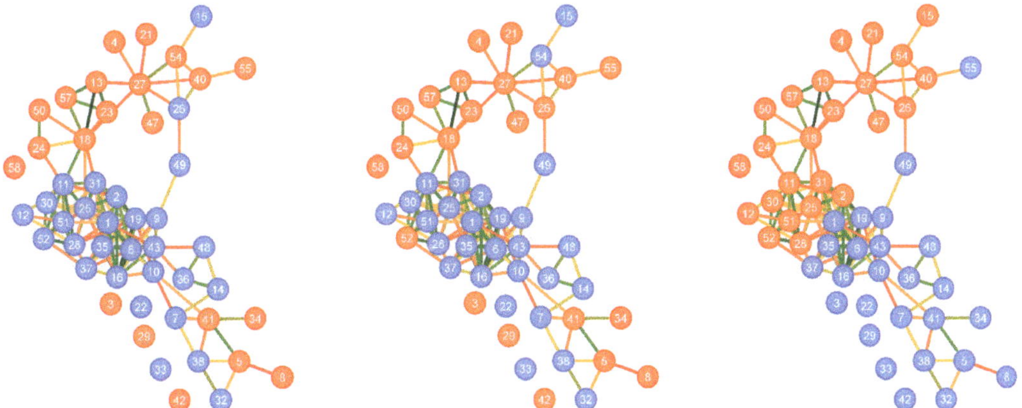

Figure 9. Clusters resulting from the three different approaches: k-means (**left**), clustering of the marginals (**center**) and clustering of the multi-dimensional histograms (**right**).

The resulting clusters using the standard k-means approach and the approach that considers just the marginals are visually similar, while the approach that consider the whole distributions of KPIs bring to different groups. Therefore, using the multi-dimensional histogram representations of the stores allows one to capture the entire distribution of the KPIs and their correlations, thus bringing different insight.

5.4. Nonlinear Structures in Data

A key assumption in this paper is that large datasets can exhibit a nonlinear structure, which is not easily captured by a Euclidean space. A key conjecture of this paper is that the WST space of histograms is a non-linear manifold. As a consequence, one can expect that embedding the problem in a Wasserstein space and using barycenters can provide a better synthesis of the dataset than the Euclidean mean.

To test this conjecture, the difference between the Euclidean mean and the barycenter is analyzed. First, a single KPI is considered, and the Euclidean mean and the barycenter of the histograms associated with the 50 stores are computed. The same process is also repeated in the cases of two, three and four KPIs to consider multi-dimensional histograms.

The computational results support the initial hypothesis. Figure 10 shows the Wasserstein distances between the Euclidean means of the histograms and the barycenters. This distance monotonically increases with the dimension of the support space of the histograms.

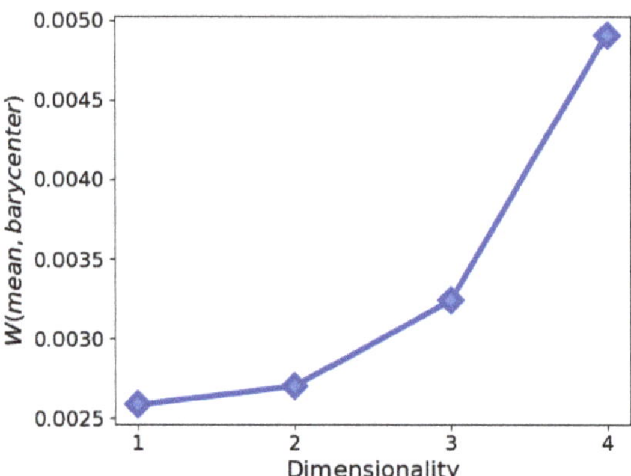

Figure 10. Distance between the Euclidean mean and the Wasserstein barycenter as the histograms' dimensionality increases. The dimensionality of the histograms is on the x-axis, and the Wasserstein distances between the Euclidean mean of the histograms and their Wasserstein barycenters are on the y-axis.

6. Conclusions, Limitations and Perspectives

The analytics proposed in this paper, based on the Wasserstein distance and barycenters, enables one to capture the quality of the customer experiences and to provide performance measures for the entire network of stores. It is the authors' opinion that the growing diversity and heterogeneity of customers makes a distributional approach more effective for analyzing samples of customer behavior than relying only on parameters such as average and variance. The Wasserstein distance (also known as the optimal transport distance) is shown to uncover nonlinear dependencies in the dataset without requiring the alignment of the distributions' support. This is demonstrated by the growing gap between the Euclidean average and the barycenter as the dimensionality of the support increases. The histograms can also be clustered in the Wasserstein space.

These features are demonstrated in a challenging business problem: the performance evaluation of the Italian store network (50 stores) of a multination retailer. Assessing the relative performance of each store with respect to the others is a critical decision for a company as a basis for the distribution of a performance-related bonus. The results enable the company to move towards a different evaluation platform. The analytics proposed in this paper, based on the Wasserstein distance and barycenters, is suitable to obtain a credible ranking system for the stores.

In terms of limitations, it is fair to remark that, although univariate distributions can be easily handled using the quantile-based closed formula, computational problems may hinder the application of the WST distance to large-scale multivariate problems. This problem is amplified in the computation of the barycenter and in the clustering of histograms in the Wasserstein space.

In terms of perspectives, it should be remarked that a byproduct of the computation of the WST distance between two stores is an optimal transport plan that indicates how much of the "probability mass" is to be moved between each couple of bins in the multivariate histograms representing the two stores. This result can be read as the impact of an improvement of each KPI on the overall score of a store.

Author Contributions: All authors contributed equally to this paper. All authors have read and agreed to the published version of the manuscript.

Funding: This research received no external funding.

Data Availability Statement: The data are available upon request to Ilaria Giordani (giordani@oaks.cloud). The data are built on a real word project and were randomized during the study.

Acknowledgments: The authors greatly acknowledge the Data Science Lab, Department of Economics Management and Statistics (DEMS), for supporting this work by providing computational resources.

Conflicts of Interest: The authors declare no conflict of interest.

References

1. Reichheld, F.F. The One Number You Need to Grow. *Harv. Bus. Rev.* **2003**, *81*, 46–55.
2. Fisher, N.I. *Analytics for Leaders. A Performance Measurement System for Business Success*, 1st ed.; Cambridge University Press: Cambridge, UK, 2013.
3. Fisher, N.I. A Comprehensive Approach to Problems of Performance Measurement. *J. R. Stat. Soc. Ser. A Stat. Soc.* **2019**, *182*, 755–803. [CrossRef]
4. Baehre, S.; O'Dwyer, M.; O'Malley, L.; Lee, N. The Use of Net Promoter Score (NPS) to Predict Sales Growth: Insights from an Empirical Investigation. *J. Acad. Mark. Sci.* **2022**, *50*, 67–84. [CrossRef]
5. Markoulidakis, I.; Rallis, I.; Georgoulas, I.; Kopsiaftis, G.; Doulamis, A.; Doulamis, N. A Machine Learning Based Classification Method for Customer Experience Survey Analysis. *Technologies* **2020**, *8*, 76. [CrossRef]
6. Markoulidakis, I.; Rallis, I.; Georgoulas, I.; Kopsiaftis, G.; Doulamis, A.; Doulamis, N. Multiclass Confusion Matrix Reduction Method and Its Application on Net Promoter Score Classification Problem. *Technologies* **2021**, *9*, 81. [CrossRef]
7. Monge, G. Mémoire Sur La Théorie Des Déblais et Des Remblais. In *Histoire de l'Académie Royale des Sciences de Paris*; Nabu Press: Charleston, NC, USA, 1781; pp. 666–704.
8. Kantorovitch, L. On the Translocation of Masses. *Manag. Sci.* **1958**, *5*, 1–4. [CrossRef]
9. Bonneel, N.; Peyré, G.; Cuturi, M. Wasserstein Barycentric Coordinates: Histogram Regression Using Optimal Transport. *ACM Trans. Graph.* **2016**, *35*, 71-1. [CrossRef]
10. Huang, G.; Quo, C.; Kusner, M.J.; Sun, Y.; Weinberger, K.Q.; Sha, F. Supervised Word Mover's Distance. In Proceedings of the 30th International Conference on Neural Information Processing Systems, Barcelona, Spain, 5–10 December 2016; pp. 4869–4877.
11. Arjovsky, M.; Chintala, S.; Bottou, L. Wasserstein Generative Adversarial Networks. In Proceedings of the 34th International Conference on Machine Learning, Sydney, Australia, 6–11 August 2017; pp. 214–223.
12. Villani, C. *Optimal Transport: Old and New*; Springer: Berlin, Germany, 2008.
13. Peyré, G.; Cuturi, M. Computational Optimal Transport. *Found. Trends Mach. Learn.* **2019**, *11*, 355–607. [CrossRef]
14. Panaretos, V.M.; Zemel, Y. *An Invitation to Statistics in Wasserstein Space*; Springer: Berlin, Germany, 2020.
15. Bigot, J. Statistical Data Analysis in the Wasserstein Space. *ESAIM Proc. Surv.* **2020**, *68*, 1–19. [CrossRef]
16. Cohen, S.; Arbel, M.; Deisenroth, M.P. Estimating Barycenters of Measures in High Dimensions. *arXiv* **2020**, arXiv:2007.07105.
17. Verdinelli, I.; Wasserman, L. Hybrid Wasserstein Distance and Fast Distribution Clustering. *Electron. J. Stat.* **2019**, *13*, 5088–5119. [CrossRef]
18. Galichon, A. *Optimal Transport Methods in Economics*; Princeton University Press: Princeton, NJ, USA, 2018.
19. Galichon, A. The Unreasonable Effectiveness of Optimal Transport in Economics. *arXiv* **2021**, arXiv:2107.04700.
20. Kiesel, R.; Rühlicke, R.; Stahl, G.; Zheng, J. The Wasserstein Metric and Robustness in Risk Management. *Risks* **2016**, *4*, 32. [CrossRef]
21. Backhoff-Veraguas, J.; Bartl, D.; Beiglböck, M.; Eder, M. Adapted Wasserstein Distances and Stability in Mathematical Finance. *Financ. Stoch.* **2020**, *24*, 601–632. [CrossRef]
22. Horvath, B.; Issa, Z.; Muguruza, A. Clustering Market Regimes Using the Wasserstein Distance. *arXiv* **2021**, arXiv:2110.11848. [CrossRef]
23. Kuhn, D.; Esfahani, P.M.; Nguyen, V.A.; Shafieezadeh-Abadeh, S. Wasserstein Distributionally Robust Optimization: Theory and Applications in Machine Learning. *arXiv* **2019**, arXiv:1908.08729. [CrossRef]
24. Mohajerin Esfahani, P.; Kuhn, D. Data-Driven Distributionally Robust Optimization Using the Wasserstein Metric: Performance Guarantees and Tractable Reformulations. *Math. Program.* **2018**, *171*, 115–166. [CrossRef]
25. Lau, T.T.-K.; Liu, H. Wasserstein Distributionally Robust Optimization via Wasserstein Barycenters. *arXiv* **2022**, arXiv:2203.12136.
26. Chen, Z.; Kuhn, D.; Wiesemann, W. Data-Driven Chance Constrained Programs over Wasserstein Balls. *Oper. Res.* **2022**. [CrossRef]
27. Xie, W. Tractable Reformulations of Distributionally Robust Two-Stage Stochastic Programs With∞- Wasserstein Distance. *arXiv* **2019**, arXiv:1908.08454.
28. Ma, C.; Ma, L.; Zhang, Y.; Tang, R.; Liu, X.; Coates, M. Probabilistic Metric Learning with Adaptive Margin for Top-K Recommendation. In Proceedings of the 26th ACM SIGKDD International Conference on Knowledge Discovery & Data Mining, Virtual Event, 6–10 July 2020; pp. 1036–1044.
29. Rakotomamonjy, A.; Traoré, A.; Berar, M.; Flamary, R.; Courty, N. Distance Measure Machines. *arXiv* **2018**, arXiv:1803.00250.
30. Le, T.; Cuturi, M. Adaptive Euclidean Maps for Histograms: Generalized Aitchison Embeddings. *Mach. Learn.* **2015**, *99*, 169–187. [CrossRef]

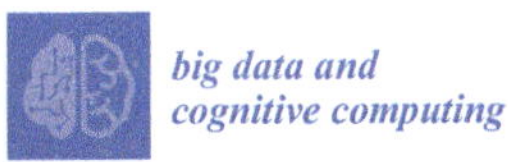
big data and cognitive computing

MDPI

Review

Explore Big Data Analytics Applications and Opportunities: A Review

Zaher Ali Al-Sai [1,2,*], **Mohd Heikal Husin** [2], **Sharifah Mashita Syed-Mohamad** [2], **Rasha Moh'd Sadeq Abdin** [2], **Nour Damer** [3], **Laith Abualigah** [2,4,5,6,7] **and Amir H. Gandomi** [8,9,*]

1   Department of Management Information Systems, Faculty of Business, Al-Zaytoonah University of Jordan, Amman 11733, Jordan
2   School of Computer Sciences, Universiti Sains Malaysia, Pulau Pinang 11800, Malaysia
3   King Talal School of Business Technology, Princess Sumaya University for Technology, Amman 11941, Jordan
4   Prince Hussein Bin Abdullah College for Information Technology, Al Al-Bayt University, Mafraq 25113, Jordan
5   Faculty of Information Technology, Al-Ahliyya Amman University, Amman 19328, Jordan
6   Faculty of Information Technology, Middle East University, Amman 11831, Jordan
7   Faculty of Information Technology, Applied Science Private University, Amman 11931, Jordan
8   Faculty of Engineering and Information Technology, University of Technology Sydney, Sydney 2007, Australia
9   University Research and Innovation Center (EKIK), Óbuda University, 1034 Budapest, Hungary
*   Correspondence: z.alsai@zuj.edu.jo (Z.A.A.-S.); gandomi@uts.edu.au (A.H.G.)

Abstract: Big data applications and analytics are vital in proposing ultimate strategic decisions. The existing literature emphasizes that big data applications and analytics can empower those who apply Big Data Analytics during the COVID-19 pandemic. This paper reviews the existing literature specializing in big data applications pre and peri-COVID-19. A comparison between Pre and Peri of the pandemic for using Big Data applications is presented. The comparison is expanded to four highly recognized industry fields: Healthcare, Education, Transportation, and Banking. A discussion on the effectiveness of the four major types of data analytics across the mentioned industries is highlighted. Hence, this paper provides an illustrative description of the importance of big data applications in the era of COVID-19, as well as aligning the applications to their relevant big data analytics models. This review paper concludes that applying the ultimate big data applications and their associated data analytics models can harness the significant limitations faced by organizations during one of the most fateful pandemics worldwide. Future work will conduct a systematic literature review and a comparative analysis of the existing Big Data Systems and models. Moreover, future work will investigate the critical challenges of Big Data Analytics and applications during the COVID-19 pandemic.

Keywords: big data; big data analytics; big data applications; big data opportunities; COVID-19 pandemic; medical applications; healthcare; education

Citation: Al-Sai, Z.A.; Husin, M.H.; Syed-Mohamad, S.M.; Abdin, R.M.S.; Damer, N.; Abualigah, L.; Gandomi, A.H. Explore Big Data Analytics Applications and Opportunities: A Review. *Big Data Cogn. Comput.* **2022**, *6*, 157. https://doi.org/10.3390/bdcc6040157

Academic Editors: Domenico Talia and Fabrizio Marozzo

Received: 11 November 2022
Accepted: 12 December 2022
Published: 14 December 2022

Publisher's Note: MDPI stays neutral with regard to jurisdictional claims in published maps and institutional affiliations.

1. Introduction

The COVID-19 pandemic has drastically changed nation's worldwide routine life and operations. People have been forced to study and work from home, commuting and traveling to local and overseas destinations have become impossible, and governments have been forced to close cities and countries' borders [1,2].

There is undoubtedly a need for the transfer/exchange the big data systems since decision-makers must be able to react swiftly to changes or trends in markets, investments, interest rates, and other crucial happenings [3]. Decision-makers should be thoroughly aware of the type of inputs they have and the best structure for exchange or analysis if they are thinking about making significant investments in KM systems or big data/business analytics systems [3].

The COVID-19 pandemic paralyzed most vital industries globally. Recently, this is the presented fact; however, a real opportunity is hidden in the new oil in the digital economy, which is Big Data. From a theoretical point of view, researchers have identified different BD-related capabilities and resources as a solid and potential foundation to enhance organizational performance. Most current works in the BD Analytics (BDA) domain cover the technology dimensions, talent, and management that can impact organizational performance [4]. The organization's ability to benefit from different forms of massive data is highly required, and the willingness to invest in BD is now at the center of interest [5,6].

Recently, it has been normal for organizations to be under pressure to remain in their positions in fiercely competitive markets and identify strategies of expenditure reduction, quality enhancement, and reduced time to market [7]. The new era of BD transformation needs next-generation technologies to attain success [8–13].

Organizations will be required to manage it appropriately for competitive advantage and durability in the modern digital market [14]. Organizations should be capable of identifying vital data resources, structure, needed skills, and architecture. Moreover, organizations must define and describe the underlying infrastructure of the process that supports BD analysis, formulate and applicable BD strategy, and measure applications and technologies that support the organization's requirements regarding their BD investments. Particularly, organizations should migrate their data collection and analysis from just being product or service orientated to a future-oriented platform [14]. To grow the adoption rate, ensure the successful implementation, and minimize the risk after implementation, it is crucial to assess and measure BD readiness and maturity level using a maturity assessment model and tool [15,16].

For instance, in the education sector, big data analytics played a key role in overcoming the negative consequences of the pandemic on the educational sector. It supported tutors and instructors to personalize the remote learning experience for educators. Additionally, it helped bridge the unemployment gap that resulted from COVID-19 major economic losses globally. The importance of big data applications and analytics in the transportation field of COVID-19 has been explicitly shown to decision-makers. For instance, regulators supported their decisions and judgments based on the data captured and analyzed via AI techniques and predictive models. Based on the results, precautionary measures were clearly defined, and any violations were easily detected. Furthermore, predictive models guided decision-makers on citizens' movement within and among cities and metropolitans; consequently, they were able to detect and predict future endemic areas.

Existing literature review papers have covered the topic of BD applications during COVID-19. However, this review paper presents new insights into how big data analytics is integrated into the picture in four critical industries. More specifically, this paper will present how big data applications and their aligned data analytics can pave the road for industries to survive an uncontrolled and unpredictable situation. This paper explains these applications in detail. A systematic comparison between the use of BD applications before and after COVID-19 is presented. The paper focuses on four highly impacted industries: Healthcare, Education, Transportation, and Banking. Additionally, this study analyzes the alignment of big data applications with their relevant data analytics models in the era of COVID-19.

The structure of this review paper will be presented as follows: The introduction Section 1, then the literature review Section 2, which highlights the definition and characteristics of Big Data. Additionally, it highlights the Big Data Analytics and types of analytics. Then big data applications and opportunities are presented in Section 3. Sections 4 and 5 review the Big Data applications before and during COVID-19, specifically. Finally, some future work suggestions will be presented in the conclusion and future work in Section 6.

2. Literature Review

Big Data is a critical asset in the competitive market of the digital economy. The benefits of Big Data allow organizations to achieve various objectives under the umbrella of Big Data insights [17]. The following sub-sections present the overall review of Big Data and its applications.

2.1. Big Data and Analytics

There has not been a standardized definition for BD among industry, business, media, academia, and various stakeholders. Absence of a systematic definition for BD concept leads to a sort of confusion [12,18,19]. BD is usually defined by individuals. It is different from one industry to another, and according to the types of available sizes of datasets and the software tools are common in a particular industry [8,20–22].

There have been remarkable thoughts from both industry and academia on BD definition [23]. By coupling the concept of BD with current grounded academic research, the BD concept can be more understandable. A clear view of BD concept will enhance the awareness about BD phenomenon for both practitioners and academics, resulting in faster growth and more efficient value obtained from BD [24]. In spite of the fact that there is no identified definition for BD, from a technical and business point of view, BD is identified as the increasing flow of various types of data from different resources [25].

The first BD definition was written by scientists from NASA. The paper published in 1997, by NASA referred to the data volume as an exciting challenge for computer systems to increase the demand for the big volume of main memory, local disk, and in addition to a remote disk. It was identified by NASA as the problem of BD that required to obtain more resources [8–13,26]. The META Group analyst Dough Laney (now Gartner) has defined data growth challenges and opportunities in to three-dimensional (velocity, volume, variety) [18,27].

The researchers have defined BD concepts from different point of views (BD characteristics, technology, business, Innovation, etc.). One of the definitions had been updated by Gartner in 2013, who defined BD concept as "high-volume, high velocity and/or high variety information assets that demand cost-effective innovative forms of information processing for enhanced insight, decision making, and process optimization" [26,28,29]. The Statistical Analysis System Institute (SAS) defined BD as "Popular term used to describe the exponential growth, availability, and use of information, both structured and unstructured" [30]. IBM also added a definition for BD, "Data is coming from everywhere; sensors that gather climate information, social media posts, digital videos and pictures, purchase transaction record, and GPS signal of mobile phone to name a few", "BD can be defined as large set of very unstructured and disorganized data", "BD is a form of data that oversteps the processing power of traditional database infrastructures or engines" [30–32].

BD was referred from more than one perspective (BD as technology, entity, and process) [33]. The definition of BD analytics consists of the technologies (database and data mining tools) and techniques (analytical methods and techniques) that organizations can utilize to analyze vast amount and complex data for a variety of applications prepared to increase the performance of organizations in many perspectives. BD can be considered as both entity and process. BD as an entity includes a volume of data captured from a variety of resources (internal and external) and consists of structured, semi-structured, and unstructured data that cannot be processed using traditional databases and software techniques. BD as a process refers to both the organizations' infrastructure and the technologies used to capture, store and analyze numerous types of data [10–13,33].

New insights are provided by BD to discover new values, supporting organizations to get the benefit of a deep understanding of the hidden values [23]. BD is pointed out as a technology that enables the processing of unstructured data; and BD technologies are the systems and tools used to process BD such as NoSQL databases, the Hadoop Distributed File System, and MapReduce [34,35].

According to [14], different theories and definitions on what shape BD exist in are provided. The most often referred definition is BD oversteps the capabilities of popularly and currently used software tools and hardware platforms to capture, manage, and process it within an acceptable and bounded time. The concept of BD has been promoted to define the novel and powerful computational technologies that have been provided to process an enormous volume of data. BD has been described in various ways, however, fundamentally is a modern technology that is primarily characterized and derived from Business Analytics

(BA) and Business Intelligence (BI). It is capable of creating business values via its predictive analytics, and decision support abilities, which results in the potency to deal with data that traditional techniques cannot process [25,34].

According to the studies by [13,36], BD is defined as "a term that describes large volumes of high velocity, complex and variable data that requires advanced techniques and technologies to enable the capture, storage, distribution, management, and analysis of the information".

2.2. Characteristics of Big Data

Existing work characterized BD as novel technologies and architectures which are designed for extracting value from enormous volumes of a wide range of data, by empowering high-velocity capture, discovery, and analysis in a cost-effective way [28]. Since BD is relatively new, it is significant for organizations to know what makes this trend valuable and they should identify the "Vs" that describe the key characteristics of BD [37]. Still, a lot of confusion and obscurity among the Vs of BD exists. Some pioneering studies pointed out that there are three, four, five, and sometimes even seven characteristics of BD [38].

The large-scale feature of BD is reflected in three different characteristics of volume, variety, and velocity. Traditional technologies do not have the ability to successfully deal with the enormous data volume, which is generated at a growing velocity, via online streaming and a variety of other different resources such as transactional systems, sensors, social media, product/service instrumentation, and web platforms [38]. META Group analyst Doug Laney (now Gartner) presented 3Vs of BD to characterize the data management in 3 dimensions represented by three main Vs of Volume, Velocity, and Variety [39]. Volume represents the amount of data. Velocity represents the speed of data generation and process. Variety refers to the diversity of resources and data types. Variety refers to the diversity of resources and data types [40–42]. The three Vs have been mentioned by NIST and Gartner in 2012 and extended by IBM to involve the 4th V representing "Veracity ". Contrarily, Oracle avoided using the paradigm of "Vs" in its BD definition. Instead, it is highly believed that BD is the derivation of values from traditional relational database-driven business decision making, grown with new resources of unstructured data [18].

The 4Vs (volume, variety, velocity and value) model was presented by [14,33,41,43,44]. Excluding the 4Vs mentioned, another V which is veracity is identified to represent the uncertainties of BD and data analysis outcome. Another research conducted by [41,42], pointed out the four major Vs of BD namely volume, velocity, variety, and value that pertains to the insight obtained by organizations from BD which not only require scalability, but also for preferable operational procedures and strategies [41,44–46] pointed out five key characteristics of BD as 5Vs (Volume, Velocity, Variety, Veracity, and Value). "Complexity" is a "C" feature added to the 4-Vs (Volume, Variety, Velocity, Value) of BD by [47–49] to formulate another 5 characteristics of BD. Security and management are additional characteristics to the 3Vs (Volume, Variety, and Value) [48]. A study by [48] also presented a critical problem of technical research that requires more investigation by scholars.

Recently, other Vs which are (Visualization/Visibility, Variability/Volatility, Validity, Virtual, and Complexity) are added to BD characteristics by [26]. Another work done by [50], defined the 7 Vs of BD namely Volume, Velocity, Variety, Value, Veracity, Variability which implies inconstancy and heterogeneity; and visualization which implies the illustrative character of data. Volume, Velocity, Variety, Veracity, and Value are the widely accepted and common Vs by stakeholders. However, the other Vs are important for BD paradigm too. By comparing existing definitions of BD and its related aspects, the 5Vs (volume, velocity, variety, veracity, and value) characteristics are extracted and formulated to point out how different traditional data and BD are [24,51,52] as illustrated in Figure 1.

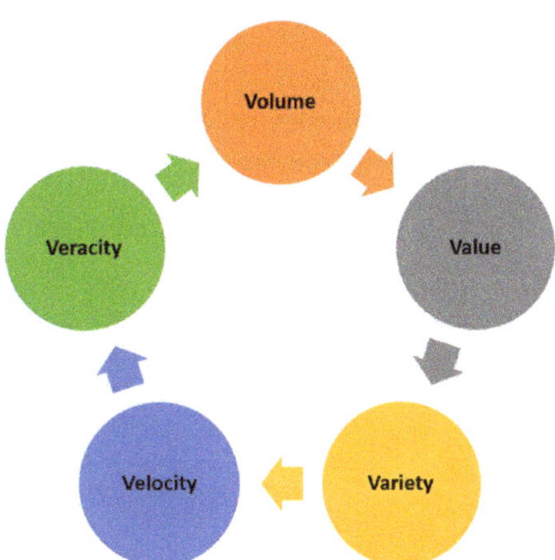

Figure 1. The Five Features of Big Dat.

Big data is more of a concept than an exact term. Some classify big data as a volume problem only for petabyte-scale (>1 million GB) data collection. Some people associate big data with different data types, even if the volume is measured in terabytes. These interpretations made the big data problem situational [51].

2.3. The Types of Data Analytics

Big Data Analytics refers to the process of collecting, organizing, and analyzing high volume, velocity, variety of data to discover the valued patterns that could use for making decisions. Analyzing the big data need new tools, methods, and technologies such as data mining, predictive analytics, and perspective analytics [52].

Most of existing literature identified the use of big data applications defined in the presence of the four types of data analytics. The four types of big data analytics that can be implemented in governments are: (i) Descriptive, (ii) Diagnostic, (iii) Predictive, (iv) Prescriptive [53].

The following section will describe each type with their related examples in governments and more specifically during COVID-19:

- Descriptive

Descriptive analytics is the preliminary stage in the analytics categorization. Descriptive analytics is known as business reporting, as such stage emphasize in creating summary reports to highlight business activities, and to illustrate the answers of questions of "what is happening or happened?" [54–56].

This type of data analysis depends on analyzing past data, visualize and understand historical trends. An example of BDA during COVID-19 are Dashboards used in the health care sector to monitor live data about the spread of COVID-19 in a particular area. Such dashboards track, illustrate and statistically explain the historical records captured about COVID-19 cases in a specific area, city or country [29].

- Diagnostic

The second data analytics type is Diagnostic data analysis. This type focuses on illustrating the correlation, hidden patters, cause-effect relation and interrelationships between different variables. An example would be the data captured from job portals. Such data is used to analyze and visualize potential market sectors and match it with the relevant workforce in the country [54].

Diagnostic analytics figure out answers to questions of "why did it happen?'. The main goal in Diagnostic Analytics is to highlight the root causes of a challenge or problem.

Such root causes identification depends on specialized techniques such as visualization, drill-down, data discovery, and data mining [54–56].

- Predictive

Predictive analytics is categorized in the third level on the data analytics hierarchy. More specifically it is the stage residing after the descriptive analytics. Based on the Data Analytics maturity model, organizations that have matured in descriptive analytics can move forward to the next stage to answer "What will happen?" [55,56].

The third data analysis focuses on patterns from past existing data and predict what will happen when changes occur in such set of data. The example here is the vaccine distribution prioritization mechanism. Data analysts predict through machine learning model who is next in need to the vaccine and prepare patient priority list accordingly [57].

- Prescriptive

The last data analysis type Prescriptive analytics. It is where the best alternative among many–that are usually created/identified by predictive and/or descriptive analytics–courses of action is determined using sophisticated mathematical models. Therefore, in a sense, this type of analytics tries to answer the question of "What should I do?". Prescriptive analytics uses optimization, simulation, and heuristics-based decision modelling techniques [58].

Perspective analytics is ranked as the highest level in data analytics maturity model, it is also viewed as the most sophisticated and complex data analysis type. Both AI and big data analysis techniques are used in Prescriptive analytics. Utilizing such techniques facilitate decision makers to frame the optimal strategic decision. Decision makers will reach to these decisions via selected optimization models. For example, Prescriptive analytics were used during COVID-19 pandemic to understand citizens' reactions towards the vaccine, and support decision makers to structure the optimal strategic decisions to control citizens' hesitant towards the vaccine [55,56].

To illustrate how the four data analytics types are classified based on the level of sophistication and data complexity, researchers have introduced the following two categorize as shown in Figure 2:

- Business Intelligent, which consist of both Descriptive analytics and Diagnostic analytics
- Advanced Analytics, which consider the higher data analytics types in maturity level, namely predictive and prescriptive analytics [55,56,59].

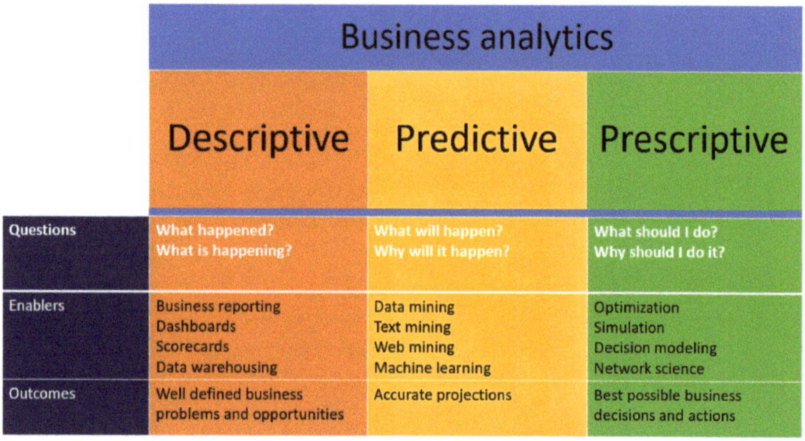

Business analytics		
Descriptive	**Predictive**	**Prescriptive**
Questions What happened? What is happening?	What will happen? Why will it happen?	What should I do? Why should I do it?
Enablers Business reporting Dashboards Scorecards Data warehousing	Data mining Text mining Web mining Machine learning	Optimization Simulation Decision modeling Network science
Outcomes Well defined business problems and opportunities	Accurate projections	Best possible business decisions and actions

Figure 2. A simple taxonomy for analytics.

3. Big Data Analytics Opportunities and Applications

Big data analytics can be described as the use of mathematical and statistical techniques, to find the hidden patterns and variances in large amount of data from multiple sources, and from different type of data (structure, semi-structured, unstructured) to gain future insight and faster decision making [60]. Such findings will be the base for organizations to provide them with valuable knowledge and support them in their strategic decisions [61]. The utilization of big data analytics has shown an added value to governments and firms during COVID-19. Consequently, those who have implemented big data analytics, outperform others. For instance, they were able to map their current status and structure better strategic decisions [55].

In a Mckinsey's report it was highlighted that big data analytics empowered those who applied it, by incrementing their annual economic value between $9.5 trillion and $15.4 trillion [62]. Furthermore, as the COVID-19 outbreak, big data analytics has emphasized its effectiveness in detecting the spread of COVID-19, and supported governments to reach optimal decisions against it [63].

The main goal for organizations is the bottom line represented in their profits, market share and customer loyalty and satisfaction levels [64]. This fact is applied for both business firms and governmental entities. With the exponential increase in the volume of data, the speed in which it is generated, the variety of sources generating it, and the importance of its quality and relevance. The vital role of big data applications in various business sectors and governmental entities have been a necessity for their success [65]. The implementation of big data applications has supported organizations to enhance their customers experience, improve cost savings, and facilitate strategic decision making [66]. Consequently, organizations' processes and operations become achieve a higher level of effectiveness and efficiency [67].

New, advanced and tactical digital technologies were considered recently as a response to the COVID-19 pandemic, such as big data applications. Countries such as Taiwan, South Korea, Hong Kong, and Singapore have demonstrated the significant positive impact from adopting such applications. Those countries proved the seamless of controlling the pandemic expected risks effectively [61].

Big Data Applications can derive insights from various data sources to provide ideal solutions for several sectors [52]. Organizations from a variety of industries have started using MapReduce-based solutions for processing enormous amounts of data [68]. To meet their needs for handling large-scale data processing, many businesses rely on MapReduce. As businesses from a variety of sectors embrace MapReduce together with parallel databases. new MapReduce workloads have appeared that contain a large number of brief interactive tasks [68].

Table 1 highlights the alignment of each big data application to its respective big data analytics model. It provides an explanation on how such an implementation has supported organizations and governments to cope with COVID-19 pitfalls. Furthermore, such an implementation provided an optimal solution to harness its operations and decision-making process. This categorization has been developed based on the description of each application in their relevant fields, and on the definition highlighted in the section on the four big data analytics types.

Table 1. How to utilize Big Data Analytics in Healthcare, Education, Transportation, and Banking.

Field	Data Analytics Type	How BDA Has Been Utilized	Data Processing Models Used to Analyse Big Data	Reference
Healthcare	Descriptive and Predictive Data Analytics	Proactive actions and interventions based on predictive models to trigger any noncommunicable diseases.	Predictive models based on search engines and social media data. Smart phone applications tracking system to identify infection hot spots	[69,70]
	Perspective Data Analytics	Vaccine distribution	Sentiment analysis to reduce community resistance towards the vaccine.	[69–71]
	Diagnostic and Predictive Data Analytics	Vaccine distribution	Machine learning models to prioritize the citizens' need and urgency to the vaccine	
	Diagnostic and Prescriptive Data Analytics	Monitoring live and frequent data on the spread of the disease Provide more personalized consultations by "virtual doctors"	Dashboards AI Chabot	[72,73]
Education	Descriptive Data Analytics	Enhance online educational platform experience	Analyzing data captured from online educational platforms can ease educators remote leaning experience	[69,74]
	Diagnostic Data Analytics	Bridge the gap of unemployment	Analysis of data captured from job portals	[69,75]
Transportation	Descriptive and Prescriptive Data Analytics	implementation of precautionary measures-Ensure social distancing in public transportation	Capturing relevant data and use machine learning techniques to detect incompliance actions	[76]
		Detect citizens' commute route to store their travel history.	Use both AI and Big data applications to capture, track and predict valuable insights about citizens movement within and across cities and countries	[77]
Banking		Fraud Detection	Use AI and ML techniques to describe and detect real-time abnormal activities and online transaction, and build ML models based on classification algorithims to predict any suspecious case.	[78]
	Descriptive and Predictive Data Analytics	Risk Assessment	Use both diagnositic and prescriptuve data analytics models to analyze real-time data and asses the creditworthiness to customers. Consequenlty developing the appropriate cutomer portfolio and tailor clients needs to their services. Cossequently boosting customers' satisfaction, loayality and enhance banks botom line records.	[78]

4. Big Data Applications Pre the COVID-19 Pandemic

In the following section, a demonstration of how big data applications have been applied, and the opportunities captured from it will be illustrated. The section focuses on certain fields before COVID-19, such as healthcare, education, transportation, and banks.

4.1. Big Data in Healthcare

The secret behind utilizing Big Data in the healthcare segment is its powerful ability to highlight the correlation and patterns between different variables rather than finding the casual inference between them. Hence, its capability to predict for the future, and therefore facilitating the e government health sector in its decision-making process [79]. For example, it can support building predictive models for risk and resource use, study the behavioral patterns for patients, analyze the population health, facilitate diagnostic and treatment decisions, use medical images as an input to the clinical decision support system [80]. Assure the safety of the drug and medical devices use on patients and serve individuals health better through analyzing, predicting and monitoring the disease patterns [81].

The sources of data in the healthcare field have elevated exponentially, ranging from the records captured from public hospitals, drug research studies, pharmacists, pathologists, medical laboratories and radiologist. Furthermore, recently other indirect sources are considered such as vital sources such as medical newsletters, websites, social media platforms, health reports, and discussion forums. Additionally, mobile phone applications such as medical smart watches can be considered in the big data process in the healthcare segment [80]. All of these sources of data are the fuel used to enhance performance in health institutes such as in vaccinations, cure of diseases, insurance procedures, and hospital management operations [82].

Big data utilization in healthcare is focused on delivering superior value to individual patients rather than on delivering analysis on general disease cases and volumes of data [29, 80]. Hence, the main goal of big data applications in the health care industry is to serve efficiently considering both value and costs to individual cases [83].

As explained in this section, the use of BDA has been emphasized throughout the medical procedure cycle, affecting the various stakeholders. From patients, medical providers, medical insurance entities, and medical researchers [29].

4.2. Big Data in Education

The educational system is one of the main civilization pillars. Its development can characterize the advancement level of any society. Big data has played a vital role in restructuring the educational system. It enabled educational institutes and professionals to personalize the educational experience for students [84]. The main goal for educators and trainers is to provide a high-quality educational scheme and teaching system. This can only happen by understanding that each student has different way of learning, level of competence, readiness to learn, and interests [85]. How this process can be personalized? Big data is the answer. Big data can analyze, find correlation between the data, highlight patterns, provide insights and predict for the ultimate teaching-learning process. Hence, educators and professionals in the educational field, will provide intelligent decisions to enhance the educational regime [86].

Sources of data in the educational field can be categorized into three main levels Micro-level data, Meso-level data, and Macrolevel data [87]. Micro-level data or what is known as clickstream data, consists of the interactions between millions of learners and their learning environment [88]. This includes the learners' interaction with the virtual gamification, simulations, online platforms, and intelligent tutoring systems. Such actions can predict students' interests [87]. Meso-level data (text data) predict the cognitive ability of students through analyzing the computerized text-oriented writing activities [87]. Such data will be analyzed through NLP techniques [89].

Macrolevel data (institutional data) are sets of data that are captured once a year and represents students' demographics, all educational institutes relevant data (admission data, courses enrolled in, major prerequisites) [90]. Done

When considering big data applications in the educational field, all the above categorization of data sources will overlap. For instance, students' interactions through social media represents both microlevel (duration spent, location of the student) and their meso-level (written posts and text-oriented interaction) [87]. Another example is specific simulation games offered by the educational institute, were the three levels of data will be represented miso/micro/and macro [91].

Applying big data techniques have unleashed several opportunities. For example, big data can improve the learning process, by optimizing the selection, of the prior teaching techniques and newly proposed ones to meet the student actual needs and interests [92]. In addition, big data can facilitate choosing the best bundle of resources, tools, and skills that of higher priority to each teaching-learning case, away from human subjectivity [93]. Moreover, big data can support educators in providing real time feedback and construct development plans based on the student interaction within the virtual learning environment [87]. Furthermore, big data can facilitate constructing a more personalized learning environment. It can track, analyze and predict every action and interaction taken by the students in their virtual environment. By collecting data on students' preferences, performance and results, a more comprehensive picture of the student will be developed. For instance, every click in the virtual learning environment can ease the prediction process [94]. This can be tracked from their interests, their doubts, the time spent in each program, their grades, and their preferred learning style [87]. Thus, big data will result in a more satisfactory learning environment for the students [95].

Enriching the learning environment through understanding the student actual performance level, areas of improvement and difficulties. For instance, big data can detect the questions which the student may fail in or struggle on solving it. Hence, big data can generate progress metrics to provide in depth analysis of the student performance [87]. Furthermore, big data provide a great tool to predict the students who may pass successfully or fail. Another crucial opportunity of applying big data in the educational field is to utilize it in the marketing research, were educational institutes can attract outstanding students [86].

4.3. Big Data in Transportation

The phenomena of big data application have raised significantly in the transportation field, as a result of the endless flow of both mobility and city data that resides in digital repositories, remote and in situ sensors and mobile phones and captured accordingly in vast volumes and velocities [96]. These data are the base for researchers, economists and regulators to analyze traffic flow, congestion and their social, economic and environmental impacts [97]. Moreover, applying a combination of new methods of analysis such as artificial intelligent approaches, paves the way for predicting and providing innovative solutions for the future. Hence, creating a new revolution in big data in the transportation field. [30].

For example, big data plays a vital role in predicting the cause effect relation between the driving restriction policies and traffic congestion [98]. Big data through its predictive capabilities and the incorporation of economic insights can exceed the ability to understand and analyze the past and real time data, to predict the optimal legislations for traffic congestion issues in smart cities [99].

To understand how big data applications used in transportation, we will illustrate the categorization of various sources of data:

1. First source of data which is the primary source is the direct physical sensing. Represented, in road-side static sensors such as LiDAR, microwave Radars, and sensors that measure speed, noise, and traffic flow known as acoustic sensors [100]. Other examples are the use of mobile phone technologies such as GPS, GSM, and Bluetooth [97].

2. The second source of data is the social media sources "human & social Sensing" highlighted in the use of motorists to the smartphone-compatible platforms [101]. For instance Instagram, twitter and others [97].

3. The third category of data source is urban sensing which is generated by transportation operators. In this category data captured can analyze urban mobility in terms of congestion and traffic flows [102]. This can be performed via credit cards and smart cards scanned through urban sensors from public transit, retail scanners and digital toll systems [97].

4.4. Big Data in Banking

In recent years, the massive use of information technology and more specifically, big data, has reshaped the banking sector intensely. This has been remarked by the introduction of digital banking operations and virtual banking systems [103]. The banking sector is a highly competitive environment. To survive in such a competitive environment a proactive strategy and better strategic decisions must be adapted by management. Big data applications are utilized in the banking sector and supported by data mining techniques to transfer customer semi-structured and un-structured data into meaningful insights and derive the ultimate strategic decisions. Such decisions can support banks to increase customer satisfaction, detect fraud cases, ease the merge and acquisition operations [95], optimize banking supply chain performance [104], outperform annual profits and expand market share. An example of how big data applications harness strategic decisions and meet strategic goals is through applying sophisticated algorithms to categorize clients and group them into clusters based on the analysis and interpretation of clients' behaviors. Such technique can facilitate banks to provide valued and satisfactory services to different clients' categories. Moreover, the ability of big data applications to integrate internal and external sources play a vital role in detecting fraud activities [105]. Furthermore, the capability of big data to analyze, predict, and visualize both external market conditions and internal clients' trends and preferences can empower management in considering the ultimate decision to invest in new markets, hence increasing their market share and enhancing profitability [106].

Table 2 depicts a summary of the Big Data opportunities. Moreover, Table 3 provides examples of Big Data applications in certain fields before COVID-19.

Table 2. The Big Data Opportunities before COVID-19 Pandemic.

Field	Opportunities	Description	Reference
Healthcare	Serve efficiently considering both value and costs to individual cases	BDA have powerful ability to highlight the correlation and patterns between different variables rather than finding the casual inference between them and serve individual patients' cases.	[79–81,83,107]
Education	Improve the learning process Provide real time feedback and construct development plans Construct a more personalized learning environment Enrich the learning environment Utilize BDA in marketing research purposes for institutions	BDA enables educational institutes and professionals to personalize the educational experience for students	[84,86,87,92–95,108]
Transportation	The base for researchers, economists and regulators to analyze traffic flow, congestion and their social, economic and environmental impacts. Apply a combination of new methods of analysis such as AI approaches, to pave the way for predicting and providing innovative solutions for the future in the field of transportation.	BDA predictive capabilities and the incorporation of economic insights can exceed the ability to understand and analyze the past and real time data, to predict the optimal legislations for traffic congestion issues in smart cities.	[30,96–99,109]
Banks	Detect fraud cases Ease the merge and acquisition operations Optimize banking supply chain performance Interpret clients' behaviors. Provide valued and satisfactory services to clients. Analyze, predict, and visualize both external market conditions and internal clients' trends and preferences Increase market share and enhance profitability.	BDA supported the introduction of digital banking operations and virtual banking systems	[103,105,106]

Table 3. Examples of Big Data applications by field before COVID-19.

Field in Charge	Application Name	Description	Reference
Health	Ebola Open Data Initiative	West Africa-data has been utilized to develop an open-source global model for tracking the cases of Ebola cases in in 2014	[29,110,111]
	HealthMap	a platform used to visualize diseases trends and provides an early trigger on the proper response	[110,112]
	Proactive listening, mobile phone-based system	Brazil-to govern the issue of bribes in the health services, and handle any related issues and take an immediate and effective action against corruption.	[110]
Education	ENOVA	Mexico, through the utilization of data and data analytics can analyze and predict students' interactions. Consequently, boosts the educational strategies and enhances the used tools and techniques in the teaching-learning process.	[113,114]
	(PASS) Personalized Adaptive Study Success	The Open University Australia-Predicts course material, beside a more personalized studying environment. The predictive data analytics model is based on analyzing students, individual characteristics, beside other student related data captured from other systems. The main goal of the application is to develop a more customized environment that ensures students involvement, engagement, and retention in an e-learning environment.	[115]
Transportation		An application to support in urban infrastructure decisions, based on data captured from both vehicles and smartphones, to analyze it and visualize it into both historic and real-time traffic situations.	[110,116]
	OpenTraffic platform	Seoul, South Africa-the application is used to support night bus drivers to ease their journey from origin to destination. This will occur through capturing data from tremendous number of calls and text data points, as well as private and corporate taxi data sources.	[110]
Banks	Avaloq, Finnova, SAP, Sungard and Temenos	OCBC is the largest bank in terms of market capitalization in Singapore. It operates in more than 15 countries globally. It is a success example of the utilization of BDA. For instance, the bank responded to customer actions, customers' personalized events and their demographic profiles. Hence, OCBC Bank succeed in achieving higher customer engagement and increasing the level of customer satisfaction by 20% in comparison to a control group. These core banking applications, such as Avaloq, Finnova, SAP, Sungard or Temenos for example, were designed to handle large amounts of transactions in back-office processes for basic financial products and services, such as bank accounts, deposits, etc.	[104,117]

5. Big Data Applications Peri the COVID-19 Pandemic

In 2020, the world has been experiencing a critical pandemic, COVID-19. Most governments were not expecting such a drastic change in their citizens daily routine and life. From cities in lock down, individuals' quarantine, people working from home to the emphasize on online services [97,118]. Moreover, many of the government's portals, e services and applications were not up to the required standard to fight against such a disaster. That triggered the importance of data analytics and the utilization of Big Data Applications. Many governments were forced to react in a short period of time [97,119]. A variety of applications have been introduced in different fields, to ease individuals' lives, support governments decisions and control the pandemic effect globally [120]. Furthermore, big data analytics, have facilitated governments to embrace remarkable strategic decisions efficiently and effectively. Moreover, data analytics proved its importance in predicting and managing risks associated to supply chain safety, and to external economic, social and legal risks [55,118].

According to a study by EY in 2021, governments are reconsidering the importance of big data to overcome the pitfalls of the pandemic and to recover from it. For instance, nations all around the globe have invested in a visionary action towards utilizing BDA. Example of countries such as, Hong Kong, US, Switzerland, and India [121].

In 2020, a study by United Nations illustrated some of the most important applications used worldwide during COVID-19. The main goal for governments was to share reliable and transparent information about COVID-19, to enhance citizens' awareness about the situation and allow policy makers to plan appropriate actions accordingly. This has been empowered by dashboards, such as in Vancouver and Australia, to track the number of cases and allocate the required community resources accordingly [122]. Furthermore, to ensure social distancing, governments in India and New York has urged their citizen to rely more on online services such as online parking payment in New York City and e- Doctor tele-video consultation to prevent crowds in hospitals in India. Also, China monitored its citizens commuting to work, grocery stores, and shopping malls via the QR health code. Many other BDA were offered by governments such as platforms for e leaning wither for schools or universities. Not to mention the countless services offered for entertainment online for citizens in quarantine periods [72].

The following sections describe the utilization of big data applications during COVID-19 pandemic in four vital sectors: Healthcare, Education, Transportation and Banking. It highlights the significant results approached in each sector and its role during COVID-19 pandemic.

5.1. Big Data in Healthcare

The first application of BDA in health care sector post COVID-19, is to support government agencies to detect a specific disease in particular area, monitor the health condition of the citizens and provide a preventive action accordingly. All of such actions will be based on predictive models which will be supported by input from smart phone connected to thermometers and tracking systems, search engines and social media data [118].

Another use of BDA post COVID-19 is the management and control of vaccine distribution. For example, governments will easily understand the community reaction towards the vaccine [71]. This will be figured through applying sentiment analysis to the data captured from social media platforms, and develop strategies that will control the community resistance towards the vaccine [69]. Furthermore, applying machine learning techniques will anticipate and prioritize who will be more vulnerable to the disease, and who should be provided with the vaccine first. Also, BDA guarantee a better technique to store the vaccine. This will be through monitoring the optimal temperature level [72].

Finally, big data solutions helped governmental entities in their vaccine distribution efforts. For instance, big data facilitated in the storage mechanism of the vaccine, since they were kept and stored within precise temperature range. Hence, ensuring the quality level of the vaccine won't be affected by any environmental circumstances through the distribution chain. Furthermore, machine learning was applied to highlight analyses of the populations. For example, a categorization of the population with health vulnerabilities were easily distinguished. Consequently, a prioritization mechanism and plan for vaccine delivery was prepared [69]. Also, sentiment analysis on citizens' casual conversation on social media were performed by governmental entities. Such large text-data, helped in understanding the public view on immunization. As a result, governments were able to develop the proper communication strategies, to persuade citizens about vaccinations and overcome any hesitancy from it [123].

5.2. Big Data in Education

COVID-19 has forced many schools, and educational institutes to shift their physical presence to online educational platforms [74]. BDA supported educators via analyzing data captured from such platforms, to analyze and predict students current and future learning abilities and develop the educators' teaching styles accordingly [69]. Furthermore, an instant need to bridge the gap of unemployment required the implementation of BDA. This has been evident through analyzing the data captured from job portals, communicating the job market needs to educators and thus develop the appropriate curriculum, and communicating it to the targeted segments [75].

5.3. Big Data in Transportation

COVID-19 has stimulated governments to reconsider its transportation decision management systems and empower it with big data applications [77]. For instance, Dubai is a leading example in the use of big data applications to ensure social distancing between bus passengers and detect any incompliance. It invested both in using AI and big data applications to capture relevant data such as, data and time of the trip, driver details, the frequency of the vehicle incompliance, and the route number. Hence facilitate applying disciplinary actions accordingly [76].

Another example is to detect citizens commute route in order to store their travel history. This will ease the regulators to detect whom infected patients with COVID-19 virus have contacted. Hence, government regulators can predict which areas might be potentially more affected than others. Therefore, preventive actions will be taken on a more methodical base. Therefore, in a broader context, countries can predict the flow of infected citizens between cities and countries and consequently declare travelling constraints and guidance [78].

5.4. Big Data in Banking

The incident of the global COVID-19 pandemic has exponential increased banks' clients use for online transactions using big data applications [124]. A study prepared by the world bank on 29 June 2022, depicted global financial figures as follow: around 76% of adults created personalized accounts wither with financial institutes or mobile money providers compared to 51% in 2011. Also, the increase has been applied to the use of digital payments. For instance, since the hit of the pandemic more than 80 million adults conducted their first digital purchase and payment in India, and more than 100 million adults in China [125]. Additionally, Big data applications and Analytics crucial role was evident to bankers in their strategic and daily operations during COVID-19. Examples in banking are the use of descriptive and predictive data analytics models in Fraud Detection, and the diagnostic and prescriptive data analysis models such as in Risk Assessment [78]. Moreover, financial intermediaries use AI-based systems for fraud detection and analyze the degree of interconnectedness between borrowers, which in turn allows them to better manage their lending portfolio [126]. Banks are increasingly using big data and analytics to assess the creditworthiness of prospective borrowers and make underwriting decisions, where both functions at the core of finance [126].

5.5. Big Data Analytics across Industry

Big Data Applications can derive insights from various data sources to provide ideal solutions for several sectors [52]. Table 4 highlights the alignment of each big data application to its respective big data analytics model. It provides an explanation on how such an implementation has supported organizations and governments to cope with COVID-19 pitfalls. Furthermore, such an implementation provided an optimal AI solution to harness its operations and decision-making process. This categorization has been developed based on the description of each application in their relevant fields, and on the definition highlighted in the section on the four big data analytics types.

Table 4. How to utilize Big Data Analytics in Healthcare, Education, Transportation, and Banking.

Field	Data Analytics Type	How BDA Has Been Utilized	Method/Model	Reference
Healthcare	Descriptive and Predictive Data Analytics Models	Proactive actions and interventions based on predictive models to trigger any noncommunicable diseases.	Predictive models based on search engines and social media data. Smart phone applications tracking system to identify infection hot spots	[69,70]
	Perspective Data Analytics	Vaccine distribution	Sentiment analysis to reduce community resistance towards the vaccine.	[69,71]
	Diagnostic and Predictive Data Analytics Models	Vaccine distribution	Machine learning models to prioritize the citizens' need and urgency to the vaccine	
	Diagnostic and Prescriptive Data Analytics Models	Monitoring live and frequent data on the spread of the disease Provide more personalized consultations by "virtual doctors"	Dashboards AI Chabot	[72,73]
Education	Descriptive Data Analytics Model	Enhance online educational platform experience	Analyzing data captured from online educational platforms can ease educators remote leaning experience	[69,74]
	Diagnostic Data Analytics Model	Bridge the gap of unemployment	Analysis of data captured from job portals	[69,75]
Transportation	Descriptive and Prescriptive Data Analytics Models	implementation of precautionary measures-Ensure social distancing in public transportation	Capturing relevant data and use machine learning techniques to detect incompliance actions	[76]
	Descriptive and Predictive Data Analytics Models	Detect citizens' commute route to store their travel history.	Use both AI and Big data applications to capture, track and predict valuable insights about citizens movement within and across cities and countries	[77]
Banking		Fraud Detection	Use AI and ML techniques to describe and detect real-time abnormal activities and online transaction, and build ML models based on classification algorithims to predict any suspecious case.	[78]
		Risk Assessment	Use both diagnositic and prescriptuve data analytics models to analyze real-time data and asses the creditworthiness to customers. Consequenlty developing the appropriate cutomer portfolio and tailor clients needs to their services. Cossequently boosting customers' satisfaction, loayality and enhance banks botom line records.	[78]

6. Conclusions

The unstable status resulting from COVID-19 forced organizations to realize the real importance of big data applications. It has been evident during pandemics that Big Data adoption enables decision-makers to make smarter decisions in real time. The technologies behind Big Data support organizations to gain valuable insights from their data. Big Data facilitates transforming organizations' practices to a new generation of digital services ensuring that added value for customers will be achieved. Organizations utilize Big Data to detect and analyze the trends and patterns of people's behavior on social networking. Hence, an organization's decision-makers can provide optimal decisions and better, effective, and efficient services and products for the public. This review paper investigated the existing literature to define Big Data, and the types of Analytics, and compared the Big Data applications before and after COVID-19. The comparison was supported by examples from four vital sectors in the industry of Healthcare, Education, Transportation, and Banking as examples of sectors affected by COVID-19. The paper presented a detailed description of the role of data analytics and its alignment with specific big data applications in those fields. Such applications supported organizations and nations to navigate through the COVID-19 pandemic confidently. Hence, they could not only overcome challenges but also unleash opportunities and create value. The limitation of this paper is related to the limited previous studies that investigated the applications and opportunities of big data during the COVID-19 Pandemic. The future work will start by investigating the challenges faced by organizations on different levels, it will also investigate the critical success factors of Big Data and their categories toward developing a conceptual model for Big Data implementation.

Author Contributions: Conceptualization, Z.A.A.-S., M.H.H., S.M.S.-M., R.M.S.A., N.D., L.A. and A.H.G.; methodology, Z.A.A.-S.; formal analysis, Z.A.A.-S.; writing—original draft preparation, Z.A.A.-S., M.H.H., S.M.S.-M., R.M.S.A., N.D., L.A. and A.H.G.; writing—review and editing, Z.A.A.-S., M.H.H., S.M.S.-M., R.M.S.A., N.D., L.A. and A.H.G.; visualization, L.A.; supervision, L.A. and A.H.G.; project administration, Z.A.A.-S., M.H.H., S.M.S.-M., R.M.S.A., N.D., L.A. and A.H.G. All authors have read and agreed to the published version of the manuscript.

Funding: This research received no external funding.

Institutional Review Board Statement: Not applicable.

Data Availability Statement: Not applicable.

Conflicts of Interest: The authors declare no conflict of interest.

References

1. Alhomdy, S.; Thabit, F.; Abdulrazzak, F.A.H.; Haldorai, A.; Jagtap, S. The role of cloud computing technology: A savior to fight the lockdown in COVID-19 crisis, the benefits, characteristics and applications. *Int. J. Intell. Netw.* **2021**, *2*, 166–174. [CrossRef]
2. Alsunaidi, S.J.; Almuhaideb, A.M.; Ibrahim, N.M.; Shaikh, F.S.; Alqudaihi, K.S.; Alhaidari, F.A.; Khan, I.U.; Aslam, N.; Alshahrani, M.S. Applications of Big Data Analytics to Control COVID-19 Pandemic. *Sensors* **2021**, *21*, 2282. [CrossRef] [PubMed]
3. Rothberg, H.N.; Erickson, G.S. Big data systems: Knowledge transfer or intelligence insights? *J. Knowl. Manag.* **2017**, *21*, 92–112. [CrossRef]
4. Adrian, C.; Adrian, C.; Abdullah, R.; Atan, R.; Jusoh, Y.Y. Conceptual Model Development of Big Data Analytics Implementation Assessment Effect on Article in Press Conceptual Model Development of Big Data Analytics Implementation Assessment Effect on Decision-Making. *Int. J. Interact. Multimed. Artif. Intell.* **2018**, *5*, 101–106. [CrossRef]
5. Gupta, M.; George, J.F. Toward the development of a big data analytics capability. *Inf. Manag.* **2016**, *53*, 1049–1064. [CrossRef]
6. Kalema, B.M.; Mokgadi, M. Developing countries organizations' readiness for Big Data analytics. *Probl. Perspect. Manag.* **2017**, *15*, 260–270. [CrossRef]
7. De Bruin, T.; Kulkarni, U.; Rosemann, M.; Freeze, R. *Understanding the Main Phases of Developing a Maturity Assessment Model*; ACIS: Sydney, Australia, 2005.
8. Rialti, R.; Marzi, G.; Ciappei, C.; Busso, D. Big data and dynamic capabilities: A bibliometric analysis and systematic literature review. *Manag. Decis.* **2019**, *57*, 2052–2068. [CrossRef]
9. Al-sai, Z.A.; Abdullah, R.; Husin, M.H.; Syed-mohamad, S.M. A Preliminary Systematic Literature Review On Critical Success Factors Categories For Big Data. In Proceedings of the AiIC2019, Toyama, Japan, 7–11 July 2019.

10. Al-Sai, Z.A.; Abdullah, R.; Husin, M.H. Big Data Impacts and Challenges: A Review. In Proceedings of the 2019 IEEE Jordan International Joint Conference on Electrical Engineering and Information Technology, Amman, Jordan, 9–11 April 2019; pp. 150–155. [CrossRef]

11. Al-Sai, Z.A.; Abdullah, R.; Husin, M.H. A review on big data maturity models. In Proceedings of the 2019 IEEE Jordan International Joint Conference on Electrical Engineering and Information Technology, Amman, Jordan, 9–11 April 2019; pp. 156–161.

12. Zulkarnain, N.; Meyliana, M.; Prabowo, H.; Nizar Hidayanto, A. The critical success factors for big data adoption in government. *Int. J. Mech. Eng. Technol.* **2019**, *10*, 864–875. [CrossRef]

13. Al-Sai, Z.A.; Abualigah, L.M. Big Data and E-government: A review. In Proceedings of the 2017 8th International Conference on Information Technology, Amman, Jordan, 17–18 May 2017; pp. 580–587. [CrossRef]

14. Malik, P. Governing Big Data: Principles and practices. *IBM J. Res. Dev.* **2013**, *57*, 1:1–1:13. [CrossRef]

15. Big Data Analytics and Fi Nancial Reporting Quality: Qualitative Evidence from Canada. Available online: https://doi.org/10.1108/JFRA-12-2021-0489 (accessed on 1 January 2021).

16. Measuring Your Big Data Maturity. Available online: https://michaelskenny.com/points-of-view/measuring-your-big-data-maturity/ (accessed on 1 January 2021).

17. Davenport, T.; Dyché, J. Big Data in Big Companies. *Baylor Bus. Rev.* **2013**, *32*, 20–21.

18. Ward, J.S.; Barker, A. Undefined By Data: A Survey of Big Data Definitions. *arXiv* **2013**, arXiv:1309.5821.

19. Bertot, J.C.; Choi, H. Big data and e-government: Issues, policies, and recommendations. In Proceedings of the 14th Annual International Conference on Digital Government Research, New York, NY, USA, 17 June 2013; pp. 1–10.

20. Braun, H. *Evaluation of Big Data Maturity Models—A Bench- Marking Study To Support Big Data Maturity Assessment In Organizations*; Tampere University of Technology: Tampere, Finland, 2015.

21. Manyika, J.; Chui, M.; Brown, B.; Bughin, J.; Dobbs, R.; Roxburgh, C.; Byers, A.H. *Big Data: The Next Frontier for Innovation, Competition, and Productivity*; McKinsey Global Institute: Chicago, IL, USA, 2011.

22. Henke, N.; Bughin, J.; Chui, M.; Manyika, J.; Saleh, T.; Wiseman, B.; Sethupathy, G. *The Age of Analytics: Competing in a Data-Driven World*; McKinsey Global Institute: Chicago, IL, USA, 2016; Volume 12, pp. 904–920. [CrossRef]

23. Chen, M.; Mao, S.; Liu, Y. Big data: A survey. *Mob. Netw. Appl.* **2014**, *19*, 171–209. [CrossRef]

24. Romijn, B.-J. Big Data in the Public Sector: Uncertainties and Readiness in the Dutch Public Executive Sector. *Inf. Syst. Frontiers.* **2017**, *19*, 267–283.

25. Sun, S.; Cegielski, C.G.; Jia, L.; Hall, D.J. Understanding the Factors Affecting the Organizational Adoption of Big Data. *J. Comput. Inf. Syst.* **2016**, *58*, 193–203. [CrossRef]

26. Zainal, N.Z.; Hussin, H.; Nazri, M.N.M. Big Data Initiatives by Governments —Issues and Challenges: A Review. In Proceedings of the 2016 6th International Conference on Information and Communication Technology for The Muslim World (ICT4M), Jakarta, Indonesia, 22–24 November 2016; pp. 304–309. [CrossRef]

27. Esteves, J.; Curto, J. A risk and benefits behavioral model to assess intentions to adopt big data. *J. Intell. Stud. Bus.* **2013**, *3*, 37–46. [CrossRef]

28. Kaka, E.S. E-Government Adoption and Framework for Big Data Analytics. In Proceedings of the Second Covenant University Conferenced on E-Governance in Nigeria (CUCEN 2015), Covenant University Canaanland, Ota Ogun State, Nigeria, 10–12 June 2015; pp. 1–28.

29. Batko, K.; Ślęzak, A. The use of Big Data Analytics in healthcare. *J. Big Data* **2022**, *9*, 3. [CrossRef]

30. Al Nuaimi, E.; Al Neyadi, H.; Mohamed, N.; Al-Jaroodi, J. Applications of big data to smart cities. *J. Internet Serv. Appl.* **2015**, *6*, 25. [CrossRef]

31. Lutfi, A.; Alrawad, M.; Alsyouf, A.; Almaiah, M.A.; Al-Khasawneh, A.; Al-Khasawneh, A.L.; Alshira'h, A.F.; Alshirah, M.H.; Saad, M.; Ibrahim, N. Drivers and impact of big data analytic adoption in the retail industry: A quantitative investigation applying structural equation modeling. *J. Retail. Consum. Serv.* **2023**, *70*, 103129. [CrossRef]

32. Big Data Analytics. Available online: https://www.ibm.com/analytics/big-data-analytics (accessed on 1 January 2021).

33. Brock, V.; Khan, H.U. Big data analytics: Does organizational factor matters impact technology acceptance? *J. Big Data* **2017**, *4*, 21. [CrossRef]

34. Chen, J.; Chen, Y.; Du, X.; Li, C.; Lu, J.; Zhao, S.; Zhou, X. Big Data Challenge: A Data Management Perspective. *Front. Comput. Sci.* **2013**, *7*, 157–164. [CrossRef]

35. Hood-Clark, S.F. Influences On The Use And Behavioral Intention To Use Big Data. Ph.D. Thesis, Capella University ProQuest Dissertations Publishing, Minneapolis, MN, USA, 2016.

36. Gandomi, A.; Haider, M. Beyond the hype: Big data concepts, methods, and analytics. *Int. J. Inf. Manag.* **2015**, *35*, 137–144. [CrossRef]

37. Munné, R. Big data in the public sector. In *New Horizons for a Data-Driven Economy*; Springer: Cham, Switzerland, 2016; pp. 195–208.

38. Comuzzi, M.; Patel, A. How organisations leverage Big Data: A maturity model. *Ind. Manag. Data Syst.* **2016**, *116*, 1468–1492. [CrossRef]

39. Laney, D. META Delta. *Appl. Deliv. Strateg.* **2001**, *949*, 4. [CrossRef]

40. Kanan, T.; Mughaid, A.; Al-Shalabi, R.; Al-Ayyoub, M.; Elbe, M.; Sadaqa, O. Business intelligence using deep learning techniques for social media contents. *Cluster Comput.* **2022**, 1–12. [CrossRef]

41. Singh, S.; Singh, N. Big Data analytics. In Proceedings of the 2012 International Conference on Communication, Information & Computing Technology, Mumbai, India, 19–20 October 2012; pp. 1–4. [CrossRef]

42. Where Big Data Projects Fail. Available online: https://www.forbes.com/sites/bernardmarr/2015/03/17/where-big-data-projects-fail/?sh=22d01455239f (accessed on 1 January 2021).

43. Cato, P.; Golzer, P.; Demmelhuber, W. An investigation into the implementation factors affecting the success of big data systems. In Proceedings of the 2015 11th International Conference on Innovations in Information Technology, Dubai, United Arab Emirates, 1–3 November 2015; pp. 134–139. [CrossRef]

44. Motau, M.; Kalema, B.M. Big Data Analytics Readiness: A South African Public Sector Perspective. In Proceedings of the 2016 IEEE International Conference on Emerging Technologies and Innovative Business Practices for the Transformation of Societies, Balaclava, Mauritius, 3–6 August 2016.

45. Big Security for Big Data: Addressing Security Challenges for the Big Data Infrastructure. Available online: https://doi.org/10.1007/978-3-319-06811-4 (accessed on 1 January 2021).

46. Soon, K.W.K.; Lee, C.A.; Boursier, P. A study of the determinants affecting adoption of big data using integrated Technology Acceptance Model (TAM) and diffusion of innovation (DOI) in Malaysia. *Int. J. Appl. Bus. Econ. Res.* **2016**, *14*, 17–47.

47. Kaisler, S.; Armour, F.; Espinosa, J.A.; Money, W. Big Data: Issues and Challenges Moving Forward. In Proceedings of the 2013 46th Hawaii International Conference on System Sciences, Wailea, HI, USA, 7–10 January 2013; pp. 995–1004. [CrossRef]

48. Khan, N.; Yaqoob, I.; Hashem, I.A.; Inayat, Z.; Ali, W.M.; Shiraz, M.; Gani, A.; Member, S. Big Data: Survey, Technologies, Opportunities, and Challenges. *Sci. World J.* **2014**, *2014*, 712826. [CrossRef]

49. Sagiroglu, S.; Sinanc, D. Big data: A review. In Proceedings of the 2013 International Conference on Collaboration Technologies and Systems, San Diego, CA, USA, 20–24 May 2013; pp. 42–47. [CrossRef]

50. Saxena, S. Integrating Open and Big Data via e-Oman: Prospects and issues—Read. *Contemp. Arab Aff.* **2016**, *9*, 607–621. [CrossRef]

51. Mohanty, S.K.; Jagadeesh, M.; Srivatsa, H.K. Big Data Imperatives: Enterprise Big Data Warehouse, BI Implementations and Analytics. Available online: https://www.ptonline.com/articles/how-to-get-better-mfi-results (accessed on 1 January 2021).

52. Harnessing the Potential of Big Data in Post-Pandemic Southeast Asia. Available online: https://www.adb.org/publications/potential-big-data-post-pandemic-southeast-asia (accessed on 1 January 2021).

53. Long, C.K.; Agrawal, R.; Trung, H.Q.; Van Pham, H. A big data framework for E-Government in Industry 4.0. *Open Comput. Sci.* **2021**, *11*, 461–479. [CrossRef]

54. Sivarajah, U.; Kamal, M.M.; Irani, Z.; Weerakkody, V. Critical analysis of Big Data challenges and analytical methods. *J. Bus. Res.* **2017**, *70*, 263–286. [CrossRef]

55. Sheng, J.; Amankwah-Amoah, J.; Khan, Z.; Wang, X. COVID-19 Pandemic in the New Era of Big Data Analytics: Methodological Innovations and Future Research Directions. *Br. J. Manag.* **2021**, *32*, 1164–1183. [CrossRef]

56. Delen, D.; Zolbanin, H.M. The analytics paradigm in business research. *J. Bus. Res.* **2018**, *90*, 186–195. [CrossRef]

57. Rustagi, V.; Bajaj, M.; Tanvi; Singh, P.; Aggarwal, R.; AlAjmi, M.F.; Hussain, A.; Hassan, M.I.; Singh, A.; Singh, I.K. Analyzing the Effect of Vaccination Over COVID Cases and Deaths in Asian Countries Using Machine Learning Models. *Front. Cell. Infect. Microbiol.* **2022**, *11*, 806265. [CrossRef] [PubMed]

58. Lepenioti, K.; Bousdekis, A.; Apostolou, D.; Mentzas, G. Prescriptive analytics: Literature review and research challenges. *Int. J. Inf. Manag.* **2020**, *50*, 57–70. [CrossRef]

59. Delen, D.; Ram, S. Research challenges and opportunities in business analytics. *J. Bus. Anal.* **2018**, *1*, 2–12. [CrossRef]

60. Sekli, G.F.M.; De La Vega, I. Adoption of big data analytics and its impact on organizational performance in higher education mediated by knowledge management. *J. Open Innov. Technol. Mark. Complex.* **2021**, *7*, 221. [CrossRef]

61. Nageshwaran, G.; Harris, R.C.; El Guerche-Seblain, C. Review of the role of big data and digital technologies in controlling COVID-19 in Asia: Public health interest vs. privacy. *Digit. Health* **2021**, *7*, 20552076211002953. [CrossRef]

62. Henke, N.; Puri, A.; Saleh, T. Accelerating analytics to navigate COVID-19 and the next normal. *McKinsey Anal.* **2020**, 9.

63. Sözen, M.E.; Sarlyer, G.; Ataman, M.G. Big data analytics and COVID-19: Investigating the relationship between government policies and cases in Poland, Turkey and South Korea. *Health Policy Plan.* **2022**, *37*, 100–111. [CrossRef]

64. Nwanga, M.E.; Onwuka, E.N.; Aibinu, A.M.; Ubadike, O.C. Impact of Big Data Analytics to Nigerian mobile phone industry. In Proceedings of the 2015 International Conference on Industrial Engineering and Operations Management, Dubai, United Arab Emirates, 3–5 March 2015; pp. 1314–1319. [CrossRef]

65. Mathrani, S.; Lai, X. Big data analytic framework for organizational leverage. *Appl. Sci.* **2021**, *11*, 2340. [CrossRef]

66. Akter, S.; Wamba, S.F. Big data analytics in E-commerce: A systematic review and agenda for future research. *Electron. Mark.* **2016**, *26*, 173–194. [CrossRef]

67. Naik, K.; Joshi, A. Role of Big Data in various sectors. In Proceedings of the 2017 International Conference on I-SMAC (IoT in Social, Mobile, Analytics and Cloud) (I-SMAC), Palladam, India, 10–11 February 2017; pp. 117–122. [CrossRef]

68. Chen, Y.; Alspaugh, S.; Katz, R. Interactive analytical processing in big data systems: A crossindustry study of mapreduce workloads. *Proc. VLDB Endow.* **2012**, *5*, 1802–1813. [CrossRef]

69. Chakraborty, S.; Saha, A.K.; Ezugwu, A.E.; Agushaka, J.O.; Zitar, R.A.; Abualigah, L. Differential Evolution and Its Applications in Image Processing Problems: A Comprehensive Review. *Arch. Comput. Methods Eng.* **2022**, 1–56. [CrossRef]

70. Yousefinaghani, S.; Dara, R.; Mubareka, S.; Papadopoulos, A.; Sharif, S. An analysis of COVID-19 vaccine sentiments and opinions on Twitter. *Int. J. Infect. Dis.* **2021**, *108*, 256–262. [CrossRef] [PubMed]
71. Mellado, B.; Wu, J.; Kong, J.D.; Bragazzi, N.L.; Asgary, A.; Kawonga, M.; Choma, N.; Hayasi, K.; Lieberman, B.; Mathaha, T.; et al. Leveraging artificial intelligence and big data to optimize covid-19 clinical public health and vaccination roll-out strategies in Africa. *Int. J. Environ. Res. Public Health* **2021**, *18*, 7890. [CrossRef]
72. E-Government Survey 2020—Digital Government in the Decade of Action for Sustainable Development: With Addendum on COVID-19. Available online: https://www.scienceopen.com/book?vid=bc74a872-5582-485a-aafe-260bd9a415bd. (accessed on 1 January 2021).
73. REal-Time Data Monitoring for Shared, Adaptive, Multi-Domain and Personalised Prediction and Decision Making for Long-Term Pulmonary Care Ecosystems (RE-SAMPLE). Available online: https://clinicaltrials.gov/ct2/show/NCT04955080 (accessed on 1 January 2021).
74. Gherheș, V.; Stoian, C.E.; Fărcașiu, M.A.; Stanici, M. E-learning vs. Face-to-face learning: Analyzing students' preferences and behaviors. *Sustainability* **2021**, *13*, 4381. [CrossRef]
75. OECD. *An Assessment of the Impact of COVID-19 on Job and Skills Demand Using Online Job Vacancy Data*; OECD: Paris, France, 2021; pp. 1–19.
76. Innovations From The Nation. Available online: https://www.mbrcgi.gov.ae/en/enrich/innovations-from-the-nation (accessed on 1 January 2021).
77. Haleem, A.; Javaid, M.; Khan, I.H.; Vaishya, R. Significant Applications of Big Data in COVID-19 Pandemic. *Indian J. Orthop.* **2020**, *54*, 526–528. [CrossRef] [PubMed]
78. Perspective, A.W. Winning in the Next Normal with Insights: How Banks & FIs Are Preparing. 2022. Available online: https://www.wns.com/%0Aperspectives/blogs/blogdetail/932/%0Awinning-in-the-next-normal-with-insights-how-banks--fis-are-preparing%0A (accessed on 1 January 2021).
79. Big Data Analytics in Healthcare. Available online: https://www.hindawi.com/journals/jhe/si/971905/ (accessed on 1 January 2021).
80. Strickland, N.H. PACS (picture archiving and communication systems): Filmless radiology. *Arch. Dis. Child.* **2000**, *83*, 82–86. [CrossRef] [PubMed]
81. Dash, S.; Shakyawar, S.K.; Sharma, M.; Kaushik, S. Big data in healthcare: Management, analysis and future prospects. *J. Big Data* **2019**, *6*, 54. [CrossRef]
82. Dayrit, M.M.; Lagrada, L.P.; Picazo, O.F.; Pons, M.C.; Villaverde, M.C. The Philippines Health System Review. *Health Syst. Transit.* **2018**, *8*, 2.
83. Wu, J.; Wang, J.; Nicholas, S.; Maitland, E.; Fan, Q. Application of big data technology for COVID-19 prevention and control in China: Lessons and recommendations. *J. Med. Internet Res.* **2020**, *22*, e21980. [CrossRef]
84. Berendt, B.; Littlejohn, A.; Kern, P.; Mitros, P.; Shacklock; Blakemore, M. *Big Data for Monitoring Educational Systems*; Publications Office of the European Union: Luxembourg, 2017.
85. Dishon, G. New data, old tensions: Big data, personalized learning, and the challenges of progressive education. *Theory Res. Educ.* **2017**, *15*, 272–289. [CrossRef]
86. Ruiz-Palmero, J.; Colomo-Magaña, E.; Ríos-Ariza, J.M.; Gómez-García, M. Big data in education: Perception of training advisors on its use in the educational system. *Soc. Sci.* **2020**, *9*, 53. [CrossRef]
87. Fischer, C.; Pardos, Z.A.; Baker, R.S.; Williams, J.J.; Smyth, P.; Yu, R.; Slater, S.; Baker, R.; Warschauer, M. Mining Big Data in Education: Affordances and Challenges. *Rev. Res. Educ.* **2020**, *44*, 130–160. [CrossRef]
88. Ochoa, X.; Worsley, M. Editorial: Augmenting Learning Analytics with Multimodal Sensory Data. *J. Learn. Anal.* **2016**, *3*, 213–219. [CrossRef]
89. Crossley, S.; Ocumpaugh, J.; Labrum, M.; Bradfield, F.; Dascalu, M.; Baker, R.S. Modeling math identity and math success through sentiment analysis and linguistic features. In Proceedings of the International Conference on Educational Data Mining (EDM), Raleigh, NC, USA, 16–20 July 2018.
90. Chaturapruek, S.; Dee, T.S.; Johari, R.; Kizilcec, R.F.; Stevens, M.L. How a data-driven course planning tool affects college students' GPA: Evidence from two field experiments. In Proceedings of the 5th Annual ACM Conference on Learning at Scale, London, UK, 26–28 June 2018. [CrossRef]
91. Lukosch, H.K.; Bekebrede, G.; Kurapati, S.; Lukosch, S.G. A Scientific Foundation of Simulation Games for the Analysis and Design of Complex Systems. *Simul. Gaming* **2018**, *49*, 279–314. [CrossRef]
92. Teaching, E.; Educational, L.T.; Mining, D.; Sin, K.; Muthu, L.; Prakash, B.R.; Hanumanthappa, M.; Kavitha, V. Enhancing Teaching and Learning Through Educational Data Mining and Learning Analytics: An Issue Brief. *ICTACT J. Soft Comput.* **2015**, *5*, 1035–1049.
93. Anaya, A.R.; Boticario, J.G. A data mining approach to reveal representative collaboration indicators in open collaboration frameworks. In Proceedings of the International Conference on Educational Data Mining (EDM), Cordoba, Spain, 1–3 July 2009; pp. 210–219.
94. Wang, X.; Guo, B.; Shen, Y. Predicting the At-Risk Online Students Based on the Click Data Distribution Characteristics. *Sci. Program.* **2022**, *2022*, 9938260. [CrossRef]
95. Zhu, Z.T.; Yu, M.H.; Riezebos, P. A research framework of smart education. *Smart Learn. Environ.* **2016**, *3*, 4. [CrossRef]

96. Torre-Bastida, A.I.; Del Ser, J.; Laña, I.; Ilardia, M.; Bilbao, M.N.; Campos-Cordobés, S. Big Data for transportation and mobility: Recent advances, trends and challenges. *IET Intell. Transp. Syst.* **2018**, *12*, 742–755. [CrossRef]

97. Selod, H.; Soumahoro, S. *Big Data in Transportation: An Economics Perspective*; World Bank: Washington, DC, USA, 2020.

98. Hou, Y.; Chen, J.; Wen, S. The effect of the dataset on evaluating urban traffic prediction. *Alex. Eng. J.* **2021**, *60*, 597–613. [CrossRef]

99. A Research Agenda for Transport Policy. Available online: https://www.e-elgar.com/shop/gbp/a-research-agenda-for-transport-policy-9781788970198.html (accessed on 1 January 2021).

100. New Traffic Data Sources—An Overview. Available online: https://www.bitre.gov.au/sites/default/files/2019-12/NewDataSources-BackgroundPaper-April%202014.pdf. (accessed on 1 January 2021).

101. Mining the Datasphere: Big Data, Technologies, and Transportation Disaster Management. Available online: https://sbenrc.com.au/app/uploads/2021/03/SBEnrc-Project-1.45-Milestone-1-Congestion-v2.pdf (accessed on 1 January 2021).

102. Blazquez, D.; Domenech, J. Big Data sources and methods for social and economic analyses. *Technol. Forecast. Soc. Chang.* **2018**, *130*, 99–113. [CrossRef]

103. Nobanee, H.; Dilshad, M.N.; Al Dhanhani, M.; Al Neyadi, M.; Al Qubaisi, S.; Al Shamsi, S. Big Data Applications the Banking Sector: A Bibliometric Analysis Approach. *SAGE Open* **2021**, *11*, 4. [CrossRef]

104. Gasser, L.Z.U.; Gassmann, O.; Hens, T.; Leifer, L.; Puschmann, T. Digital Banking 2025. 2017. Available online: http://www.dv.co.th/blog-th/digital-banking-trend/ (accessed on 1 January 2021).

105. Bhasin, M.L. Combatting Bank Frauds by Integration of Technology: Experience of a Developing Country. *Br. J. Res.* **2016**, *3*, 64–92.

106. Vives, X. *Digital Disruption in Banking and Its Impact on Competition*; OECD: Paris, France, 2020; pp. 1–50.

107. Alexandru, A.G.; Radu, I.M.; Bizon, M.-L. Big Data in Healthcare—Opportunities and Challenges. *Inform. Econ.* **2018**, *22*, 43–54. [CrossRef]

108. Bourdeaux, M. Reimagining the Role of Technology in Education. *Relig. Communist Lands* **2017**, *9*, 2–3. [CrossRef]

109. Modeling the Big Data Challenges in Context of Smart Cities—An Integrated Fuzzy ISM-DEMATEL Approach. Available online: https://doi.org/10.1108/IJBPA-02-2021-0027 (accessed on 1 January 2021).

110. World Bank. *Data Big in Action for Government*; World Bank: Washington, DC, USA, 2017; p. 18.

111. Use of Technology in the Ebola Response in West Africa. Available online: https://pdf.usaid.gov/pdf_docs/PA00K99H.pdf (accessed on 1 January 2021).

112. Oussous, A.; Benjelloun, F.Z.; Ait Lahcen, A.; Belfkih, S. Big Data technologies: A survey. *J. King Saud Univ.—Comput. Inf. Sci.* **2018**, *30*, 431–448. [CrossRef]

113. ENOVA Annual Report 2013. Available online: https://www.enova.no/upload_images/5649E609BFEA4B2A890777583DD1654D.pdf (accessed on 1 January 2021).

114. Data Analytics Tools in Higher Education. Available online: https://ceur-ws.org/Vol-3061/ERIS_2021-art10(sh).pdf (accessed on 1 January 2021).

115. Learning Analytics in Higher Education: A Review of UK and International Practice Full Report. Available online: https://www.jisc.ac.uk/sites/default/files/learning-analytics-in-he-v2_0.pdf%0Ahttps://www.jisc.ac.uk/reports/learning-analytics-in-higher-education (accessed on 1 January 2021).

116. Alsrehin, N.O.; Klaib, A.F.; Magableh, A. Intelligent Transportation and Control Systems Using Data Mining and Machine Learning Techniques: A Comprehensive Study. *IEEE Access* **2019**, *7*, 49830–49857. [CrossRef]

117. Big Data in Banking for Marketers—How to Derive Value from Big Data. Available online: https://dataanalytics.report/Resources/Whitepapers/be309286-97b2-497d-9c6d-af9de5f620e1_bank-2020---big-data---whitepaper.pdf (accessed on 1 January 2021).

118. Corsi, A.; de Souza, F.F.; Pagani, R.N.; Kovaleski, J.L. Big data analytics as a tool for fighting pandemics: A systematic review of literature. *J. Ambient Intell. Humaniz. Comput.* **2021**, *12*, 9163–9180. [CrossRef]

119. Gigauri, I. Effects of COVID-19 on Human Resource Management from the Perspective of Digitalization and Work-life-balance. *Int. J. Innov. Technol. Econ.* **2020**, *31*, 1–8. [CrossRef]

120. OCED. The Territorial Impact of COVID-19: Managing The Crisis across Levels of Government. 2020. Available online: https://www.oecd.org/coronavirus/policy-responses/the-territorial-impact-of-covid-19-managing-the-crisis-across-levels-of-government-d3e314e1/ (accessed on 1 January 2021).

121. Big Data, Big Outcomes: How Analytics Can Transform Public Services and Improve Citizens' Lives. Available online: https://assets.ey.com/content/dam/ey-sites/ey-com/en_gl/topics/future-of-government/ey-future-of-gov-digital-analytics-report.pdf?download#:~{}:text=By%20combining%20data%20from%20a,%2C%20well%2Dbeing%20and%20safety (accessed on 1 January 2021).

122. E-Government Survey 2020. Available online: https://publicadministration.un.org/egovkb/en-us/Reports/UN-E-Government-Survey-2020 (accessed on 1 January 2021).

123. Mihalis, K. Ten technologies to fight coronavirus. *Eur. Parliam. Res. Serv.* **2020**, 1–20.

124. Central Bank of the Russian Federation. *Using Big Data in The Financial Sector and Risk to Financial Stability*; Central Bank of the Russian Federation: Moscow, Russia, 2021.

125. Asli Demirgüç-Kunt, J.H.; Klapper, L.; Singer, D.; Ansar, S. *The Global Findex Database 2017: Measuring Financial Inclusion and the Fintech Revolution*; World Bank: Washington, DC, USA, 2017; ISBN 9781464812590.

126. OECD. Artificial Intelligence, Machine Learning and Big Data in Finance: Opportunities, Challenges, and Implications for Policy Makers. 2021. Available online: https://www.oecd.org/finance/financial-markets/Artificial-intelligence-machine-learning-big-data-in-finance.pdf (accessed on 1 January 2021).

93

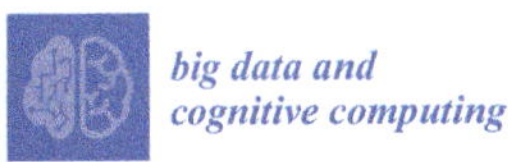

Review

A Survey on Big Data in Pharmacology, Toxicology and Pharmaceutics

Krithika Latha Bhaskaran [1,*], **Richard Sakyi Osei** [2], **Evans Kotei** [3], **Eric Yaw Agbezuge** [3], **Carlos Ankora** [4] and **Ernest D. Ganaa** [2]

1   School of Information Technology and Engineering, Vellore Institute of Technology, Vellore 632014, India
2   Information and Communication Technology Department, Faculty of Applied Science and Technology, Dr. Hilla Limann Technical University, Wa P.O. Box 553, Ghana
3   Computer Science Department, Faculty of Applied Science, Kumasi Campus, Kumasi Technical University, Kumasi 00233, Ghana
4   Department of Computer Science, Faculty of Applied Sciences and Technology, Ho Technical University, Ho P.O. Box HP 217, Ghana
*   Correspondence: krithika.lb@vit.ac.in

Abstract: Patients, hospitals, sensors, researchers, providers, phones, and healthcare organisations are producing enormous amounts of data in both the healthcare and drug detection sectors. The real challenge in these sectors is to find, investigate, manage, and collect information from patients in order to make their lives easier and healthier, not only in terms of formulating new therapies and understanding diseases, but also to predict the results at earlier stages and make effective decisions. The volumes of data available in the fields of pharmacology, toxicology, and pharmaceutics are constantly increasing. These increases are driven by advances in technology, which allow for the analysis of ever-larger data sets. Big Data (BD) has the potential to transform drug development and safety testing by providing new insights into the effects of drugs on human health. However, harnessing this potential involves several challenges, including the need for specialised skills and infrastructure. In this survey, we explore how BD approaches are currently being used in the pharmacology, toxicology, and pharmaceutics fields; in particular, we highlight how researchers have applied BD in pharmacology, toxicology, and pharmaceutics to address various challenges and establish solutions. A comparative analysis helps to trace the implementation of big data in the fields of pharmacology, toxicology, and pharmaceutics. Certain relevant limitations and directions for future research are emphasised. The pharmacology, toxicology, and pharmaceutics fields are still at an early stage of BD adoption, and there are many research challenges to be overcome, in order to effectively employ BD to address specific issues.

Keywords: big data; drug development; healthcare pharmacology; pharmaceutics; toxicology

Citation: Latha Bhaskaran, K.; Osei, R.S.; Kotei, E.; Agbezuge, E.Y.; Ankora, C.; Ganaa, E.D. A Survey on Big Data in Pharmacology, Toxicology and Pharmaceutics. *Big Data Cogn. Comput.* **2022**, *6*, 161. https://doi.org/10.3390/bdcc6040161

Academic Editors: Domenico Talia and Fabrizio Marozzo

Received: 13 October 2022
Accepted: 2 December 2022
Published: 19 December 2022

1. Introduction

The field of research involving analysis of the functioning of drugs in the human body is referred to as pharmacology. It details a class of medical science intended to address the employment of drugs in preventing, analysing, and treating diseases. As such, pharmacologists research the chemical properties of drugs and their impacts on the human body, in order to develop novel drugs and test them for efficacy and safety. Toxicology is the study of poisons, and relevant research helps to identify the effects of toxins and toxicants on the human body. It is a branch of pharmacology that aids in addressing the characterisation, identification, and quantification of the biological agents and chemicals that are responsible for creating adverse effects of the chemical agents on the human body. They develop novel methods to test for toxicity, and identify and quantify the toxicants in provided samples [1,2]

Pharmaceutics is a branch of pharmacy that manages the process of turning new chemical agents or old drugs into medications that can be used safely and efficiently by patients. It is also referred to as the science of dosage, which informs the design. Many chemicals with pharmacological properties require special measures to assist in attaining therapeutically related amounts at their sites of action. Pharmaceutics also helps in relating the formulations of drugs to their disposition and delivery in the body. Pharmacology, pharmaceutics, and toxicology are all categorised as interdisciplinary sciences [3,4]. They involve the extraction of knowledge from several disciplines, such as chemistry, biology, mathematics, and physics. BD has been one of the most researched topics in recent decades. BD denotes large or complex data sets that render the use of existing data-processing methods inadequate. Challenges associated with BD analysis include data storage, data capturing, sharing, searching, visualising, transferring, information privacy, and data source updating.

BD in health and medical care has attracted the attention of researchers owing to its various benefits. BD-based solutions for clinical decision support systems have revealed promising results in treating diseases such as Alzheimer's disease [5]. BD approaches have also been used for optimising electronic medical records [6]. The data generated in pharmacology, toxicology, and pharmaceutics include outcomes regarding the clinical behaviours, pharmacokinetics, chemical properties, associated toxicity of drugs. Data from cell culture experiments and animal studies are also included in this category. Thus, the volume of data generated in pharmaceutics, pharmacology, and toxicology has been increasing rapidly. This is primarily due to the employment of next-generation sequencing (NGS) and high-throughput screening (HTS). HTS is a technology that enables the simultaneous testing of millions of chemical elements. Additionally, NGS enables the efficient sequencing of RNA or DNA molecules.

It has been estimated that the global data volume generated by the toxicology, pharmaceutics, and pharmacology fields is approximately 2.5 zettabytes, where one zettabyte is equal to one sextillion bytes. BD is generally useful in pharmacology, pharmaceutics, and toxicology, as it can help to improve the prediction rate and accuracy of the effects of the researched drugs. It has helped to enhance the accuracy and speed of drug discovery and development. Although there are certain associated advantages of using BD in pharmacology, toxicology, and pharmaceutics, there are also certain drawbacks. BD can be challenging and overwhelming to navigate, and it may be difficult to trace useful data from the vast database. In addition, the implementation of BD is generally expensive, due to the overheads related to data collation, transformation, and analyses/modelling. The challenges and the overwhelming nature of BD can be resolved through the use of a data visualisation tool. Such an approach allows users to see the data and filter the necessary data, making it easier to understand, navigate, and extract the specific necessary information. Figure 1 shows a generic workflow representation of BD in the Hospital and Pharmacology ecosystem, based on the studies [7–9].

Hospital and clinics are the touchpoints for patients, that provide the symptom analysis, pre-diagnosis, physician advice, case history, and preliminary investigations from both the patient and physician perspectives. The data repository is the data store that collates data from all entities in the ecosystem, which are stored for further analytics, and as data sets used for prediction. In the scenarios presented in Figure 1, hospitals, clinics, and pharmacies provide the data that will eventually be stored in the big data repository. The repository possesses a big data nature, due to the data velocity and the heterogeneity of the data that are collated. The data from the BD repository are used for analytics such as identifying illness patterns, trends, and pre-emptive prediction of pandemics. Furthermore, BD analytics can be used to develop predictive models, which may be used to identify high -risk patients. Predictive model and pattern analytics can be used to model and develop targeted interventions. The use of a monitoring system coupled with BD models can form a proactive monitoring platform that can provide feedback to physicians. Based on Figures 1 and 2, a graph-based representation of Scenario 1—Drug efficacy monitoring system using BD—was derived.

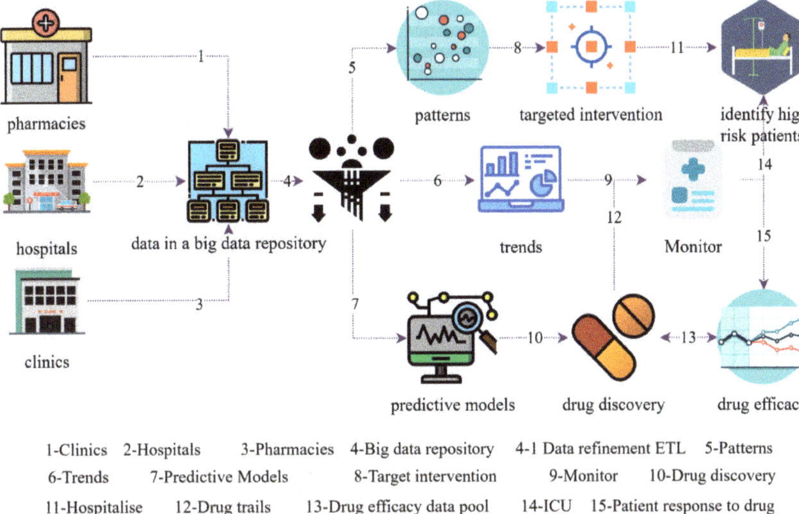

Figure 1. Generic representational workflow of big data in the Hospital and Pharmacology ecosystem.

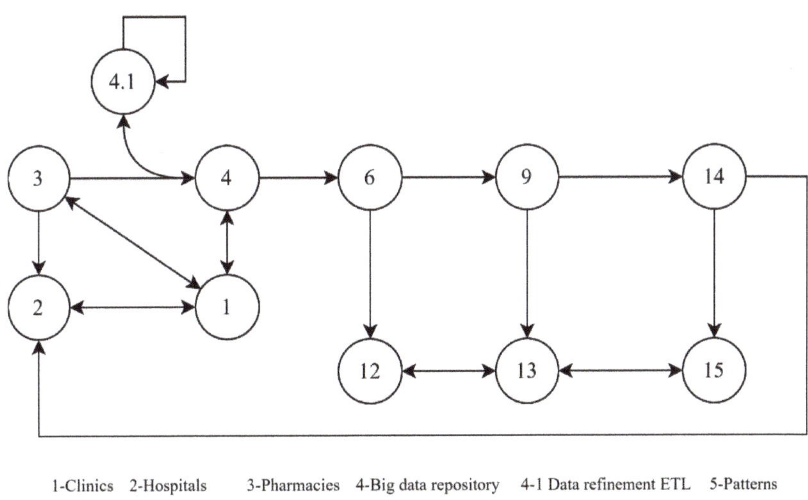

Figure 2. Flowchart for drug efficacy monitoring system using big data.

Scenario 1 considers a dataflow graph path for the drug efficacy monitoring system, one of the applications of BD in the healthcare domain. 1. The patient is attended at the clinic for pre-investigation; 2. the patients referred for specialist consultation are received at the hospital; 3. the required prescribed drug is collected from the pharmacy; 4. data of all patient activities are collected in the BD repository; 4.1. data cleaning and transformation are carried out as a continuous process; 6. the trend of the patient is analysed; 9. the patient is monitored in real-time during the drug course; 14. check whether hospitalisation is required; 15. drug efficacy is improved based on all the data that is collected; 13. an efficacy report is shared with the drug discovery team, in order to improve the drugs; 14. the patient is recoursed with an improved drug; and 2. feedback is sent to the physician for recommendation of a new prescription and dosage. This is one example scenario of the use of BD in the healthcare and pharmaceutical ecosystem. BD has extensive uses, and its potential has still not been fully discovered and practically implemented in real scenarios.

Another scenario based on Figure 1 is shown in Figure 3, which depicts the representation of Scenario 2: Drug discovery for a pandemic situation using BD.

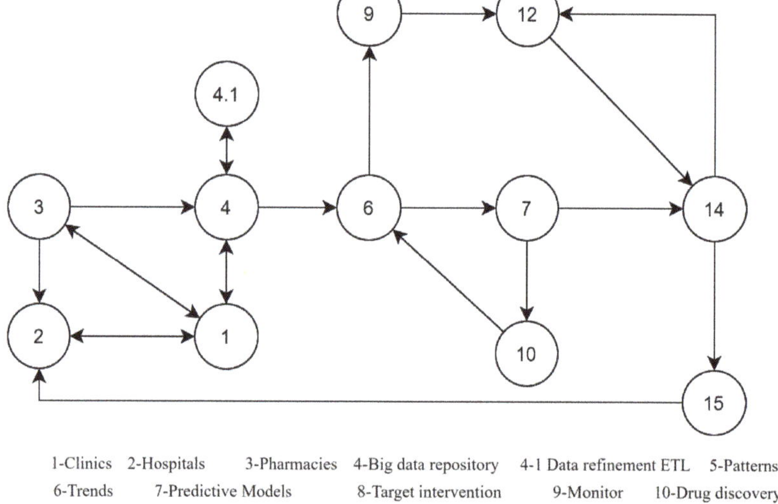

1-Clinics 2-Hospitals   3-Pharmacies 4-Big data repository 4-1 Data refinement ETL 5-Patterns

6-Trends   7-Predictive Models   8-Target intervention   9-Monitor   10-Drug discovery

11-Hospitalise   12-Drug trails   13-Drug efficacy data pool   14-ICU 15-Patient response to drug

Figure 3. Flowchart for drug discovery in pandemic situation using big data.

Scenario 2—Drug discovery for a pandemic situation—uses BD, following the path 3–2–4–6–7–10–6–9–12–14–15–2. First, when a sudden surge of patients with unknown illness is reported at (3.) clinics and (2.) hospitals, (4.) a new set of big data is rapidly created for diagnosis. Prescriptions and pathological reports are generated, (6.) the trends are matched with existing pool to find similar of any historic pandemic; and (7.) the data are quickly modelled to present a pandemic containment prediction predicated on the speed for the contagion vector, as well as its time to mutate, time to outgrow the available medical facilities, and similar data useful for prediction of pandemic containment. Then, the data from 9, 12, and 10 are used recursively used for prediction and drug discovery and provided to (14.) and monitored at (15.) These scenarios represent the application of BD in healthcare and related domains. As data plays the dominant role in the era of data analytics, BD has great scope in health science and related fields.

Through extensive research, it was confirmed that very few studies have attempted to review existing works to analyse the implementation of BD in the pharmacology, toxicology, and pharmaceutics fields. Thus, the present study is expected to greatly contribute to upcoming research, by providing clear knowledge regarding the implementation of BD in the field of drug development, and will also encourage the development of different big data-based models to serve the medical community. Therefore, the main goal of the present study is to review the literature regarding the employment of BD in pharmaceutics, pharmacology, and toxicology.

1.1. Objectives of the Study

The present study has the following objectives:

- To review the implementation of BD in the toxicology, pharmacology, and pharmaceutics fields;
- To offer a comparative analysis regarding the implementation of BD in pharmacology, toxicology, and pharmaceutics;
- To provide directions for future researchers and end-users to facilitate the usage of BD.

1.2. Paper Organization

The introduction section describes the importance of the topic, and the remainder of the article is organised as follows: Section 2 investigates the literature related to the work. Section 3 discusses the benefits of BD. Sections 4 and 5 present the survey analyses. Section 6 presents the limitations of the paper. Finally, Section 7 concludes our survey.

1.3. Definitions and Concepts of BD

BD can be defined as a huge and complex database that stores data that are heterogeneous and featuring multiple scales of information retrieved from many sources. BD can be related to healthcare in terms of electronic healthcare reports, clinical trial data, and administrative claims. The processing of BD includes feeding the data to the system, data preservation for storage, data analysis, and visualization of outcomes. Grouping the BD and smaller machine resource, offers many advantages, such as high availability, pooling of resources, and scalability [10]. As healthcare information is becoming digitalized, there has been widespread development in healthcare BD, and value-based care has motivated the healthcare sector to use BD analytics to make strategic professional decisions. The healthcare sector is handling many challenges based on the variety, volume, and veracity of data in this sector. Thus, BD plays a huge role by motivating healthcare innovation, influenced by many financial systems, considering factors such as the requirements of patients, motivations of the developers, and technical development. It has been observed that BD can offer optimal treatment decisions for patients and healthcare providers, based on population statistics [11].

1.3.1. Why BD?

Large volumes of data are generally available in two formats: Structured or unstructured. Structured data can be generated by machines and humans using a particular model or schema, and are usually accumulated in a database. Structured data are ordered around outlines with the data types that are clearly defined. Certain examples that characterise structured data include data, time, numbers, and strings stored in the database's columns. On the other hand, unstructured data do not possess any pre-defined model or schema. Associated examples of unstructured data are log files, mobile data, social media posts, text files, and other media. These media do not have any pre-defined schema set, so they are categorised as unstructured data [12].

The amount of data generated by popular corporations, small-scale industries, and scientific projects has been growing at an extraordinary level. These high volumes of data produced present incredible processing, storage, and analytical challenges that must be carefully dealt with and considered. Furthermore, traditional relational database management systems (RDBMSs) and the associated data processing tools are inadequate in dealing with huge data effectively, where the data size is typically measured in petabytes or terabytes. These existing tools lack the ability to deal with a large amount of data effectively when the size is enormous. Fortunately, paradigms and BD tools such as Hadoop and MapReduce are available to solve these BD challenges.

Certain features of BD are explained in the following.

Value

This allows for the extraction of beneficial information from large data sets [13]. The mechanism is designed based on how the data are added to create the knowledge. It has been stated that having access to the data is good, but it may be useless if it cannot be converted into values. Thus, it is the most important feature of BD that many institutions and enterprises invest the most into, in order to generate income and knowledge [14].

Variability

This particular characteristic represents the consistency of the data over time [15].

Variety

This represents the kinds of information associated with structured, unstructured, or semi-structured data. Key values include web clicks, relational tables, articles, e-mail messages, streamed audio and videos, and other media. This information may be gathered through sensors, smartphones, and social networks. In the healthcare sector, the information is gathered from unstructured and semi-structured sources, such as clinical trial outcomes, electronic health records, and physiological and chemical sensors [16].

Volume

This refers to the amount of data available from the various related resources. The data volume in BD typically starts at the Terabyte level. An example of this characteristic associated with the biomedical field is the proteomics database generated by the University of Munich, which has collected a data volume of approximately 5.17 TB, possessing 92% of unknown genes. In medical imaging, the visible human project has archived 5189 female anatomical images and 1871 male cryosections [16].

Velocity

This is the speed of data processing, transfer, generation, and collection. The content of the data is constantly changing with the addition of new data and various forms of streamed data from many sources at varying speed levels. Sequencing technologies have recently allowed for the production of billions of DNA sequences at low cost; this information is stored on desktop computers and shared within institutions worldwide.

Veracity

This denotes the accuracy and reliability of the information, the correctness of the data, quality, and data governance. This particular attribute is completely dependent on the data source.

1.4. Growth of BD

There has recently been a huge shift in the volume and speed of the data, beyond the comprehension of human minds. In 2013, the total volume of data in the world was estimated at 4.4 Zettabytes. This volume experienced an enormous increase, up to 44 Zettabytes by 2020. Although there has been a steady rise in technology, at present, it is not easy to analyse such enormous data. The demand for analysis of large data sets has paved the way for the rise of BD over the past decade. Data analytics, data analysis, and BD originate from the long-standing database management domain, which is completely dependent on the extraction, storage, and optimisation methods that are usually used for data stored in RDBMSs. Since the early 20th century, the internet has offered unique data analysis and data collection opportunities [17]. With the expansion of web traffic and online stores, companies such as Amazon, Yahoo, and eBay began analysing customer behaviours by investigating their clicking rates and tracking customer locations through their IP addresses, revealing a new world of possibilities. In addition, HTTP-based web traffic has increased the volume of unstructured and semi-structured data. To analyse these data, organisations require new approaches and solutions for storage issues, in order to investigate these new data efficiently.

1.5. Development of BD in the Medical Sector

There has been a constant increase in the demand for solutions regarding efficient analytical tools. This trend has also been noticed with regard to analysing large volumes of data. Organisations and institutions are searching for approaches to make use of the power of BD to enhance their competitive advantage, decision making, or business performance. BD provides potential solutions for private and public organisations; however, regarding outcomes, the practical employment of BD in various kinds of organisations requires domain-level adoption and re-structuring. Specifically, the healthcare industry has started shifting from a disease-centred to a patient-centred model, which is applicable in value-based healthcare delivery systems. To meet the demand and provide efficient patient-centred care, it is important to address and investigate a large amount of data from the healthcare sector. Many issues arise when healthcare data are considered. Healthcare has always produced large amounts of data. In addition, the introduction of electronic medical records and the large amount of data collected by different sensors or the data that the patients generate through social media has created many data streams. The appropriate use of such data can enable healthcare organisations to support clinical decision-making, public health management, and disease surveillance [18].

Classification provides a significant approach for bringing intelligence to medical data. Due to the simplicity of the kNN classification algorithm, it has been widely employed in several sectors. However, when the sample size is large and the features of the attributes are large, the effectiveness of the kNN algorithm will be reduced. A study [19] has proposed a novel kNN algorithm and compared it with the other existing kNN algorithms. In particular, the classification was made in the query instance neighbourhood of the existing kNN classifiers, and weights were allocated to each class. The recommended algorithm considered the class distribution around the query instance, in order to ensure that the assigned weights do not impact the outliers. The results of the considered study revealed that the recommended algorithm could efficiently enhance the effectiveness of the classification of the kNN algorithm when processing large data sets while maintaining the classification accuracy of the KNN algorithm, as well as providing better performance in terms of classification. However, the considered study only researched single-class classification while, in terms of application, multi-class classification is more popular and necessary. Additionally, healthcare data typically have a high missing rate, where these missing fields have been shown to greatly impact the classification results in existing works.

Similarly, another study [20] has developed a BD analytics-enabled transformation system based on the practice-based view. This revealed the causal relationships among BD capabilities, benefit dimensions, IT-enabled business values, and transformation practices. This model was then validated in a medical setting, offering a strategic view of BD analysis. Three vital paths for value chains were detected for medical organisations, through implementing a model that offers practical insights for managers. This study revealed the important elements and links for understanding the transformation of BD. One major limitation of the considered study was the data source. Additionally, better validation could have been performed by collecting and investigating primary data.

To date, the healthcare sector has not completely utilised the potential of BD. While the constantly developing academic research on the concepts of BD analytics has been technically oriented, there is an increasing demand for understanding the strategic implications of BD. Intending to address this lack, the study [21] has attempted to investigate the historical development, component functionalities, and architectural design of BD analytics. They identified 5 BD analytical capabilities from 26 BD implementations, including unstructured data, analytical capability for pattern, decision support capability, traceability, and predictive capability. The main limitation of the considered study was that IT adoption usually lags, when compared with other sectors, which is one of the main reasons why such cases are difficult to find. Although many cases have been found from various sources, the majority of cases were detected from vendors.

Wearable medical tools with sensors continuously generate a large amount of data, which can be considered as BD, in the form of unstructured and semi-structured data. Due to the complexity of the data, it is not easy to investigate valuable information that could help in decision making. Alternately, data security is another major requirement of BD in the healthcare sector. To address this issue, traditional research [22] has attempted to recommend novel architectures for implementing IoT, in order to accumulate and process scalable sensor data for healthcare applications. The recommended architecture consists of two main frameworks: Grouping and choosing (MC) and metafog redirection (MF-R) frameworks. MF-R frameworks employ BD technologies such as Apache HBase and Apache Pig to collect and store the sensor data produced from various sensor devices.

On the other hand, various security frameworks have been studied in the attempt to build models that combine multi-variate and non-stationary data. The obtained models utilize a log-normal distribution for the margins with linear trends and peak series [23].

2. Applications of BD

This section briefly reviews the body of related work that is available and indexed by reliable databases such as SCOPUS and WoS. The keywords used were under the subject categories of 'BD', 'pharmacology', 'toxicology' and 'pharmaceutics'.

The employment of BD for safety management in various areas, such as traffic safety [24], public safety [25], food safety [26], and patient safety [27], has recently been extensively studied. In addition, the influence of BD on drug discovery and design has been explored, in terms of future developments of medicine [6]. The core points in the discussion were the challenges that arise while implementing BD technologies, preserving the quality and privacy of data sets, and how the industry should adapt to welcome the BD era. It was concluded that, while BD has a significant impact on the advancement of pharmaceutical science, there are still many challenges to overcome.

The perspective of BD analytics in adapted medicine, focusing on how it could improve patient care, has been discussed in [25]. It was emphasised that the advancements in information technology have made this possible, but challenges remain to be addressed. BD analytics provide the potential to improve patient care, but more research is required to make this a reality.

The author in [26] has noted that current in vitro toxicity data could be used to develop models and tools to help in chemical toxicity research. The core points of the discussion were that the data are rich in information that can be used to evaluate complex bioactivities, and that a BD approach is necessary for relevant processing. It was found that the data are valuable for chemical toxicity research, but more tools need to be developed to help researchers use it. The pharmaceutical industry is facing a challenge in terms of productivity, in light of which BD initiatives may provide the insights needed to turn the industry around [28].

BD and translational medicine have evolved, and disruptive technology is bringing them together. The evolution of BD and translational medicine has been discussed, as well as the hindrances in applying BD techniques to translational medicine and the future of translational medicine. The author concluded that the future of translational medicine is bright and that the "Complete Health Record" concept will revolutionise the way in which translational medicine is practised [29]

BD is essential in safety sciences [27], and can be used to find similar substances and clusters of properties. Moreover, the need for safety BD [30] has been rapidly growing with constant development, and integration with science and technology has added more life to safety science research [31].

The author in [27] has sought to better understand the interactions between BD and Dynamic Simulation Modelling (DSM), as well as how incorporating them could be useful to healthcare decision-makers. The core points in the discussion were the benefits of BD and DSM, and how they can be used together to improve healthcare delivery. Integrated

BD and DSM offer complementary value in healthcare, in terms of addressing complex, systemic health economics and outcomes questions.

2.1. BD in Toxicology

The rate of data generation associated with toxicology continues to multiply, and the volume of data that is generated has been growing drastically. This is due to advancements in software solutions and the chemical-informatics method, which increase the accessibility of open resources such as biological, chemical, and toxicology data. Thus, the significant necessity for BD analytics to store and access the data associated with the toxicology domain has surged. Concerning this aspect, a conventional study [32] has proposed a machine learning method for raw HRMS-DIA (High-resolution mass spectrometry-Data independent acquisition) data. They evaluated the machine learning model by training, validating, and testing on sets of solvents and blood samples containing drugs considered to be usual in forensic toxicology, with the aim of categorical prediction using a feed-forward neural network framework. With the application of the employed machine learning approach, the specificity and sensitivity of the validation process and the test set for the prediction sample classes were observed to be in a suitable range for routine use in the laboratory. The study clearly emphasised the efficacy of employment of BD along with machine learning algorithms.

Probabilistic topic modelling has been used to analyse large-scale genomic data to uncover hidden patterns; in particular, this method was used to analyse a toxic genomic data set, and it was found that patterns related to the impact of doses and time points of treatment could be identified. The authors concluded that this method can reduce animal use in research [33].

A better understanding of how BD helps to delineate personalised approaches in severe mental illness and the provision of a quantitative synthesis of BD approaches for metabolomics in severe mental illness is necessary [34]. Notably, BD has the potential to improve our understanding of the developmental trajectories of mental disorders.

The considered existing research has used broad data utilized in clinical studies conducted from the perspectives of neurology, tumours, cardiovascular disease, psychiatric diseases, and other implementations [35]. Traditional research has emphasized the advantages of BD, in that it enables the study of diseases at the genetic level, thus offering more valuable treatments than traditional or usual treatments, as well as providing the ability to discover the evolution trajectory of humans. BD has an optimistic impact on medical studies, and its growth continues.

2.2. BD in Pharmacology

The implementation of BD in precision medicine has been welcomed. Pharmacogenomics—that is, the study of the effect of genes on a person's reaction to certain drugs—is within the realm of precision medicine. This new area combines pharmacology and genomics to improve valid and safe drugs and doses that respond to variations in individual genes. Precision medicine has a relatively limited role in daily care; however, researchers expect that this approach will encompass many healthcare sectors in the coming years. In addition, BD has the potential to facilitate personalised precision medicine [27].

Various analysis techniques [29] and tools are being implemented for genetic/genomic discovery in pharmacogenomics. However, the BD-related issues faced by pharmacogenomics need to be addressed, in order to maximise the potential in the field. Compared with applications in IT fields, such as social network analysis, the data sets used for drug discovery research are relatively small. However, with the development of combinatorial chemistry synthesis, HTS techniques, and genomics/genetics knowledge, the databases for drugs and drug candidates are growing rapidly.

New modelling approaches are needed to handle these larger data sets [36]. The existing research [37] has attempted to investigate the feasibility of BD analysis on 3290 approved drugs and formulations, for which 1,637,499 adverse events have been recorded in both human and animal species for approximately 70 years. A BD technique was utilized in this study, which is known to be a powerful analytic approach. However, it was revealed that the principle feasibility of a combined text mining and statistical method also led to numerous pitfalls, such as inadequate arrangement of pre-clinical ontologies and insufficiency of controlled vocabulary.

A conventional study [27] has attempted to identify the factors associated with the success of hypertension drug treatment, using BD approaches along with machine learning methods. As a result, it was disclosed that proton-pump inhibitors (PPIs) and hydroxymethylglutaryl coenzyme (HMGCoA) reductase inhibitors could significantly enhance the success rate of hypertension. In addition, new machine learning methodologies with BD have helped in identifying the prominent anti-hypertension therapy by re-generating medications available for new symptoms.

In a previous study [38], the author has attempted to determine standard methods that would likely help to increase the usability of (publicly available or privately produced) biological data. It was identified that data integrity is significant during pre-clinical drug development, and that investigators should use consistent methods to exploit the functions of privately and publicly created biological data. The author also emphasised that the increasing interest in and the interpretation of cross-platform approaches is significant.

BD can be used in paediatric drug [31] development. The use of BD for clinical trial design, efficiency, and safety of data has been attained in clinical trials. Therefore, exploring the current opportunities and challenges of BD in future paediatric drug development must be enriched. Although BD has the potential to play a significant role in paediatric drug development, and there are still many challenges that need to be addressed.

BD can be used in drug research to determine efficacy and safety signals [39]. The steps involve data acquisition, extraction, aggregation, analysis, modelling, and interpretation. BD can leverage and improve clinical decisions at the point of care, uncovering or validating drug efficacy and safety.

The steps of pharmacogenomics studies, [38] has considered data collection for interpretation and highlighted the bioinformatics aspects that can pose problems. The major challenges of data processing and analysis can lead to inaccurate results. Therefore, paying careful attention to these steps is important, in order to avoid mistakes and produce accurate pharmacogenomics studies.

The author in [40] have discussed the discovery of novel bromodomain BRD4 binders. It was inferred that public databases are useful for predictive model building, and that machine learning can allow for the extraction of real knowledge, despite the noise present in structure-activity data. Therefore, public databases are key assets in drug discovery, and machine learning plays a significant role in mining real data.

BD has changed the field of drug development [41]. Novel methods for therapeutic drug discovery, inference of clinical toxicity, candidate drug prioritisation, and machine learning techniques for drug discovery are becoming familiar. Experts from various platforms should conduct closer collaborations to translate the analysis results for treatment and prognosis in medical practice [42].

BD is significant for medical use and requires re-thinking, regarding the data storage infrastructure, the analysis growth, and the associated tools to drive advancements in the considered field [43]. In addition, BD is undoubtedly important for clinical practice, and physicians are responsible for developing and using BD to enhance patient care.

Machine learning has been utilized to predict psychiatric outcomes [44] in humans, where these techniques are more powerful than traditional statistical approaches. The author also discussed ways to optimise machine-learning techniques in the context of psychiatric research. BD has transformed natural product research and helped researchers both ask and answer new questions [45]. The author also highlighted the limitations regarding our current engagement with large data sets.

2.3. BD in Pharmaceutics

Clinical behaviours are important in pharmaceutics and life science, as they can be employed to evaluate whether a particular treatment is efficient and to check whether it is safe for human beings. In addition, clinical behaviours are costly and time-consuming to assess, and many clinical traits may fail to be observed during testing; furthermore, recruiting the right patients is also crucial. The entire trial process is also difficult. With the assistance of BD analytics, pharmaceutical industries can recruit the right patients for clinical traits, employing data such as genetic information, the status of the disease, and personality traits to increase the drug's success rate. This also helps in precisely determining the appropriate medicine(s) for treatment and the diagnosis of the considered disorders, performed using the most related and relevant data along with analysis of certain characteristics, such as behavioural patterns and genetic makeup. Using this BD, pharmaceutical companies can design personalized medicines in line with a particular patient's genetics and lifestyle.

The construction of medical BD involves not just a simple application and collection of medical data but, instead, is a complex systematic model. An existing research study [46] has discussed China's experience in constructing a regional medical BD ecosystem. The construction of the medical BD includes several institutions and high-level management, and cooperation was observed to enhance innovation and effectiveness. Compared with the construction of infrastructure, it is more time-consuming and challenging to develop proper data standards, data mining tools, and data integration. Similarly, another traditional study [47] has attempted to construct a proof-of-concept illustrating that BD approaches possess the capability to enhance the safety of drug monitoring in hospitals and, as such, can highly aid pharmaco-vigilance professionals to determine adverse drug events through data-driven targeted analysis of Drug–Drug Interactions (DDI). They also designed an automatic DDI detection model based on the treatment of the data and the laboratory analysis from electronic health records accumulated in a clinical data warehouse. The research results revealed that the developed DDI model worked effectively and that the time required for computation was manageable. This developed model can be used for regular monitoring processes.

Likewise, another traditional paper [48] has attempted to address data quality issues in electronic patient records using a computerized electronic patient report system with the abstraction of Map reduce and Apache HIVE of BD technology. The existing research also attempted to analyse which patients are spending more money, compared to patients with reduced maps. The data were obtained through a traditional system of Hadoop, through the functions of extract, transform, and load (ETL). The considered model was observed to resolve issues related to the use of conventional manual models. Security was also observed to be improved, as the system demands appropriate authentication for access. However, the developed model does not seem to send any alert regarding the expiration dates of drugs. In addition, factors such as assets and security were not included in the existing system.

The body of work presented in the literature survey indicates the growing importance and trend towards adapting BD in the fields of pharmacology, toxicology, and pharmaceutics. The existing literature has demonstrated that BD can solve various problems and, so, the application of BD in these fields needs to be reinforced.

3. Benefits of Big Data

The data associated with the healthcare sector are enormous. They are stored in and withdrawn from clinics, hospitals, and insurance companies, resulting in the under-use of resources, data redundancy, and inadequacy. However, stakeholders have increased their voices and requirements to improve the exploitation and exploration of traditional data. With the employment of BD:

- Healthcare organizations can construct networks to bring about extensive changes in the educational field of medicine, practice, and research;

- the sorting, storage and analysis of patient information can be supported;
- the identification of therapeutic assessments, disease identification and prevention, surgical planning, and outcome predictions can be enhanced.

With clinical semiology, computer science, advanced imaging, radiology, biochemistry, and genomics, BD has emerged as a promising tool that can assist in developing a wide range of technical devices, surgical approaches, pharmacological therapies, and others.

3.1. Economic Benefits

Although well-developed countries spend a large amount of their gross domestic products on healthcare systems, the expenditures spent may not help to boost health outcomes. Furthermore, the increases in medical care expenses and health benefits indicate that additional strategies should be incorporated to enhance the efficiency of healthcare systems and protect public investments [49]. Despite having the highest healthcare expenditures, the U.S. has reported that it has not increased its life expectancy or last-day quality of life [50]. There is a rapid increment in relative economic demands, due to the sharp elevation in the age of the population and increasing chronic diseases. It has been estimated that the senior population will increase from 14 million to 19 million in 2020 and, by 2050, it will increase to 40 million. The impact of these demands has been observed in European regions. By employing BD as a tool for forecasting models, the economy of the healthcare sector can be improved, in order to develop expenditure projections for potential medicinal hazards, discover various policies that can assist in resolving intricate circumstances, and implement the most efficient approaches against various threats. It has been reported that BD might produce more than 300 billion in savings per year for the U.S. healthcare sector [50].

3.2. Technological Benefits

Social media and portable devices have become a common source of data collection and feedback results, due to their familiarity in the present population, closeness, and portability. In the medicinal sector, physiological sensors and electronic health records (EHRs) are the main aspects for the follow-up and monitoring of patients. All of these tools have generated a movement towards the revamping of resources. Thus, the mechanism to analyse and manage the information should also evolve. This hectic demand may be met through the use of BD analytics. For example, in hospitals, BD on smartphones can create an effective tool to forward inspirational and medicinal messages to patients, in order to enhance their lifestyles and accomplish a prominent treatment that will enhance their health and welfare [51].

BD has had a significant impact on the advancement of pharmaceutical science, but there are still many challenges to overcome. Our survey indicated the impact of BD on drug discovery and design, and allowed for speculation on future developments in the field. The challenges are related to implementing and maintaining the quality and privacy of data sets, and how the industry must adapt to welcome the BD era. Especially in the pharmaceutical industry, the challenges related to BD initiatives could provide the insights needed to turn the industry around. The anticipated future of BD applications demonstrates their potential for use in drug discovery to speed up drug manufacturing, improving productivity, drug performance, drug safety, clinical analysis, clinical study, and drug personalisation in drug efficacy, as represented in Figure 4.

Drug discovery is expected to be the most benefited field. By using BD, the following advantages can be achieved: 1. BD can help to identify new drug targets; 2. identifying new drug candidates; 3. improving the efficiency of drug discovery processes; 4. improving the accuracy of drug discovery predictions; 5. identifying potential drug interactions; and 6. identifying adverse drug reactions.

As for drug efficacy and performance, there are many benefits of BD in drug efficacy, including detecting patterns in large data sets, identifying new drug targets, and improving the accuracy of predictions regarding how a drug will behave in the body. There are also many benefits of BD relating to drug performance. The prime benefit is that BD can help researchers and doctors to better understand how drugs work and how they can be improved. BD can also help doctors and patients make more informed decisions about which drugs to use and how to use them. Additionally, BD can help researchers to identify new drug targets and develop new drugs quickly and efficiently.

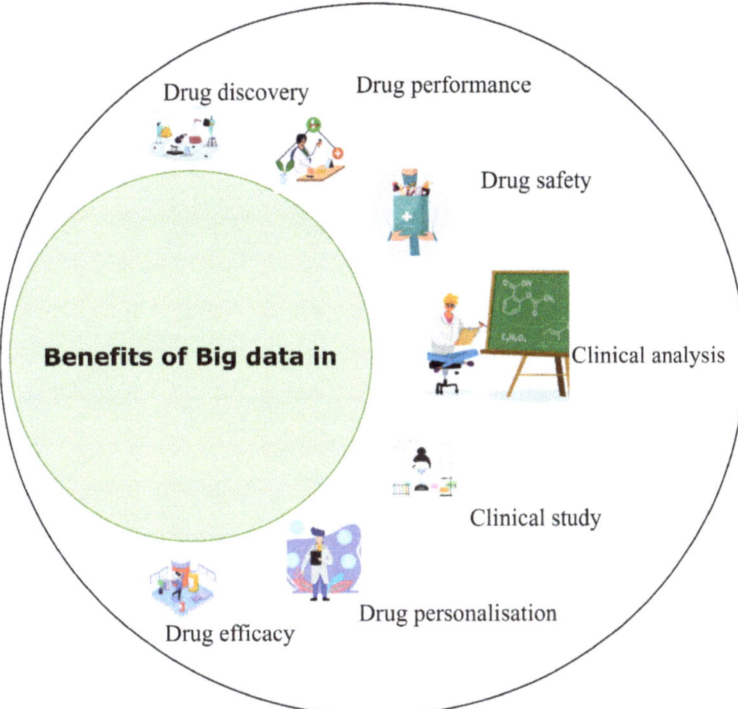

Figure 4. Benefits of BD in Pharmacology, Toxicology and Pharmaceutics.

The benefits of BD in clinical study analysis are as follows: 1. Increased data accuracy, due to the volume and variety of data sources; 2. faster identification of trends and correlations; 3. more efficient and effective clinical trial design and execution; 4. better understanding of patient populations and their needs; and 5. improved decision making, including more timely and effective interventions.

The benefits of BD in drug safety analysis are as follows: 1. Increased accuracy and precision in identifying potential safety concerns; 2. earlier detection of potential safety concerns; 3. more efficient and effective safety surveillance; and 4. better understanding the safety profiles of drug.

There are many benefits of BD in drug personalisation. The key benefit is that it can help improve the accuracy of predictions regarding how a particular drug will work in a particular person. This is because BD can help to improve our understanding of the complex interactions between drugs and the human body. It can also help identify which patients are most likely to respond to a particular drug and which patients may experience adverse effects.

4. Comparative Analysis

Based on the literature survey, Table 1 below presents the domains, the purposes, the broad areas of application, and the core advantages related to BD.

Table 1. Summary of BD in Pharmacology, Toxicology and Pharmaceutics.

	Purpose	Broad Area	Core Area
Pharmaceutical science [41]	Highlight the benefit by capturing the multi-dimensional contributions	Quality and privacy of data sets	Advancement in pharmaceutical
Biomedicine [43]	Improve patient care through personalised medicine programs.	Information technology and its impact on biomedicine.	Biomedicine to improve patient care.
Chemical toxicity [34]	Build a modern chemical toxicity research using historical data repositories.	Synthesis of bioassays and biological proteins/receptors.	Complex bioactivity evaluation
Toxicogenomics [33]	Store and channelise biological data in biomedical science.	High-throughput screening technologies	Explore hidden patterns of genomic data.
Pharmaceutics [28]	Productivity in the pharmaceutical industry by providing insights into improving output while reducing costs.	Pharmaceutical industry	Productivity
Translational Medicine [29]	Understanding the evolution of Translational Medicine.	Alternative methods	Translational medicine.
Toxicology [35]	Reveal patterns, trends, and associations of substances.	Substances exploration	Predict toxic properties.
Health Economics [27]	Informed patient-centred care and with healthcare decision-making and improving healthcare.	Dynamic simulation modelling (DSM)	Synergies
Drug development [39]	Identify novel drugs or repurposed existing drugs.	Drug development	Personalised precision medicine
Pharmacogenomics [44]	Identify genetic and genomic factors for drug treatment response.	Pharmacogenomics	Drug efficacy
Drug efficacy [45]	Machine language-based drug efficacy on patient BD sets.	Machine learning techniques	Drug performance
Drug discovery [38]	Improve pre-clinical drug discovery and development.	Life sciences	Data integrity.
Drug efficacy [52]	Improve the clinical trial design and improve safety.	Paediatric drug development	Clinical trials
Drug Safety and Efficacy [53]	Enhance clinical decisions and uncover the efficacy and safety of drugs.	Healthcare	Medication safety & effectiveness.
Pharmacogenomics/ Bioinformatics [54]	Bioinformatics aspects of pharmacogenomic.	Pharmacogenomics	BD bioinformatics.
In Silico Mining/ Inhibitor-Predictive modelling [40]	Find new Bromodomain BRD4 binders and build predictive BRD activity models.	Drug discovery	Predictive model building.
Drug development [39]	Therapeutic target discovery, candidate drug prioritisation, and inference accuracy improvement.	Drug development	Precision medicine

Table 1. *Cont.*

	Purpose	Broad Area	Core Area
Neurocritical Care [55]	Improve patient care	Healthcare industry	Neurocritical care unit
Mental illness [56]	Mental illness data analysis and inference.	Early detection and intervention strategies	Personalised approaches
Biomedicine [57]	Study human origins and migration and develop better treatments for diseases.	Medical industry	BD in medical research.
Psychiatry [58]	Uncover psychiatric disorders based on pathophysiological data	Machine learning	Deep learning
Natural products [59]	To enable discoveries that were impossible before.	Natural product sciences.	Natural product sciences.

5. Critical Analysis

The critical analysis was conducted with the aim of tracing which particular field has implemented BD. The results of the critical analysis are graphically represented in Figure 5.

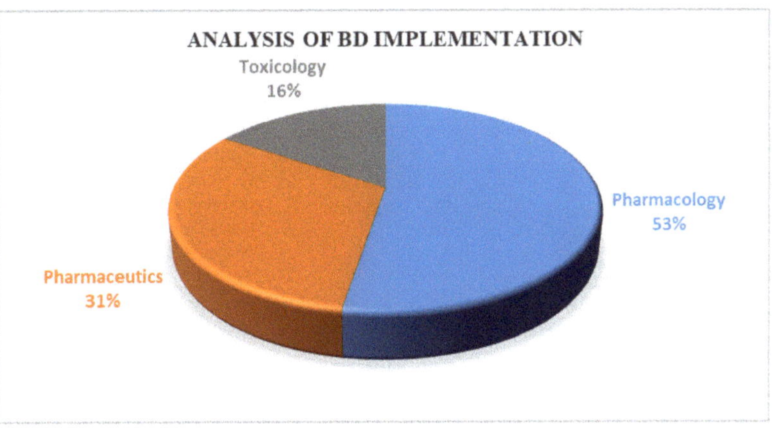

Figure 5. Analysis of BD implementation in Pharmacology, Toxicology and Pharmaceutics.

From Figure 5, it is clear that the pharmacology sector is observed to employ BD more than the other two fields. This is because this sector produces more data while developing drugs for the identified chronic diseases. Additionally, through extensive research, it has been found that very few researchers have attempted to conduct research on the implementations of BD in the considered fields. Therefore, it might be more beneficial for the medicinal community to have investigators attempt to execute research regarding the technical implementation of BD in the drug development sector.

6. Limitations of BD

The limitations of BD include cases where the quality of the data is compromised and when the users fail to utilise BD analytics approaches correctly. In addition, certain other limitations are discussed in this section.

The main limitation of BD is mostly associated with the quality of data. The main determinant of this aspect is completely dependent on the source of the data. In addition, the management and storage of data also play a vital role in the characteristics of the data. Some significant features regarding data quality are data completeness, accuracy, and adequacy. The modification of these features may pose a threat to users, especially when using BD, as it can endanger the integrity of the associated results of the analysis [51]. Thus, BD is said to return inaccurate results due to corruption of the quality of the data, resulting from the generation of false assumptions. These false assumptions might produce weak knowledge with large errors. This does not result only from the data quality, but also the data selection approach and the sample size. Large data sets with a high number of attributes can enable statistically significant results to be obtained; however, on the other hand, due to the huge data size, users may choose data arbitrarily while neglecting information regarding the data representativeness, resulting in selection bias. In both cases, the results and the accuracy of a BD-based approach might be compromised [51].

These aforementioned limitations also involve the user. It is significant to understand when to implement BD to resolve certain issues. Users should be well-aware of the features of the data and perceive compatibility among the data sets to obtain an appropriate and beneficial analysis, and should be well-aware of the underlying difficulties that arise when data are compared within domains without similar features and attributes [60]. To correctly utilise BD analytics, the main objectives and implementation results should be understood a priori. Additionally, users should educate themselves, in order to understand the possible mechanism(s) behind the researched phenomenon or object, in order to hypothesise the possible results. Finally, they should estimate the outcomes with the presumed objective at the initial step. If the users neglect or commit any mistakes in the steps above, the BD mechanism will likely produce erroneous results [60].

Table 2. Challenges and future directions.

BD Impacting Domain	Benefits	Challenges
Drug discovery	• Identify new drug targets • Identify new drug candidates • Efficiency of drug discovery processes • Drug discovery predictions • Potential drug interactions • Adverse drug reactions	• BD initiative process • Privacy protection of data sets • Data governance • Regional data compliance law • Data storage • Data security • Data sharing • Data collaboration
Drug efficacy & performance	• Detect patterns in large datasets • Identify new drug targets • Accuracy of predictions • How drugs work • Informed decisions • Faster development of new drugs	• General Data Protection Regulation • Data capturing process • Data protection • Data analytics • Data digitisation process • Data exploration and navigation
Clinical study analysis	• Increased accuracy • Identification of safety concerns • Effective safety surveillance • The safety profile of a drug	• Data authenticity • Identity governance • Human errors • Data maintenance • Data interpretation techniques
Drug safety analysis	• Increased accuracy and precision • Detection of safety concerns • Efficient safety surveillance • Understanding the profile of a drug	• Data transformation • Data benchmark • Data trend & pattern development
Drug personalisation	• Understanding human & drug interactions • Identify the patient's response to drug • Equivalent risk of adverse effects	• Real-time data inference • Real-time Data collection infrastructure • Real-time pre-processing algorithms • Real-time mining and extraction

Based on the summary presented in Table 2, future research lines to address the existing challenges may be gleaned to take the domain in new directions, helping to advance the considered fields and, thereby, indirectly helping to better humankind.

7. Conclusions and Discussion

The pharmaceutical industry is facing a challenge in productivity, and BD initiatives may provide the insights necessary to turn the industry around. Considering this, the present study detailed a substantial attempt to review the existing literature regarding the implementation of BD in the pharmacology, pharmaceutics, and toxicology sectors. The pharmacology, toxicology, and pharmaceutics fields are still in the early stage of BD adoption. Additionally, according to the critical analysis, the pharmacology sector has employed BD more than the other two sectors. Based on our survey, the key inferences were as follows: first, BD can help researchers better understand the effects of drugs and other chemicals on the human body, which can help to improve the safety and efficacy of drugs and other chemicals; second, BD can help to improve the accuracy of predictions regarding the effects of drugs and chemicals, which can improve safety in drug development and help to avoid potential adverse drug interactions; finally, BD can help improve our understanding of how the body metabolises drugs and other chemicals, which can improve the safety and efficacy of drugs and other chemicals. The domains considered in our survey are ultimately necessary for humanity, and BD may significantly impact the betterment of these domains. BD has revolutionary potential, providing new ways to understand and predict the effects of drugs. However, BD in this domain also poses new challenges, which should be taken up as key research problems. Despite these challenges, in the future, BD will likely play an important role in pharmacology, toxicology, and pharmaceutics, critically helping to improve drug safety and efficacy.

Author Contributions: Review design, Ideation, initial draft, figure illustration and conceptualization, K.L.B.; literature curation, review and editing, R.S.O., E.D.G.; Additional illustration, additional data curation E.Y.A.; Improve the presentation, validation and restructuring of the manuscript, C.A.; Proofreading the manuscript and improvements, E.K. All authors have read and agreed to the published version of the manuscript.

Funding: This research received no external funding.

Data Availability Statement: Not applicable.

Conflicts of Interest: The authors declare no conflict of interest.

References

1. Laurence, D. What is pharmacology? A discussion. *Trends Pharmacol. Sci.* **1997**, *18*, 1051–1052. [CrossRef] [PubMed]
2. Mückter, H. What is toxicology and how does toxicity occur? *Best Pract. Res. Clin. Anaesthesiol.* **2003**, *17*, 5–27. [CrossRef] [PubMed]
3. Hassan, W.; Zafar, M. Pharmacology, Toxicology, and Pharmaceutics Research Output in One Hundred and Fifty Countries for the Year 2019–2020. *Can. J. Med.* **2021**, *3*, 56–60. [CrossRef]
4. Biglu, M.; Hossein, O. Scientific Profile of Pharmacology, Toxicology and Pharmaceutics Fields in Middle East Countries: Impacts of Iranian Scientists. *Int. J. Adv. Pharm. Sci.* **2010**, *1*, 122–127.
5. Pc, S.; Sherimon, V.; Sp, P.; Nair, R.V.; Mathew, R. A Systematic Review of Clinical Decision Support Systems in Alzheimer's Disease Domain. *Int. J. Online Biomed. Eng.* **2021**, *17*, 74–90.
6. Gattan, A.M. A Knowledge Based Analysis on Big Data Analytics in Optimizing Electronic Medical Records in Private Hospitals. *Int. J. Online Biomed. Eng.*, **2021**, *17*, 119–134. [CrossRef]
7. Chan, C.L.; Chang, C.C. Big Data, Decision Models, and Public Health. *Int. J. Environ. Res. Public Health* **2020**, *17*, 6723. [CrossRef]
8. Batool, M.; Ahmad, B.; Choi, S. A Structure-Based Drug Discovery Paradigm. *Int. J. Mol. Sci* **2019**, *20*, 2783. [CrossRef]
9. Bernetti, M.; Bertazzo, M.; Masetti, M. Data-Driven Molecular Dynamics: A Multifaceted Challenge. *Pharmaceuticals* **2020**, *13*, 253. [CrossRef]
10. Price, W.N.; Cohen, I.G. Privacy in the age of medical big data. *Nat. Med.* **2019**, *25*, 37–43. [CrossRef]
11. Beam, A.L.; Kohane, I.S. Big Data and Machine Learning in Health Care. *JAMA* **2018**, *319*, 1317–1318. [CrossRef] [PubMed]
12. Li, Y.; Zhang, Y.; Li, W.; Jiang, T. Marine Wireless Big Data: Efficient Transmission, Related Applications, and Challenges. *IEEE Wirel. Commun.* **2018**, *25*, 19–25. [CrossRef]

13. Bello-Orgaz, G.; Jung, J.J.; Camacho, D. Social big data: Recent achievements and new challenges. *Inf. Fusion* **2016**, *28*, 45–59. [CrossRef] [PubMed]

14. Basha, S.A.K.; Basha, S.M.; Vincent, D.R.; Rajput, D.S. Chapter 11—Challenges in Storing and Processing Big Data Using Hadoop and Spark. In *Deep Learning and Parallel Computing Environment for Bioengineering Systems*; Academic Press: Cambridge, MA, USA, 2019; pp. 179–187.

15. Vesoulis, Z.A.; Husain, A.N.; Cole, F.S. Improving child health through Big Data and data science. *Pediatr. Res.* **2022**, 1–8. [CrossRef]

16. Venkatesh, R.; Balasubramanian, C.; Kaliappan, M. Development of Big Data Predictive Analytics Model for Disease Prediction using Machine learning Technique. *J. Med. Syst.* **2019**, *43*, 272. [CrossRef] [PubMed]

17. Singh, P.; Singh, A. Growth Trend in Global Big Data Research Publications as Seen From SCOPUS Database. *Prof. J. Libr. Inf. Technol.* **2018**, *8*, 49–61.

18. Elhoseny, M.; Abdelaziz, A.; Salama, A.S.; Riad, A.M.; Muhammad, K.; Sangaiah, A.K. A hybrid model of Internet of Things and cloud computing to manage big data in health services applications. *Future Gener. Comput. Syst.* **2018**, *86*, 1383–1394. [CrossRef]

19. Xing, W.; Bei, Y. Medical Health Big Data Classification Based on KNN Classification Algorithm. *IEEE Access* **2020**, *8*, 28808–28819. [CrossRef]

20. Wang, Y.; Kung, L.; Wang, W.Y.C.; Cegielski, C.G. An integrated big data analytics-enabled transformation model: Application to health care. *Inf. Manag.* **2018**, *55*, 64–79. [CrossRef]

21. Wang, Y.; Kung, L.; Byrd, T.A. Big data analytics: Understanding its capabilities and potential benefits for healthcare organizations. *Technol. Forecast. Soc. Chang.* **2018**, *126*, 3–13. [CrossRef]

22. Manogaran, G.; Varatharajan, R.; Lopez, D.; Kumar, P.M.; Sundarasekar, R.; Thota, C. A new architecture of Internet of Things and big data ecosystem for secured smart healthcare monitoring and alerting system. *Future Gener. Comput. Syst.* **2018**, *82*, 375–387. [CrossRef]

23. Chebana, F.; Ouarda, T.B.M.J. Multivariate non-stationary hydrological frequency analysis. *J. Hydrol.* **2021**, *593*, 125907. [CrossRef]

24. Shi, Q.; Abdel-Aty, M. Big Data applications in real-time traffic operation and safety monitoring and improvement on urban expressways. *Transp. Res. Part C Emerg. Technol.* **2015**, *58*, 380–394. [CrossRef]

25. Cejun, C.A.O.; Congdong, L.I.; Yu, W.; Ting, Q.U.; Wei, Z. Evolution and governance mechanism of urban public safety risk in big data era. *China Saf. Sci. J.* **2020**, *27*, 151.

26. Marvin, H.J.P.; Janssen, E.M.; Bouzembrak, Y.; Hendriksen, P.J.M.; Staats, M. Big data in food safety: An overview. *Crit. Rev. Food Sci. Nutr.* **2017**, *57*, 2286–2295. [CrossRef] [PubMed]

27. Marshall, D.A. Transforming Healthcare Delivery: Integrating Dynamic Simulation Modelling and Big Data in Health Economics and Outcomes Research. *Pharmacoeconomics* **2016**, *34*, 115–126. [CrossRef] [PubMed]

28. Tormay, P. Big Data in Pharmaceutical R&D: Creating a Sustainable R&D Engine. *Pharmaceut. Med.* **2015**, *29*, 87–92.

29. Jordan, L. The problem with Big Data in Translational Medicine. A review of where we have been and the possibilities ahead. *Appl. Transl. Genom.* **2015**, *6*, 3–6.

30. Wang, B. Safety intelligence as an essential perspective for safety management in the era of Safety 4.0: From a theoretical to a practical framework. *Process Saf. Environ. Prot.* **2021**, *148*, 189–199. [CrossRef]

31. Wang, B.; Wu, C. Safety informatics as a new, promising and sustainable area of safety science in the information age. *J. Clean. Prod.* **2020**, *252*, 119852. [CrossRef]

32. Streun, G.L.; Elmiger, M.P.; Dobay, A.; Ebert, L.; Kraemer, T. A machine learning approach for handling big data produced by high resolution mass spectrometry after data independent acquisition of small molecules—Proof of concept study using an artificial neural network for sample classification. *Drug Test. Anal.* **2020**, *12*, 836–845. [CrossRef] [PubMed]

33. Chung, M.H. Asymmetric author-topic model for knowledge discovering of big data in toxicogenomics. *Front. Pharmacol.* **2015**, *6*, 81. [CrossRef] [PubMed]

34. Zhu, H.; Zhang, J.; Kim, M.T.; Boison, A.; Sedykh, A.; Moran, K. Big data in chemical toxicity research: The use of high-throughput screening assays to identify potential toxicants. *Chem. Res. Toxicol.* **2014**, *27*, 1643–1651. [CrossRef] [PubMed]

35. Hartung, T. Making big sense from big data in toxicology by read-across. *ALTEX* **2016**, *33*, 83–93. [CrossRef] [PubMed]

36. Yan, X.; Sedykh, A.; Wang, W.; Yan, B.; Zhu, H. Construction of a web-based nanomaterial database by big data curation and modeling friendly nanostructure annotations. *Nat. Commun.* **2020**, *11*, 2519. [CrossRef] [PubMed]

37. Clark, M.; Steger-Hartmann, T. A big data approach to the concordance of the toxicity of pharmaceuticals in animals and humans. *Regul. Toxicol. Pharmacol.* **2018**, *96*, 94–105. [CrossRef] [PubMed]

38. Brothers, J.F., 2nd; Ung, M.; Escalante-Chong, R.; Ross, J.; Zhang, J.; Cha, Y.; Lysaght, A.; Funt, J.; Kusko, R.L. Integrity, standards, and QC-related issues with big data in pre-clinical drug discovery. *Biochem. Pharmacol.* **2018**, *152*, 84–93. [CrossRef] [PubMed]

39. Qian, T.; Zhu, S.; Hoshida, Y. Use of big data in drug development for precision medicine: An update. *Expert Rev. Precis. Med. Drug Dev.* **2019**, *4*, 189–200. [CrossRef]

40. Casciuc, I. Pros and cons of virtual screening based on public 'Big Data': In silico mining for new bromodomain inhibitors. *Eur. J. Med. Chem.* **2019**, *165*, 258–272. [CrossRef]

41. Dossetter, A.G.; Ecker, G.; Laverty, H.; Overington, J. 'Big data' in pharmaceutical science: Challenges and opportunities. *Future Med. Chem.* **2014**, *6*, 857–864.

42. Lv, Z.; Qiao, L. Analysis of Healthcare Big Data. *Future Gener. Comput. Syst.* **2020**, *109*, 103–110. [CrossRef]

43. Costa, F.F. Big data in biomedicine. *Drug Discov. Today* **2014**, *19*, 433–440. [CrossRef] [PubMed]
44. Li, R.; Kim, D.; Ritchie, M.D. Methods to analyze big data in pharmacogenomics research. *Pharmacogenomics* **2017**, *18*, 807–820. [CrossRef] [PubMed]
45. Koren, G.; Nordon, G.; Radinsky, K.; Shalev, V. Machine learning of big data in gaining insight into successful treatment of hypertension. *Pharmacol. Res. Perspect.* **2018**, *6*, 396. [CrossRef] [PubMed]
46. Li, B.; Li, J.; Jiang, Y.; Lan, X. Experience and reflection from China's Xiangya medical big data project. *J. Biomed. Inform.* **2019**, *93*, 103149. [CrossRef]
47. Bouzillé, G. An Automated Detection System of Drug-Drug Interactions from Electronic Patient Records Using Big Data Analytics. *Health Technol. Inf.* **2019**, *264*, 45–49.
48. Zhang, C.; Ma, R.; Sun, S.; Li, Y.; Wang, Y.; Yan, Z. Optimizing the Electronic Health Records Through Big Data Analytics: A Knowledge-Based View. *IEEE Access* **2019**, *7*, 136223–136231. [CrossRef]
49. Papanicolas, I.; Woskie, L.R.; Jha, A.K. Health Care Spending in the United States and Other High-Income Countries. *JAMA* **2018**, *319*, 1024. [CrossRef]
50. Bodas-Sagi, D.; Labeaga, J. Big Data and Health Economics: Opportunities, Challenges and Risks. *Int. J. Interact. Multimed. Artif. Intell.* **2018**, *4*, 47. [CrossRef]
51. Wang, W.; Krishnan, E. Big data and clinicians: A review on the state of the science. *JMIR Med. Inf.* **2014**, *2*, e2913. [CrossRef]
52. Mulugeta, L.Y.; Yao, L.; Mould, D.; Jacobs, B.; Florian, J.; Smith, B.; Sinha, V.; Barrett, J.S. Leveraging Big Data in Pediatric Development Programs: Proceedings From the 2016 American College of Clinical Pharmacology Annual Meeting Symposium. *Clin. Pharmacol. Ther.* **2018**, *104*, 81–87. [CrossRef] [PubMed]
53. Christensen, M.L.; Davis, R.L. Identifying the 'Blip on the Radar Screen': Leveraging Big Data in Defining Drug Safety and Efficacy in Pediatric Practice. *J. Clin. Pharmacol.* **2018**, *58*, 86–93. [CrossRef] [PubMed]
54. Barrot, C.C.; Woillard, J.B.; Picard, N. Big data in pharmacogenomics: Current applications, perspectives and pitfalls. *Pharmacogenomics* **2019**, *20*, 609–620. [CrossRef] [PubMed]
55. Foreman, B. Neurocritical Care: Bench to Bedside (Eds. Claude Hemphill, Michael James) Integrating and Using Big Data in Neurocritical Care. *Neurotherapeutics* **2020**, *17*, 593–605. [CrossRef] [PubMed]
56. Rajula, H.S.R.; Manchia, M.; Carpiniello, B.; Fanos, V. Big data in severe mental illness: The role of electronic monitoring tools and metabolomics. *Per. Med.* **2021**, *18*, 75–90. [CrossRef]
57. Liu, Y.; Li, N.; Zhu, X.; Qi, Y. How wide is the application of genetic big data in biomedicine. *Biomed. Pharmacother* **2021**, *133*, 111074. [CrossRef] [PubMed]
58. Koppe, G.; Meyer-Lindenberg, A.; Durstewitz, D. Deep learning for small and big data in psychiatry. *Neuropsychopharmacology* **2021**, *46*, 176–190. [CrossRef]
59. Cech, N.B.; Medema, M.H.; Clardy, J. Benefiting from big data in natural products: Importance of preserving foundational skills and prioritizing data quality. *Nat. Prod. Rep.* **2021**, *38*, 1947–1953. [CrossRef]
60. Ellaway, R.H.; Pusic, M.V.; Galbraith, R.M.; Cameron, T. Developing the role of big data and analytics in health professional education. *Med. Teach.* **2014**, *36*, 216–222. [CrossRef]

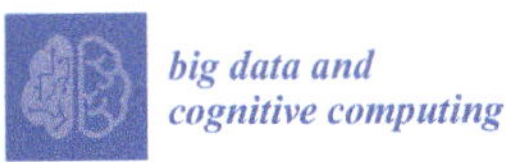

Review

Impact of Artificial Intelligence on COVID-19 Pandemic: A Survey of Image Processing, Tracking of Disease, Prediction of Outcomes, and Computational Medicine

Khaled H. Almotairi [1], Ahmad MohdAziz Hussein [2,*], Laith Abualigah [3,4,5,6,7,8], Sohaib K. M. Abujayyab [9], Emad Hamdi Mahmoud [10], Bassam Omar Ghanem [11] and Amir H. Gandomi [12,13,*]

[1] Computer Engineering Department, Computer and Information Systems College, Umm Al-Qura University, Makkah 21955, Saudi Arabia
[2] Deanship of E-Learning and Distance Education, Umm Al-Qura University, Makkah 21955, Saudi Arabia
[3] Computer Science Department, Prince Hussein Bin Abdullah College for Information Technology, Al Al-Bayt University, P.O. BOX 130040, Mafraq 25113, Jordan
[4] Hourani Center for Applied Scientific Research, Al-Ahliyya Amman University, Amman 19328, Jordan
[5] Faculty of Information Technology, Middle East University, Amman 11831, Jordan
[6] Applied Science Research Center, Applied Science Private University, Amman 11931, Jordan
[7] School of Computer Sciences, Universiti Sains Malaysia, Pulau Pinang 11800, Malaysia
[8] Center for Engineering Application & Technology Solutions, Ho Chi Minh City Open University, Ho Chi Minh 700000, Vietnam
[9] International College of Engineering and Management, Muscat 112, Oman
[10] Department of Internal Medicine, Riyadh Care Hospital, Riyadh 14214, Saudi Arabia
[11] School of Educational and Psychological Sciences, Amman Arab University, Amman 11953, Jordan
[12] Faculty of Engineering and IT, University of Technology Sydney, Ultimo, NSW 2007, Australia
[13] University Research and Innovation Center (EKIK), Óbuda University, 1034 Budapest, Hungary
* Correspondence: amihussein@uqu.edu.sa (A.M.H.); gandomi@uts.edu.au (A.H.G.); Tel.: +966-591-082-327 (A.M.H.)

Citation: Almotairi, K.H.; Hussein, A.M.; Abualigah, L.; Abujayyab, S.K.M.; Mahmoud, E.H.; Ghanem, B.O.; Gandomi, A.H. Impact of Artificial Intelligence on COVID-19 Pandemic: A Survey of Image Processing, Tracking of Disease, Prediction of Outcomes, and Computational Medicine. *Big Data Cogn. Comput.* **2023**, *7*, 11. https://doi.org/10.3390/bdcc7010011

Academic Editors: Domenico Talia and Fabrizio Marozzo

Received: 11 November 2022
Revised: 20 December 2022
Accepted: 23 December 2022
Published: 11 January 2023

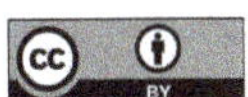

Abstract: Integrating machine learning technologies into artificial intelligence (AI) is at the forefront of the scientific and technological tools employed to combat the COVID-19 pandemic. This study assesses different uses and deployments of modern technology for combating the COVID-19 pandemic at various levels, such as image processing, tracking of disease, prediction of outcomes, and computational medicine. The results prove that computerized tomography (CT) scans help to diagnose patients infected by COVID-19. This includes two-sided, multilobar ground glass opacification (GGO) by a posterior distribution or peripheral, primarily in the lower lobes, and fewer recurrences in the intermediate lobe. An extensive search of modern technology databases relating to COVID-19 was undertaken. Subsequently, a review of the extracted information from the database search looked at how technology can be employed to tackle the pandemic. We discussed the technological advancements deployed to alleviate the communicability and effect of the pandemic. Even though there are many types of research on the use of technology in combating COVID-19, the application of technology in combating COVID-19 is still not yet fully explored. In addition, we suggested some open research issues and challenges in deploying AI technology to combat the global pandemic.

Keywords: machine learning; deep learning; artificial intelligence; COVID-19; virus; epidemic

1. Introduction

The well-known severe acute respiratory syndrome coronavirus 2 (SARS-CoV-2) contamination, dubbed coronavirus disease 2019 (COVID-19), has posed a universal healthcare issue. The pandemic has affected almost 215 nations across the continents, with more than 643,875,406 million confirmed cases of infection, including 6,630,082 deaths, at a rate of 1.59% deaths from all confirmed cases. However, 506,530,275 have recovered from the infection, at 78.6%, as of 9 December 2022 [1].

The domain of science and technology is performing an essential function in creating a cure for the virus. With the pandemic globally still raging due to the evolvement of new variants (i.e., delta variant), there has been a desperate search for ways to curtail its spread and develop a vaccine for the virus [2]. Early response to the disease in China was made by employing artificial intelligence (AI), such as tracking and tracing patients' travel history through facial recognition cameras, delivery of food and medicines using robots [3], disinfection of public buildings using drone technology [4], and dissemination of infoJessrmation to the public to remain indoors [5]. In addition, AI has been employed in the development of new molecules in the fight against COVID-19 [6], as shown in Figure 1, just as scientists are developing new drugs, along with computer experts aiming to detect people suffering from the disease via medical imaging, including CT scans and X-rays [7,8].

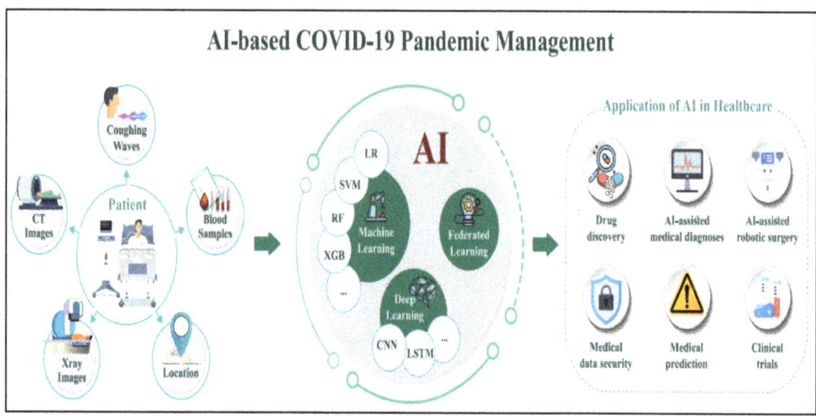

Figure 1. AI-based COVID-19 Management Architecture.

Furthermore, with the assistance of AI, tracking innovation is being developed through applications such as monitoring bracelets, which easily track patients breaching lockdown rules. The combination of AI- and mobile phone-aided cameras is also being deployed to take people's body temperature [9]. For example, the national medical insurance database in Taiwan is input with the dataset from both the custom and immigration databases to reconstruct patients' itineraries and symptoms [10,11].

Generally, AI is used to model, forecast epidemics and pandemics, diagnose [12], and validate the healthcare claims of a patient. With the help of supercomputers, different vaccines are being developed for COVID-19 [13]. In addition, drones and robots are deployed for logistics: distributing food and drugs and disinfecting public buildings.

Figure 2 represents the deadliest pandemics and data for the past 102 years. Dengue was discovered in 1950, with about a 100 million–400 million infected persons per year, which leads to about 2.5% of death. Smallpox was discovered and led to the death of about a 300 million people in the 20th century. HIV was discovered in 1920, with more than 75 million infected people and 36 million deaths. Another virus, called rabies, was discovered in 1920, with infection and death rates of 29 million and 5900 yearly, respectively. The Spanish flu was discovered in 1918, which infected more than 500 million every year and led to the deaths of about 50 million–100 million infected people. In 1973, a rotavirus virus was discovered, leading to about 0.2 million–0.5 million deaths yearly.

Afterward, an Ebola virus was discovered, which infected more than 31,000 people and led to the deaths of about 13,000 death tolls. A different virus was discovered, up until the current COVID-19, which was first discovered in 2019, with more than a 200 million infected persons and 4.4 million deaths. Several studies have been conducted to leverage the AI-centred model to enhance the COVID-19 prevention and detection process. In [14], the importance of AI was emphasized for handling the critical stage of COVID-19 prevention and detection, which is the decision-making stage. Thus, adopting AI would double up and assist in managing patient treatment efficiently in the intensive care unit (ICU).

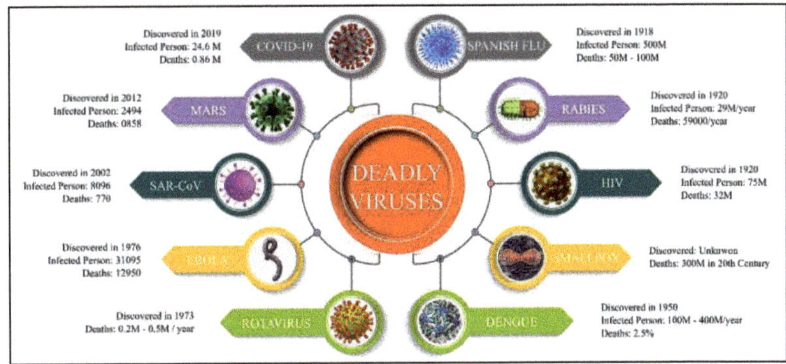

Figure 2. Deadliest Pandemics over the last 102 years (as of 25 August 2021).

Naude [10] explored several AI-related research focusing on the COVID-19 pandemic. The use areas of AI for COVID-19 include data dashboards, prognosis cures, diagnosis prediction, and tracking, warning and alert triggering [15], and social control. It is asserted that data scarcity or extensive abundant data employed in data analytics could cause an obstacle for utilizing AI for COVID-19 [16].

Motivation and Literature Gap

Several papers have proposed reviews/surveys of applications of AI for curtailing COVID-19. However, the direction and focus vary regarding the characteristics of protocols. For example, in Kumar et al. [17], improved modern technologies for handling the COVID-19 pandemic were reviewed, focusing on the functions of AI and other computer technologies for tackling the pandemic. However, related challenges and the severity of COVID-19 across different countries have not been analyzed. Further, Calandra and Favareto [18] have proposed an overview of the use of AI in combating the COVID-19 outbreak. In addition, dominant variables for AI in combating the COVID-19 outbreak were analyzed. However, current challenges concerning adopting AI for handling the pandemic have not been explored. AI application functions for fighting the spread of COVID-19 have been reviewed [19].

Similarly, a survey on AI and digital style using industry and energy for the post-COVID-19 outbreak has been proposed [20]. However, the research challenges related to security and privacy for adopting AI technologies have not been explored. Hassan et al. [21] proposed a systematic literature review for measuring the impact of AI and mathematical modeling in combating the COVID-19 outbreak. The proposal further surveyed different variants of COVID-19 and quality metrics for evaluating AI and mathematical modeling performances. However, the proposal did not look into the challenges of adopting mathematical modeling and AI paradigms.

In our proposal, we have reviewed different AI technologies and considered their impact on combating the COVID-19 outbreak. An analysis of outbreaks considering different countries is presented. Further, research challenges and open issues focusing on the application of AI for tackling the COVID-19 outbreak have also been proposed. Hence, little or no literature considered the open issues and research challenges in COVID-19 detection and control.

Considering the discussion above, this paper assesses the employment of AI in combating COVID-19. The paper comprehensively reviews the technological advancements at the forefront of the fight against the pandemic. The paper critically examines the AI-based procedures for handling COVID-19. Additionally, this paper advocates the usage of AI. In addition, the paper explains the deployment of AI and provides context on how innovation is employed against the pandemic. Figure 3 shows the top 17 countries most affected by COVID-19.

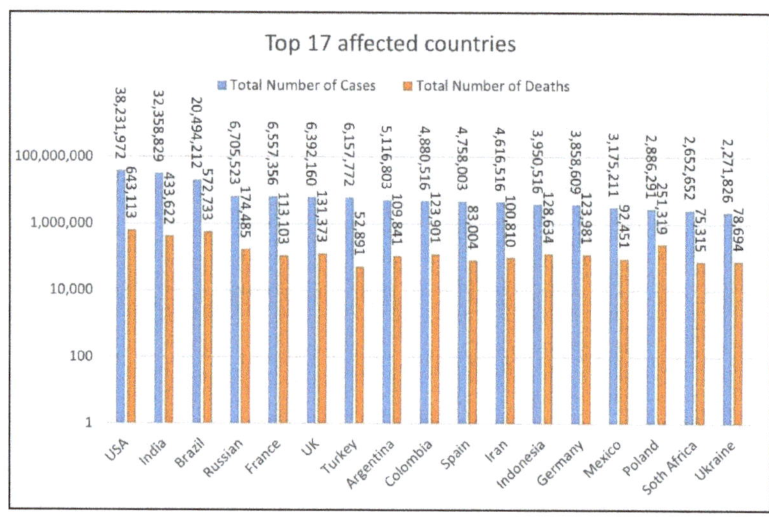

Figure 3. Top 17 most affected countries by COVID-19.

The rest of the paper is arranged as follows: Section 2 involves a comparative discussion of related surveys. In Section 3, the analysis of the impact of AI technology on COVID-19 is presented. Further, Section 4 entails a discussion on open research issues and challenges. Lastly, the conclusion and recommendations are presented in Section 5.

2. Comparative Discussion of Related Surveys

This section provides a comparative discussion of the related survey, which is further divided into two subsections. Section 2.1 is about the spread of COVID-19, and Section 2.2 involves the diagnostics of COVID-19.

2.1. Spread of COVID-19

The ravaging COVID-19 pandemic has changed the direction of research studies because researchers are given more concentration on how to alleviate the virus using various techniques in the AI-centered field. In the interim, researchers have suggested reviews based on AI's function in combating COVID-19 to support relevant authorities, such as medical practitioners [12] and policymakers, in decision-making. The related surveys can be classified into problem-centered AI solutions and AI structures implemented on various COVID-19 processes.

A survey that suggested a classification of tasks involved in predicting the COVID-19 virus has been presented [22,23]. The study outlined the use area of big data and AI. However, most of the considered papers for review are not from reputable sources. In addition, open issues and current research challenges have not been highlighted in the study. In the same direction, Bansal et al. [24] precisely highlighted the function of the AI strategies employed for detecting, predicting, and controlling COVID-19 [25].

Conversely, some COVID-19 processes have not considered some parameters, such as severity assessment and death rates. Further, Kumar et al. [26] concisely extend the function of deep learning (DL) and machine learning networks to handle the pandemic, even though research studies focusing on COVID-19 treatment via respiratory waves and clinical data have not been explored. Moreover, few studies were explored by analysis of AI-centered applications from different facets [27].

2.2. Diagnostics in COVID-19

The foundation of the AI-centered framework and big data concepts used for handling the spread of the COVID-19 pandemic have been reviewed in [28]. Discussions have been provided on the different AI-categorized learning techniques, with specific details on clinical data analysis and results about COVID-19. However, little attention has been given to analyzing the employed techniques. In a similar survey, Swapnarekha et al. [29] classified the reviewed papers into three models, i.e., ML, DL, and statistical, for handling COVID-19 and another related viruses. Further, a summarized review of COVID-19 recognition and prediction is proposed in [30].

A survey based on complicated DL has been proposed by Jamshidi et al. [31]. The survey explored DLs, such as the generative adversarial network (GAN), recurrent neural network (RNN) [32], extreme learning machine, and long short-term memory (LSTM), for a COVID-19 cure. However, the employed models are presented without critical comparative analysis. Further, a description of AI-centered forecasting and statistical model was presented in [33]. On the other hand, the only review of data mining strategies and ML for predicting COVID-19 was proposed in [34,35]. Furthermore, there was a taxonomy for complicated DL techniques for creating radiology reports [36].

Several studies reviewed a certain kind of dataset; for instance, Jalaber et al. [37] put forth the function of CT images for handling COVID-19-infected patients.

The function of the CT scan was also used for handling the presentation of lesions and severity signs. At the end of the paper, five related papers were explored to describe the AI's function for COVID-19 diagnosis. The landscape of radiographic imaging structures and AI methods was investigated. The imaging structures, such as PET, CXR, and CT, were considered for the AI data training and testing. However, the papers considered had constrained information regarding the gained results [38]. In another survey, the imaging characteristics of PET-CT and CT from several articles were presented [39], as well as a comparison of the AI techniques applied for COVID-19 prediction [40]. AI methods for diagnosing COVID-19 have been discussed by categorizing CT and CXR images [41]. In both [42,43], the domain of biosensors and IoT for handling the COVID-19 pandemic have been discussed.

Our paper surveyed articles containing AI's concept for handling COVID-19, in terms of prediction, diagnosis, survival assessment, drug discovery, recasting, and pandemic outbreak. Considering the discussion mentioned above, it is evident that a study focused on a distinct part of COVID-19 handling or described a single type of dataset. Further, many of these reviews offered fewer relative analyses and examined few papers. Conversely, there are a handful of articles that have not been surveyed.

The following section explores and presents the impact of AI in handling COVID-19.

3. Impact of AI on Repressing COVID-19

This part discusses the use of artificial intelligence (AI) techniques for handling the COVID-19 pandemic that have been discussed. AI technologies could be based on natural language processing (NLP), ML, and other applications of computer visualization. The different capabilities allow machines to use large information-based frameworks to build, show, and foretell. Table 1 presents numerous uses of technology in the fight against COVID-19. AI is often used to diagnose viruses, analyze medical images, trace, track, and carry out future disease predictions [44]. In addition, it is also used to send alerts to raise awareness and create social awareness virtually.

Table 1. Use cases of AI in CT diagnosis for COVID-19 pandemic.

Country	Authors(s)	AI Technique	Data Size	Correctness Level
China	[45]	Improved inception transfer-training system	740 viral pneumonia samples and 325 COVID-19 samples, totaling 1065 CT image data	The sensitivity test result is 0.67 The specificity test result is 0.83 The correctness test result is 79.3%
	[46]	Two-dimensional Deep CNN	The sample size for non-positive cases is 1385, with 970 CT capacity, of which 496 patients have been diagnosed with COVID-19	The specificity test result is 95.47%, The sensitivity test result is 94.06% AUC test result is 97.91% The correctness test result is 94.98%
	[47]	It is based on a three-dimensional DL system	An aggregate of 618 CT specimens was gathered of which 219 are from 110 infected persons	The correctness test result is 86.7%
	[48]	COVID-19 prediction using neural network called COVNet	An aggregate of 4356 chest CT examinations, which are from 3322 infected persons	The correctness test result is 95%
Canada (Toronto)	[49]	A deep CNN dubbed COVID-Net:	From 13,645 infected persons, the total of 16,756 CXR images were collected.	The correctness test result is 92.4%
Hong Kong and Thailand	[50]	The RT-PCR assay is real-time	From 246 infected people, 340 clinical samples were collected	From each reaction or response, more than 10 genomic copies, which is the Potential detection limit
Universal	[11]	The CXR image from 50 uninfected patients and 50 infected patients with the COVID-19 virus.	Inception ResNet V2 InceptionV3 and ResNet50	The inception-ResNet at V2 is 87%, the ResNet at 50 is 98%, and the inception at V3 is 97%.
Saudi Arabia	[51]	COVID-19 detection fuzzy analytic hierarchy process (AHP)	Saudi open data	High efficacy
	[52]	Deep learning-based convolutional CNN	Dataset of 340 DX-ray radiographs, 170 images of each Healthy and Positive COVID-19 class.	High precision with maximum accuracy of up to 94.12%
	[53]	A dilated CNN and branching design model, and VGG-16 technique	Dataset contains from 13,975 CXR images	Accuracy = 96.5% Sensitivity = 96%

AI techniques have been used to extract the exact graphical features of COVID-19 that help provide clinical treatment/diagnosis before conducting the pathogenic test, thereby minimizing the time for pandemic control. By employing radiology images in diagnoses, AI obtains radiological characteristics for the prompt and precise discovery of COVID-19 [45]. The techniques employ deep learning algorithms using a computer vision model that considers specific parameters, such as level of specificity, accuracy, sensitivity, region area under the curve (AUC), negative predictive value, and positive predictive value. Similarly, deep convolutional neural networks (CNN), which employ X-ray image data for model training and testing, have been proposed for the automatic detection and prediction of COVID-19 [54]. The proposed technique serves as a substitute treatment and diagnosis decision to avoid the spread of the coronavirus among the infected people around the globe using CNN-based models, which include ResNet50, ResNet101, ResNet152, Inception-ResNetV2, and InceptionV3 [54].

Another solution Wang et al. [49] proposed for handling the pandemic is COVID-Net. It employs the AI concept for detecting coronavirus using the data from an open-source repository of chest X-ray images. Another AI technique has been proposed to screen coronavirus using multiple CNN to classify images and find the probability of the virus infection [47]. The current CT application, and/or the above AI techniques that have been proposed, appear to help ascertain the pandemic to provide diagnosis/clinical support to a patient before conducting the pathogenic result that is ready for proper action.

Wang et al. [55] presented a somewhat effective respiratory simulation model (RSM), in order to handle the limitation between the massive volume of training data and the limited available real data. Meanwhile, the suggested deep learning model could be expanded to big-scale use areas, such as office environments, sleep scenarios, and public places. Although, the technique has faced some challenges, including adequate real-world data to realize the learning method, and the variation in different respiratory patterns is also less than average. The disease tracking procedure involves the following steps: (1) irregular respiratory sequence classifier, which can lead to mass testing of people infected with COVID-19. (2) The SIR model, which is time-bound, is employed for determining the number of infected people. (3) The gated recurrent unit (GRU) is a neural network that uses an embedded bi-directional and attentional system (BI-AT-GRU) for categorizing respiratory sequences. (4) The infectious, exposed, vulnerable, and eliminated or recovered framework is employed to predict the cause of the pandemic.

An ML-based model for predicting the survivability of patients infected with COVID-19 and the prediction result of the patient's state of health has been presented in [56,57]. In [56], the supervised XGBoost classifier gives a straightforward and spontaneous medical screening to measure the likelihood of bereavement accurately and promptly. In [57], the ML-based CT frameworks indicated the possibility and precision of forecasting the stay time of patients infected with COVID-19 at the hospital.

A model is a supporting tool for decision-making and logistical planning for the healthcare system. The technique uses different algorithms with different datasets. Richardson et al. [27] also employed Benevolent AI's knowledge graph to search for approved drugs to help minimize coronavirus infection. The authors did not discuss the detail of the algorithms and how the model performance was evaluated using the available parameters. Similarly, a novel deep-learning pipeline architecture has been proposed [58] as an alternative to COVID-19 detection. The technique uses a chest x-ray image with convolutional CNN to detect whether the patient is a carrier of COVID-19 or not, with detailed diagnosis features and a quicker diagnosis. The technique has been regarded as the most suitable in places that have advanced computing machines. However, during this pandemic, people need a solution that can be integrated with existing and/or available resources. Another technique, based on a cuckoo search optimization algorithm, has been proposed to extract basic information from the X-rays conducted on the lungs using three classification processes: called normal patients, COVID-19-infected patients, and pneumonia patients.

The approach is an alternate solution to detect COVID-19 from the X-ray images using a modified CS algorithm [59,60].

Protein structure prediction is used to extract some features from medical images. In [61], the residual learning procedure was utilized to simplify the training of considerably deep systems for image feature detection. In [62], the critical assessment of methods for protein structure prediction (CASP) by employing a deep neural network to forecast protein characteristics based on its genetic pattern was suggested. In [63], convolutional network architecture was inspected for heavy projection.

Drug innovation is an application for adversarial auto-encoders, which is employed in extracting the method and the structure of image data, dimensionality reduction, unsupervised clustering, and data conception [64]. While in [65], protein structure is used as an incorporated AI-centered drug detection conduit to award new drug mixtures.

In [66], cough-type diagnosis utilized a considerable selection of acoustic characteristics administered to the documented audio from many uninfected and infected persons. In [30], a smartphone thermometer was a simple substitute device for measuring the temperature of infected persons.

Social media has become very popular worldwide, as it is used to interact and communicate [25]. However, one problem is information overload, misinformation, and fake news. To counter this "infodemic", the World Health Organization (WHO) introduced the information network for epidemics (EPI-WIN) to distribute news and data with some major partners [67]. Social media giant Facebook analyzes posts about infections; its ad library [68] examines all ads through the tag "COVID-19" and "coronavirus", and Facebook aggregated 923 outcomes in 34 nations, the maximum of which were from the US (39%) and Europe (Italy had 25% of the ads).

A system for detecting COVID-19 utilizing data from mobile phones' sensors, including cameras, microphones, inertial sensors, and temperature, was proposed in [66]. Similarly, audio data collected from hand-held phones' microphones was employed to identify coughing [30]. It is essential for AI to be trained to predict infection threats and, as such, help identify high-risk cases for containment purposes, thereby curtailing the spread of the virus among the populace [69]. Some drones were also used to trail and detect people who were not using mouth/nose masks, and some were employed as a public address system to address the public or disinfect public places. A company from Shenzhen in China, Small-Multi-Copter, has helped dramatically with logistical support and distribution of medical supplies and lockdown materials via drones.

To curtail the transmission of the virus in India, the authorities introduced Aarogya Setu [70], a mobile phone app that could track coronavirus patients to fight the infection on an individual basis. The app also helped trace contamination using mobile phone GPSs and Bluetooth to collect data on whether a person has come into contact with a COVID-19 patient. To curtail further infection from the coronavirus in India, the authorities developed a mobile application known as Aarogya Setu [70], which tracks coronavirus infection and also aids in stopping the spread from person-to-person. It aids in tracing coronavirus infection by using mobile phones' GPS networks, as well as the Bluetooth of the phones, with which it detects whether an individual has had an interaction with a COVID-19 patient [71].

3.1. Medical Image Processing

The effectiveness of the current diagnostics at the beginning of the pandemic was challenged. Open clinical methods were ineffective against the COVID-19 virus, and with limited medical equipment and other assets, the cure needs of every patient were determined by the seriousness of their symptoms. With many outpatients with mild symptoms that could suddenly be serious, there was a need to diagnose the symptoms early enough for effective treatment and ultimately drive down the mortality rate. Therefore, AI could be effective in the prognosis, prediction [72], and curing of COVID-19 patients and drive down treatment costs [73]. Most medical uses of AI are often used for diagnosis using medical imaging. In some current studies, it was established that only a small number of the studies used AI in arriving at their CT scans. Additionally, other studies employ patients' medical records to predict the severity of the virus [5,45,54].

3.1.1. The Role of CT Scan for COVID-19 Patients Screening

The results obtained based on CT from COVID-19 scenarios include multilobar GGO and bilateral with surface or subsequent distribution. This is often in the lower lobes and with less frequency in the intermediate lobe. Subpleural, septal thickening, pleural thickening, and bronchiectasis involvement are a few of the usual outcomes, particularly in the subsequent phase of the virus. CT halo symbol, pleural effusion, lymphadenopathy, pericardial effusion, cavitation, and pneumothorax are also among the few unusual, but probable, outcomes observed from the virus evolution [3,6,7].

Bai and his team noted common features within 201 infected patients, CT irregularities and suitable RT-PCR patients, as follows: 80%, 91%, 56%, and 59% for the surface circulation, GGO, good reticular opacity, and vascular congealing, respectively. Fewer usual features for the CT photographing on the chest included the following: 14%, 2.7%, and 4.1% for the central and peripheral distribution, lymphadenopathy, and pleural effusion, respectively [10]. At an early stage, the chest film is not usually sensitive, and it can be found to be significant at a later stage during the monitoring of the disease [11]. According to Malpani et al. [74], another way of calculating the severity score is to assign the percentages of individuals of the five given lobes shown as <5% contribution, 5–25% contribution, 26–49% contribution, 50–75% contribution, and >75% contribution [8,10]. The overall CT mark contains the summation of each of the given lobar marks that cover the bound of values from 0 to 25 (for no contribution and maximum contribution, respectively), once the contribution of all the five lobes is found to be above 75% [11].

3.1.2. Diagnosis Using Radiology Images

With the application of AI, many lives could ultimately be saved, and the spread of the virus could be checked, leading to the generation of relevant data from AI models with correct diagnoses of the virus. With AI, radiologists could achieve faster, not to mention cheaper, diagnosis rates than mainstream coronavirus tests [75]. In the same vein, doctors could also use a combination of X-rays and CT scans [46]. The different AI use cases for handling COVID-19 are presented in Table 1. COVID-19 medical tests are not widely available and often expensive, but most emergency and trauma clinics usually have CT and X-ray machines. Thus, with the help of DL, a radiology expert could analyze and detect the presence of COVID-19. In another development, COVID-Net has proposed an IT-based application for examining COVID-19 signs, based on CXR, through the various information of the lungs of infected patients [76]. Using diagnostic research, AI software was developed from an inceptions migration neural network for analyzing and detecting COVID-19 symptoms with the help of CT images with an 89.5% accuracy rate [45].

A preliminary discovery model has been developed to detect the COVID-19 virus from Influenza-A and specific cases with pulmonary CT images using a DL system. The affected portions of the patients were aggregated using the 3D DL model, and the research had an 86.7% accuracy rate [47,48]. Similarly, Cao et al. [77] built a DL system to effectively diagnose the virus symptoms contracted from other lung ailments and community-acquired pneumonia (CAP). Using chest CT scans, a 3D learning method was developed using a DNN (COV-Net) [78]. Additionally, to diagnose coronavirus, a DL framework was developed that quickly uses CT data as inputs, carries out lung categorization, detects COVID-19, and diagnoses any irregular slice. In addition, the research shows that the diagnoses of AI methods could be explained using data to check the shortcoming of the DNN model as a black box [79]. Subsequently, a computerized system has been developed to quantify the different signs of the virus in patients' lungs and check the virus or response to treatment by employing a DL technique. The range of capabilities of AI clinical analyses have not yet been determined. However, some hospitals in China have been using AI-aided radiology innovations. Transcription polymerase chain reaction (RT-PCR) tests are critical for diagnosing coronavirus. However, they have their limitations regarding specimen variety and the duration needed for the research and processing [50]. Some abnormalities in CT image data of COVID-19 have been seen using the central AI concept [80,81]. Similarly, the fuzzy-based decision-making technique has been explored by [51] to assess the severity of COVID-19 in the Kingdom of Saudi Arabia (KSA), while adopting a more robust computational model for evaluating the severity using social influence to control the spread of the COVID-19 pandemic [51].

An X-ray technique with an automated system identifier for COVID-19 detection on chest images has been designed using the convoluted CNN architecture. The technique extracts the feature descriptors from the chest X-ray image using a speed-up feature robust algorithm and integrated k-means clustering algorithm to detect whether there is a presence or absence of COVID-19. The study used the dataset of 340 X-ray radiographs and 170 images of both healthy and positive COVID-19 classes [52]. Chest X-ray (CXR) has been used to detect the coronavirus infection by proposing the dilated CNN, branching design model, and VGG-16 technique. Therefore, the VGG-16 used the beginning of the ten layers in the model's front end to extract and utilize the high-level merits [53].

3.1.3. Disease Tracking

AI can be deployed for tracing and tracking COVID-19. Current studies have shown that COVID-19 is characterized by respiratory patterns, which differ from normal colds and periodic influenza, including fast breathing (tachypnea) [82]. Predicting tachypnea could become a premium diagnostic characteristic that aids the scope screening of possible patients [55]. So many proposals have been made on how best to employ mobile phones for COVID-19 diagnoses. The best way is either by using embedded sensors that detect COVID-19 symptoms or by conducting phone surveys to help vulnerable patients who depend on responding to critical questions [83].

Berlin uses a model based on epidemiological SIR, which uses curtailment actions by the relevant authorities, such as quarantines, social distance, and partial or total lockdown measures [84]. Another SIR model involves public health methods for handling the virus. It also uses data sources from China and was made available in R [85]. GLEAMviz epidemiological model could be deployed to check the spread of the virus [33]. Similarly, Metabiota [86] uses a tracker for the epidemic to detect COVID-19 [87]. It is also used as a near-tenure forecasting system for the transmission of 93infections. Information about tracking the virus is essential for public health experts to curtail the pandemic [88,89] effectively.

3.1.4. Prediction of the Infected Patient

An innovative method that depends on patients' blood tests and medical information was developed to assist doctors in determining vulnerable patients early enough. This will improve virus forecasting and reduce the mortality rate among high-risk patients [56].

Machine learning (ML) has been used extensively to solve various complex challenges in various application areas. ML can help enhance the reliability, performance, predictability, and accuracy of diagnostic systems for many diseases. This paper provides a comprehensive review of the use of ML in the medical field such as detect COVID-19. Such algorithms learn from many diagnosed samples collected from medical test reports. They can also support medical experts in predicting and diagnosing diseases in the future [90].

As an alternative, another forecast model that calculates XGBoost was developed to forecast fatality rates and differentiate the essential factors that can be determined in clinics. The researchers determined three critical factors: high-affectability C-receptive protein, lactic dehydrogenase, and lymphocyte for determining a patient's survivability. The highlight of this approach is its easy convertibility, and the triple factors recognized by the procedure are the important and critical indicators in the pathophysiological progress of COVID-19, especially cell damage, cell inflammation, immunity, and inflammation [91].

A similar study was conducted to predict whether a COVID-19 infected person may need a longer period to stay in the hospital or not, based on a U-Net AI system, which is secondarily trained using CT data [57]. While these methodologies have their shortcomings regarding scope and information, they represent important studies that can be improved with additional clinical information from other cases worldwide. Together, these methods may significantly aid in identifying infected persons needing longer stay periods at the hospital, thereby supporting hospitals in having an adequate plan.

3.2. Disease Tracking and Treatment

Computational biologists are essential in combatting the COVID-19 pandemic because of their contributions to modeling. Computational biology is called computational simulation, mathematical modeling, and data analytics for advancing biology [92]. With disease dynamics modeling, the impact of specific parameters that abet disease transmission and mediation's impact in fighting infections is better understood [93]. When a patient dies from the virus, their lungs start manifesting glass and permeating. Different data-aided medication transposition methods were developed to identify diseases, patients, or conditions that could be tackled with the medications used for different ailments [27].

3.2.1. Prediction in COVID-19

As soon as a virus RNA penetrates a particular cell, it bonds the affected host cell's protein creation, using it to produce proteins replicating RNA molecules. Proteins possess a 3D structure that can be examined through sequences prearranged by amino acid order. The 3D structure affects the character and objective of the protein [61,92]. They are usually called polymerases and proteins and are the focus of treatments [94].

The two main ways of dealing with forecasts are template modeling, which forecasts structures using the same type of proteins as a framework model succession, and prototype-free modeling, which forecasts patterns for proteins with unidentified associated patterns [62]. It is proposed that these forecasts may assist in finding a cure for the COVID-19 pandemic. Further, the AlphaFold system relies on a bigger ResNet structure and utilizes amino acid order, as well as the characteristics from the corresponding amino acid order through different order structures, to predict the length and the sparsity of gradients among amino acid remains [63]. This method could be used to determine the patterns of the six proteins related to the SARS-CoV-2 layer protein, Nsp2, Nsp4, protein 3a, Nsp6, and proteolytic-like penzyme [61].

3.2.2. Discovery of a Drug for COVID-19

At the Massachusetts Institute of Technology (MIT), some experts are currently developing a method for fighting the ravaging COVID-19 by producing a "decoy" receptor or protein, which might be used as a drug. The virus causes illness by attacking and attaching to the body's ACE2 receptors. The experts at MIT are using an AI concept, built on data related to ACE2 receptors, to mimic the link between the hooks and the virus [95]. Few studies are looking at ways to find new composites to focus on SAR-Cov2 by deploying novel conduits to determine constraints for the 3C-similar enzymes [64].

These systems employ three sets of data of the precise architecture of the enzyme, the c-clear substance, and the homogeneity template of the enzyme. Different types of information are used, including the productive automatic-encipher and the productive antipathetic matrix [65]. The researchers are investigating the possibility of utilizing a supplementing cognitive method with a large receptibility that can integrate factors such as the dosages of drugs, similarity, freshness, and different varieties.

4. Research Challenges and Open Issues

In this part, we have emphasized some research issues that require research consideration to attain efficient AI technologies for COVID-19 pandemic mitigation. The research issues cut across insufficient data for algorithm training, high computation expenses, security and privacy issues, and unclear interoperability functions. The detailed discussion is as follows:

- **Insufficient Data for Machine Training**

In some parts of the world, there are not sufficient data, such as CXR images from COVID-19-infected persons, for training the machine/algorithm. Similarly, there is no sufficient repository containing all data on the symptoms of infected COVID-19 cases. News and social media data reports may be highly unstructured, multidimensional, and low quality. Data may not be accessible from the community with limited Internet access. In addition, there are challenges in collecting patients' physiological features and therapeutic outcomes. Thus, projecting the skewed outcome of results and erroneous predictions could cause mass hysteria in the healthcare system [16,70]. Considering these challenges, there is a need to build national and global repositories for COVID-19 medical data.

- **High Computational Expenses**

Since different researchers have mainly employed deep learning (DL) concepts in the quest for combating COVID-19, the machine/algorithm has a high dependency on high-capacity hardware. This is because DL uses a neural network that depends on large datasets for training and testing the COVID-19 prediction model. The need for a large dataset for algorithm training also leads to a long training time, which may not be helpful for the early prediction of the virus [96,97]. Therefore, there is a need to develop more robust DL techniques that consider the urgent need for the COVID-19 predictive model. The model should take less training time in the model training phase.

- **Scarce Data**

The primary ingredient of machine learning techniques is the large quantity of data. Labeled data are often used to train machine models to learn and make specific predictions. However, with partial data, the whole of the AI system could become flawed. Thus, the large data set might not be readily available in some countries affected by COVID-19. Therefore, there is a need for global repositories where COVID-19 patient data can be accessed.

- **Security and Privacy**

To restrain the transmission of the virus, mobile applications for the real-time transmission trailing, detection, and observation for quick warning and alerting have been developed. However, the privacy and security of mobile phone users is not explored [76,98]. For instance, using government surveillance gadgets in public places to detect infected persons has sparked adverse reactions from people because such surveillance reveals the identity of every detected individual. Thus, there is a need to ensure that mobile phone data and other surveillance data remain anonymous in the AI technique.

- **Interoperability**

The data exchange between different nodes or neurons of the learning system is unclear. In DL, interoperability is difficult to detect or understand because it involves complex neurons and operations [99,100]. It is almost unclear how a particular set of inputs leads to a specific solution for various problems. The interoperability issue emanates from either a lack of standardized and coordinated data representation or a standardized application programming interface. In the design of the AI system for COVID-19 prediction, there is a need to design an AI system so that the reasoning behind the operation is evident.

5. Conclusions

Scientists are looking at every possible cure for the virus, and modern technology increasingly searches for a possible cure. It is pertinent that technology has become part of our everyday lives; it has additionally now been used in the fight against the coronavirus. This paper highlights the problem of the coronavirus and discusses some algorithms that are practically used in hospitals. The paper also discusses the fact that there is an interest in building a yardstick framework to examine the present methods. The present systems have precise correctness in predicting COVID-19 symptoms with various types of pneumonia using X-rays scans; however, they do not have both interpretability and transparency. Therefore, we can conclude that technology has many capabilities to overcome the medical and social problems caused by the COVID-19 pandemic. Few such capabilities are advanced and adequate for demonstrating any impact. CT investigation performs a vital function in the mitigation of COVID-19. It was used at the initial detection of the COVID-19 virus, particularly in the extremely vulnerable, asymptomatic occurrences with non-positive PCR tests; CT may perform functions in the following points: triage of patients, estimation of deteriorating, estimation of good cure, and problem handle. The triage of patients can be divided into three categories: possibly with COVID-19, without COVID-19, and seriousness of the infection.

Author Contributions: Conceptualization, K.H.A. and A.M.H.; methodology, L.A., A.M.H. and S.K.M.A.; investigation, E.H.M. and B.O.G.; resources, K.H.A. and A.M.H.; writing—original draft preparation, A.M.H. and S.K.M.A.; writing—review and editing, A.M.H.; project administration, K.H.A.; funding acquisition, K.H.A.; writing—review and editing A.H.G. All authors have read and agreed to the published version of the manuscript.

Funding: This research was funded by the Deanship of Scientific Research at Umm Al-Qura University (https://uqu.edu.sa) for supporting this work by grant code: (22UQU4320277DS15) to KA. The authors would like to thank the Deanship of Scientific Research at Umm Al-Qura University for supporting this work.

Institutional Review Board Statement: Not applicable.

Informed Consent Statement: Not applicable.

Data Availability Statement: Not applicable.

Conflicts of Interest: The authors declare no conflict of interest.

References

1. World Health Organization. Available online: https://covid19.who.int/ (accessed on 9 December 2022).
2. Salgotra, R.; Rahimi, I.; Gandomi, A.H. Artificial Intelligence for Fighting the COVID-19 Pandemic. In *Humanity Driven AI*; Springer: Cham, Switzerland, 2022; pp. 165–177.
3. Ruiz Estrada, M.A. The uses of drones in case of massive Epidemics contagious diseases relief humanitarian aid: Wuhan-COVID-19 crisis. *SSRN Electron. J.* **2020.** [CrossRef]
4. Jokisch, O.; Siegert, I.; Loesch, E. Speech communication at the presence of unmanned aerial vehicles. In Proceedings of the 46th Annual German Conference on Acoustics (DAGA 2020), Hannover, Germany, 16–19 March 2020.
5. Alalawi, H.; Alsuwat, M.; Alhakami, H. A Survey of the Application of Artifical Intelligence on COVID-19 Diagnosis and Prediction. *Eng. Technol. Appl. Sci. Res.* **2021**, *11*, 7824–7835. [CrossRef]
6. Mahanty, C.; Kumar, R.; Asteris, P.G.; Gandomi, A.H. COVID-19 Patient Detection Based on Fusion of Transfer Learning and Fuzzy Ensemble Models Using CXR Images. *Appl. Sci.* **2021**, *11*, 11423. [CrossRef]
7. Nguyen, T.T.; Waurn, G.; Campus, P. Artificial intelligence in the battle against Coronavirus (COVID-19): A survey and future research directions. *arXiv* **2020**, arXiv:2008.07343.
8. El Homsi, M.; Chung, M.; Bernheim, A.; Jacobi, A.; King, M.J.; Lewis, S.; Taouli, B. Review of Chest CT Manifestations of COVID-19 Infection. *Eur. J. Radiol. Open* **2020**, *7*, 100239. [CrossRef]
9. Maghdid, H.S.; Ghafoor, K.Z.; Sadiq, A.S.; Curran, K.; Rabie, K. A novel AI-enabled framework to diagnose coronavirus COVID-19 using smartphone embedded sensors: Design study. *arXiv* **2020**, arXiv:2003.07434.
10. Wang, C.J.; Ng, C.Y.; Brook, R.H. Response to COVID-19 in Taiwan: Big data analytics, new technology, and proactive testing. *JAMA* **2020**, *323*, 1341–1342. [CrossRef]
11. techUK. Available online: https://www.techuk.org/resource/how-taiwan-used-tech-to-fight-covid-19.html#:~{}:text=Taiwan%20has%20also%20used%20AI,risk%20of%20contracting%20COVID%2D19 (accessed on 19 December 2022).
12. Hota, L.; Dash, P.K.; Sahoo, K.S.; Gandomi, A.H. Air Quality Index Analysis of Indian Cities During COVID-19 Using Machine Learning Models: A Comparative Study. In Proceedings of the 2021 8th International Conference on Soft Computing & Machine Intelligence (ISCMI), Cairo, Egypt, 26–27 November 2021; pp. 27–31.
13. Bullock, J.; Alexandra, L.; Pham, K.H.; Lam, C.S.N.; Luengo-Oroz, M. Mapping the landscape of artificial intelligence applications against COVID-19. *arXiv* **2020**, arXiv:2003.11336. [CrossRef]
14. Rahmatizadeh, S.; Valizadeh-Haghi, S.; Dabbagh, A. The role of Artificial Intelligence in Management of Critical COVID-19 patients. *J. Cell. Mol. Anesth.* **2020**, *5*, 16–22.

15. Fayyoumi, E.; Idwan, S.; AboShindi, H. Machine Learning and Statistical Modelling for Prediction of Novel COVID-19 Patients Case Study: Jordan. *Mach. Learn.* **2020**, *11*. [CrossRef]
16. Naudé, W. *Artificial Intelligence against COVID-19: An Early Review*; Institute of Labor Economics: Bonn, Germany, 2020.
17. Kumar, A.; Gupta, P.K.; Srivastava, A. A review of modern technologies for tackling COVID-19 pandemic. *Diabetes Metab. Syndr. Clin. Res. Rev.* **2020**, *14*, 569–573. [CrossRef]
18. Calandra, D.; Favareto, M. Artificial Intelligence to fight COVID-19 outbreak impact: An overview. *Eur. J. Soc. Impact Circ. Econ.* **2020**, *1*, 84–104.
19. Piccialli, F.; Di Cola, V.S.; Giampaolo, F.; Cuomo, S. The role of artificial intelligence in fighting the COVID-19 pandemic. *Inf. Syst. Front.* **2021**, *23*, 1467–1497. [CrossRef]
20. Sharifi, A.; Ahmadi, M.; Ala, A. The impact of artificial intelligence and digital style on industry and energy post-COVID-19 pandemic. *Environ. Sci. Pollut. Res.* **2021**, *28*, 46964–46984. [CrossRef]
21. Hassan, A.; Prasad, D.; Rani, S.; Alhassan, M. Gauging the Impact of Artificial Intelligence and Mathematical Modeling in Response to the COVID-19 Pandemic: A Systematic Review. *BioMed Res. Int.* **2022**, *2022*, 7731618. [CrossRef]
22. Pham, Q.V.; Nguyen, D.C.; Huynh-The, T.; Hwang, W.J.; Pathirana, P.N. Artificial intelligence (AI) and big data for coronavirus (COVID-19) pandemic: A survey on the state-of-the-arts. *IEEE Access* **2020**, *8*, 130820–130839. [CrossRef]
23. Rasheed, J.; Jamil, A.; Hameed, A.A.; Al-Turjman, F.; Rasheed, A. COVID-19 in the Age of Artificial Intelligence: A Comprehensive Review. *Interdiscip. Sci. Comput. Life Sci.* **2021**, *13*, 153–175. [CrossRef]
24. Bansal, A.; Padappayil, R.P.; Garg, C.; Singal, A.; Gupta, M.; Klein, A. Utility of artificial intelligence amidst the COVID-19 pandemic: A review. *J. Med. Syst.* **2020**, *44*, 1–6. [CrossRef]
25. Rahimi, I.; Gandomi, A.H.; Asteris, P.G.; Chen, F. Analysis and prediction of COVID-19 Using SIR, SEIQR, and machine learning models: Australia, Italy, and UK Cases. *Information* **2021**, *12*, 109. [CrossRef]
26. Kumar, S.; Raut, R.D.; Narkhede, B.E. A proposed collaborative framework by using artificial intelligence-internet of things (AI-IoT) in COVID-19 pandemic situation for healthcare workers. *Int. J. Healthc. Manag.* **2020**, *13*, 337–345. [CrossRef]
27. Richardson, P.; Griffin, I.; Tucker, C.; Smith, D.; Oechsle, O.; Phelan, A.; Rawling, M.; Savory, E.; Stebbing, J. Baricitinib as potential treatment for 2019-nCoV acute respiratory disease. *Lancet* **2020**, *395*, e30. [CrossRef] [PubMed]
28. Hussain, A.A.; Bouachir, O.; Al-Turjman, F.; Aloqaily, M. AI techniques for COVID-19. *IEEE Access* **2020**, *8*, 128776–128795. [CrossRef] [PubMed]
29. Swapnarekha, H.; Behera, H.S.; Nayak, J.; Naik, B. Role of intelligent computing in COVID-19 prognosis: A state-of-the-art review. *Chaos Solitons Fractals* **2020**, *138*, 109947. [CrossRef] [PubMed]
30. Nemati, E.; Rahman, M.M.; Nathan, V.; Vatanparvar, K.; Kuang, J. Poster abstract: A comprehensive approach for cough type detection. In Proceedings of the 4th IEEE/ACM International Conference on Connected Health: Applications, Systems and Engineering Technologies (CHASE), Arlington, VA, USA, 25–27 September 2019; pp. 15–16.
31. Jamshidi, M.B.; Roshani, S.; Talla, J.; Lalbakhsh, A.; Peroutka, Z.; Roshani, S.; Sabet, A.; Dehghani, M.; Lotfi, S.; Hadjilooei, F.; et al. A Review on Potentials of Artificial Intelligence Approaches to Forecasting COVID-19 Spreading. *AI* **2022**, *3*, 493–511. [CrossRef]
32. Salgotra, R.; Gandomi, M.; Gandomi, A.H. Evolutionary modelling of the COVID-19 pandemic in fifteen most affected countries. *Chaos Solitons Fractals* **2020**, *140*, 110118. [CrossRef]
33. Shinde, G.R.; Kalamkar, A.B.; Mahalle, P.N.; Dey, N.; Chaki, J.; Ssanien, A.E. Forecasting models for coronavirus disease (COVID-19): A survey of the state-of-the-art. *SN Comput. Sci.* **2020**, *1*, 1–15. [CrossRef]
34. Albahri, O.S.; Zaidan, A.A.; Albahri, A.S.; Zaidan, B.B.; Abdulkareem, K.H.; Al-Qaysi, Z.T.; Alamoodi, A.H.; Aleesa, A.M.; Chyad, M.A.; Alesa, R.M.; et al. Systematic review of artificial intelligence techniques in the detection and classification of COVID-19 medical images in terms of evaluation and benchmarking: Taxonomy analysis, challenges, future solutions and methodological aspects. *J. Infect. Public Health* **2020**, *13*, 1381–1396. [CrossRef]
35. Ahmad, F.; Almuayqil, S.N.; Mamoona, H.; Shahid, N.; Wasim Ahmad, K.; Kashaf, J. Prediction of COVID-19 cases using machine learning for effective public health management. *Comput. Mater. Contin.* **2020**, *66*, 2265–2282. [CrossRef]
36. Monshi, M.M.A.; Poon, J.; Chung, V. Deep learning in generating radiology reports: A survey. *Artif. Intell. Med.* **2020**, *106*, 101878. [CrossRef]
37. Jalaber, C.; Lapotre, T.; Morcet-Delattre, T.; Ribet, F.; Jouneau, S.; Lederlin, M. Chest CT in COVID-19 pneumonia: A review of current knowledge. *Diagn. Interv. Imaging* **2020**, *101*, 431–437. [CrossRef]
38. Shaikh, F.; Andersen, M.B.; Sohail, M.R.; Mulero, F.; Awan, O.; Dupont-Roettger, D.; Kubassova, O.; Dehmeshki, J.; Bisdas, S. Current landscape of imaging and the potential role for artificial intelligence in the management of COVID-19. *Curr. Probl. Diagn. Radiol.* **2021**, *50*, 430–435. [CrossRef]
39. Dong, J.; Wu, H.; Zhou, D.; Li, K.; Zhang, Y.; Ji, H.; Tong, Z.; Lou, S.; Liu, Z. Application of big data and artificial intelligence in COVID-19 prevention, diagnosis, treatment and management decisions in China. *J. Med. Syst.* **2021**, *45*, 1–11. [CrossRef]
40. Asteris, P.G.; Gavriilaki, E.; Touloumenidou, T.; Koravou, E.E.; Koutra, M.; Papayanni, P.G.; Anagnostopoulos, A. Genetic Prediction of ICU hospitalization and mortality in COVID-19 patients using artificial neural networks. *J. Cell. Mol. Med.* **2022**, *26*, 1445–1455. [CrossRef]
41. Shi, F.; Wang, J.; Shi, J.; Wu, Z.; Wang, Q.; Tang, Z.; He, K.; Shi, Y.; Shen, D. Review of artificial intelligence techniques in imaging data acquisition, segmentation, and diagnosis for COVID-19. *IEEE Rev. Biomed. Eng.* **2020**, *14*, 4–15. [CrossRef]

42. Merkoçi, A.; Li, C.Z.; Lechuga, L.M.; Ozcan, A. COVID-19 biosensing technologies. *Biosens. Bioelectron.* **2021**, *178*, 113046. [CrossRef]

43. Maheshwari, V.; Mahmood, M.R.; Sravanthi, S.; Arivazhagan, N.; ParimalaGandhi, A.; Srihari, K.; Sagayaraj, R.; Udayakumar, E.; Natarajan, Y.; Bachanna, P.; et al. Nanotechnology-Based Sensitive Biosensors for COVID-19 Prediction Using Fuzzy Logic Control. *J. Nanomater.* **2021**, *2021*, 3383146. [CrossRef]

44. Salgotra, R.; Gandomi, M.; Gandomi, A.H. Time series analysis and forecast of the COVID-19 pandemic in India using genetic programming. *Chaos Solitons Fractals* **2020**, *138*, 109945. [CrossRef]

45. Wang, S.; Kang, B.; Ma, J.; Zeng, X.; Xiao, M.; Guo, J.; Cai, M.; Yang, J.; Li, Y.; Meng, X.; et al. A deep learning algorithm using CT images to screen for Corona Virus Disease (COVID-19). *Eur. Radiol.* **2021**, *31*, 6096–6104. [CrossRef]

46. Jin, W.; Stokes, J.M.; Eastman, R.T.; Itkin, Z.; Zakharov, A.V.; Collins, J.J.; Jaakkola, T.S.; Barzilay, R. Deep learning identifies synergistic drug combinations for treating COVID-19. *Proc. Natl. Acad. Sci. USA* **2021**, *118*, e2105070118. [CrossRef]

47. Xu, X.; Jiang, X.; Ma, C.; Du, P.; Li, X.; Lv, S.; Yu, L.; Ni, Q.; Chen, Y.; Su, J.; et al. Deep learning system to screen coronavirus disease 2019 pneumonia. *Engineering* **2020**, *6*, 1122–1129. [CrossRef]

48. Li, L.; Qin, L.; Xu, Z.; Yin, Y.; Wang, X.; Kong, B.; Bai, J.; Lu, Y.; Fang, Z.; Song, Q.; et al. Artificial intelligence distinguishes COVID-19 from community acquired pneumonia on chest CT. *Radiology* **2020**, 200905. [CrossRef]

49. Wang, L.; Wong, A. COVID-net: A tailored deep convolutional neural network design for detection of COVID-19 cases from chest radiography images. *Sci. Rep.* **2020**, *10*, 19549. [CrossRef] [PubMed]

50. Emery, S.L.; Erdman, D.D.; Bowen, M.D.; Newton, B.R.; Winchell, M.; Meyer, F.; Tong, S.; Cook, T.; Holloway, P.; McCaustland, K.A.; et al. Real-time reverse transcription-polymerase Chain reaction assay for SARS-associated Coronavirus. *Emerg. Infect. Dis.* **2004**, *10*, 311–316. [CrossRef]

51. Baz, A.; Alhakami, H. Fuzzy based decision-making approach for evaluating the severity of COVID-19 pandemic in cities of kingdom of saudi arabia. *Comput. Mater. Contin.* **2021**, *66*, 1155–1174. [CrossRef]

52. Khan, M.A. An automated and fast system to identify COVID-19 from X-ray radiograph of the chest using image processing and machine learning. *Int. J. Imaging Syst. Technol.* **2021**, *31*, 499–508. [CrossRef]

53. Binsawad, M.; Albahar, M.; Sawad, A.B. VGG-CovidNet: Bi-branched dilated convolutional neural network for chest X-ray-based COVID-19 predictions. *Comput. Mater. Contin.* **2021**, *68*, 2791–2806. [CrossRef]

54. Narin, A.; Kaya, C.; Pamuk, Z. Automatic detection of coronavirus disease (COVID-19) using x-ray images and deep convolutional neural networks. *Pattern Anal. Appl.* **2021**, *24*, 1207–1220. [CrossRef]

55. Wang, Y.; Hu, M.; Li, Q.; Zhang, X.-P.; Zhai, G.; Yao, N. Abnormal respiratory patterns classifier may contribute to large-scale screening of people infected with COVID-19 in an accurate and unobtrusive manner. *E3S Web Conf.* **2021**, *271*, 01039.

56. Yan, L.; Zhang, H.; Goncalves, J.; Xiao, Y.; Wang, M.; Guo, Y.; Sun, C.; Tang, X.; Jin, L.; Zhang, M.; et al. A machine learning-based model for survival prediction in patients with severe COVID-19 infection. *medRxiv Prepr.* **2020**. [CrossRef]

57. Qi, X.; Jiang, Z.; Yu, Q.; Liu, C.; Huang, Y.; Jiang, Z.; Shao, C.; Zhang, H.; Ma, B.; Wang, Y.; et al. Machine Learning based CT radiomics model for predicting hospital stay in patients with pneumonia associated with SARS-CoV-2 infection: A multicentre study. *Ann. Transl. Med.* **2020**, *8*, 859. [CrossRef]

58. Yousri, D.; Abd Elaziz, M.; Abualigah, L.; Oliva, D.; Al-Qaness, M.A.; Ewees, A.A. COVID-19 X-ray images classification based on enhanced fractional-order cuckoo search optimizer using heavy-tailed distributions. *Appl. Soft Comput.* **2021**, *101*, 107052. [CrossRef]

59. Mousavi, M.; Salgotra, R.; Holloway, D.; Gandomi, A.H. COVID-19 time series forecast using transmission rate and meteorological parameters as features. *IEEE Comput. Intell. Mag.* **2020**, *15*, 34–50. [CrossRef]

60. Sumari, P.; Syed, S.J.; Abualigah, L. A Novel Deep Learning Pipeline Architecture based on CNN to Detect COVID-19 in Chest X-ray Images. *Turk. J. Comput. Math. Educ. (TURCOMAT)* **2021**, *12*, 2001–2011.

61. Jumper, J.; Hassabis, D.; Kholi, P. Alpha Fold Using AI for Scientific Discovery What Is the Protein Folding Problem? Why Is Protein Folding Important? 2018. Available online: https://deepmind.com/blog/article/alphafold-casp13 (accessed on 4 April 2018).

62. Yu, F.; Koltun, V. Multi-scale context aggregation by dilated convolutions. In Proceedings of the ICLR 2016, San Juan, Puerto Rico, 2–4 May 2016.

63. He, K.; Zhang, X.; Ren, S.; Sun, J. Deep residual learning for image recognition. In Proceedings of the IEEE Conference on Computer Vision and Pattern Recognition, Las Vegas, NV, USA, 27–30 June 2016; pp. 770–778.

64. Zhavoronkov, A.; Aladinskiy, V.; Zhebrak, A.; Zagribelnyy, B.; Terentiev, V.; Bezrukov, D.S.; Polykovskiy, D.; Shayakhmetov, R.; Filimonov, A.; Orekhov, P.; et al. Potential COVID-2019 3C-like protease inhibitors designed using generative deep learning approaches. *Chem. Biol.* **2020**. [CrossRef]

65. Makhzani, A.; Shlens, J.; Jaitly, N.; Goodfellow, I.; Frey, B. Adversarial autoencoders. *arXiv* **2015**, arXiv:1511.05644.

66. Maddah, E.; Beigzadeh, B. Use of a smartphone thermometer to monitor thermal conductivity changes in diabetic foot ulcers: A pilot study. *J. Wound Care* **2020**, *29*, 61–66. [CrossRef]

67. Facebook. Available online: https://www.facebook.com/ads/library/?active_status=all&ad_type=all&country=GB&impression_search_field=has_impressions_lifetime (accessed on 24 April 2020).

68. Allam, Z.; Jones, D.S. On the Coronavirus (COVID-19) outbreak and the smart city network: Universal data sharing standards coupled with artificial intelligence (AI) to benefit urban health monitoring and management. *Healthcare* **2020**, *8*, 46. [CrossRef]

69. Available online: https://economictimes.indiatimes.com/tech/software/how-to-use-aarogya-setu-app-and-find-out-if-you-have-covid-19-symptoms/articleshow/75023152.cms (accessed on 24 April 2020).

70. Chen, J.; See, K.C. Artificial intelligence for COVID-19: Rapid review. *J. Med. Internet Res.* **2020**, *22*, e21476. [CrossRef]

71. Abualigah, L.; Diabat, A.; Sumari, P.; Gandomi, A.H. A novel evolutionary arithmetic optimization algorithm for multilevel thresholding segmentation of COVID-19 ct images. *Processes* **2021**, *9*, 1155. [CrossRef]

72. Rahimi, I.; Chen, F.; Gandomi, A.H. A review on COVID-19 forecasting models. *Neural Comput. Appl.* **2021**, 1–11. [CrossRef]

73. Baz, M.; Khatri, S.; Baz, A.; Alhakami, H.; Agrawal, A.; Khan, R.A. Blockchain and artificial intelligence applications to defeat COVID-19 pandemic. *Comput. Syst. Sci. Eng.* **2022**, *40*, 691–702. [CrossRef]

74. Malpani Dhoot, N.; Goenka, U.; Ghosh, S.; Jajodia, S.; Chand, R.; Majumdar, S.; Ramasubban, S. Assigning computed tomography involvement score in COVID-19 patients: Prognosis prediction and impact on management. *BJR Open* **2020**, *2*, 20200024. [CrossRef] [PubMed]

75. Maghraby, A.; ALsakiti, F.; Alsubhi, A.; Alghamdi, R. Software to Assist a Health Practitioner in Caring of COVID-19 Home Isolated Patients. In Proceedings of the 2021 National Computing Colleges Conference (NCCC), Taif, Saudi Arabia, 27–28 March 2021; pp. 1–4.

76. Bai, X.; Wang, H.; Ma, L.; Xu, Y.; Gan, J.; Fan, Z.; Yang, F.; Ma, K.; Yang, J.; Bai, S.; et al. Advancing COVID-19 diagnosis with privacy-preserving collaboration in artificial intelligence. *Nat. Mach. Intell.* **2021**, *3*, 1081–1089. [CrossRef]

77. Cao, Y.; Xu, Z.; Feng, J.; Jin, C.; Han, X.; Wu, H.; Shi, H. Longitudinal assessment of COVID-19 using a deep learning–based quantitative CT pipeline: Illustration of two cases. *Radiol. Cardiothorac. Imaging* **2020**, *2*, e200082. [CrossRef] [PubMed]

78. Jin, C.; Chen, W.; Cao, Y.; Xu, Z.; Zhang, X.; Deng, L. Development and evaluation of an AI system for COVID-19 diagnosis. *Nat. Commun.* **2020**, *11*, 5088. [CrossRef] [PubMed]

79. Huang, L.; Han, R.; Ai, T.; Yu, P.; Kang, H.; Tao, Q.; Xial, L. Serial quantitative chest CT assessment of COVID-19: Deep-learning approach. *Radiol. Cardiothorac. Imaging* **2020**, *2*, e200075. [CrossRef]

80. Ai, T.; Yang, Z.; Xia, L. Correlation of chest CT and RT-PCR testing in coronavirus disease. *Radiology* **2019**, *296*, E32–E40. [CrossRef]

81. Alafif, T.; Tehame, A.M.; Bajaba, S.; Barnawi, A.; Zia, S. Machine and deep learning towards COVID-19 diagnosis and treatment: Survey, challenges, and future directions. *Int. J. Environ. Res. Public Health* **2021**, *18*, 1117. [CrossRef]

82. Lalmuanawma, S.; Hussain, J.; Chhakchhuak, L. Applications of machine learning and artificial intelligence for COVID-19 (SARS-CoV-2) pandemic: A review. *Chaos Solitons Fractals* **2020**, *139*, 110059. [CrossRef]

83. Rao, A.; Vazquez, J.A. VazquezIdentification of COVID-19 can be quicker through artificial intelligence framework using a mobile phone-based survey in the populations when cities/towns are under quarantine. *Infect. Control Hosp. Epidemiol.* **2020**, *41*, 826–830.

84. Hamzah, F.A.B.; Lau, C.H.; Nazri, H.; Ligot, D.; Lee, G.; Bin Mohd Shaib, M.K.; Binti Zaidon, U.H.; Abdullah, A. Worldwide COVID-19 outbreak data analysis and Prediction. *Bull. World Health Organ.* **2020**. [CrossRef]

85. gleamviz. Available online: http://www.gleamviz.org/ (accessed on 19 December 2022).

86. Metabiota. Available online: https://www.metabiota.com/ (accessed on 24 April 2020).

87. Epidemictracker. Available online: https://www.epidemictracker.com (accessed on 24 April 2020).

88. Shuja, J.; Alanazi, E.; Alasmary, W.; Alashaikh, A. COVID-19 open source data sets: A comprehensive survey. *Appl. Intell.* **2021**, *51*, 1296–1325. [CrossRef]

89. Chen, T.; Guestrin, C. Xgboost: A scalable tree boosting system. In Proceedings of the 22nd ACM SIGKDD International Conference on Knowledge Discovery and Data Mining, San Francisco, CA, USA, 13–17 August 2016; pp. 785–794.

90. Shehab, M.; Abualigah, L.; Shambour, Q.; Abu-Hashem, M.A.; Shambour MK, Y.; Alsalibi, A.I.; Gandomi, A.H. Machine learning in medical applications: A review of state-of-the-art methods. *Comput. Biol. Med.* **2022**, *145*, 105458. [CrossRef]

91. Ferguson, N.M.; Laydon, D.; Nedjati-Gilani, G.; Imai, N.; Ainslie, K.; Baguelin, M.; Bhatia, S.; Boonyasiri, A.; Cucunubá, Z.; Cuomo-Dannenburg, G.; et al. *Impact of Non-Pharmaceutical Interventions (NPIs) to Reduce COVID-19 Mortality and Healthcare Demand*; Imperial College London: London, UK, 2020; pp. 3–20.

92. GJoynt, M.; Wu, W.K. Understanding COVID-19: What does viral RNA load really mean? *Lancet Infect. Dis.* **2020**, *3099*, 19–20.

93. Atawneh, S.H.; Ghaleb, O.A.; Hussein, A.M.; Al-Madi, M.; Shehabat, B. A Time Series Forecasting for the Cumulative Confirmed and Critical Cases of the COVID-19 Pandemic in Saudi Arabia using Autoregressive Integrated Moving Average (ARIMA) Model. *J. Comput. Sci.* **2020**, *16*, 1278–1290. [CrossRef]

94. Busse, L.W.; Chow, J.H.; McCurdy, M.T.; Khanna, A.K. COVID-19 and the RAAS—A potential role for angiotensin II? *Crit. Care* **2020**, *24*, 1–4. [CrossRef]

95. Zarocostas, J. How to fight an infodemic. *Lancet* **2020**, *395*, 676. [CrossRef]

96. Rodriguez, C.R.; Luque, D.; La Rosa, C.; Esenarro, D.; Pandey, B. Deep learning applied to capacity control in commercial establishments in times of COVID-19. In Proceedings of the 2020 12th International Conference on Computational Intelligence and Communication Networks (CICN), Nainital, India, 25–26 September 2020; pp. 423–428.

97. Sharma, N.; Sharma, R.; Jindal, N. Machine Learning and Deep Learning Applications-A Vision. *Glob. Transit. Proc.* **2021**, *2*, 24–28. [CrossRef]

98. Mbunge, E.; Akinnuwesi, B.; Fashoto, S.G.; Metfula, A.S.; Mashwama, P. A critical review of emerging technologies for tackling COVID-19 pandemic. *Hum. Behav. Emerg. Technol.* **2021**, *3*, 25–39. [CrossRef]

99. Liang, S.H.; Saeedi, S.; Ojagh, S.; Honarparvar, S.; Kiaei, S.; Mohammadi Jahromi, M.; Squires, J. An Interoperable Architecture for the Internet of COVID-19 Things (IoCT) Using Open Geospatial Standards—Case Study: Workplace Reopening. *Sensors* **2021**, *21*, 50. [CrossRef]
100. Biswas, S.; Li, F.; Latif, Z.; Sharif, K.; Bairagi, A.K.; Mohanty, S.P. GlobeChain: An Interoperable Blockchain for Global Sharing of Healthcare Data-A COVID-19 Perspective. *IEEE Consum. Electron. Mag.* **2021**. [CrossRef]

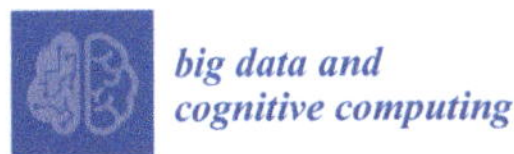

Article

Detecting Multi-Density Urban Hotspots in a Smart City: Approaches, Challenges and Applications

Eugenio Cesario [1,*,†], Paolo Lindia [2,†] and Andrea Vinci [3,†]

1 DiCES Department, University of Calabria, Via Pietro Bucci 18B, 87036 Rende, CS, Italy
2 DIMES Department, University of Calabria, Via Pietro Bucci 42c, 87036 Rende, CS, Italy
3 Institute for High-Performance Computing and Networking (ICAR), CNR—National Research Council of Italy, Via Pietro Bucci, Cubo 8/9C, 87036 Rende, CS, Italy
* Correspondence: eugenio.cesario@unical.it
† These authors contributed equally to this work.

Abstract: Leveraged by a large-scale diffusion of sensing networks and scanning devices in modern cities, huge volumes of geo-referenced urban data are collected every day. Such an amount of information is analyzed to discover data-driven models, which can be exploited to tackle the major issues that cities face, including air pollution, virus diffusion, human mobility, crime forecasting, traffic flows, etc. In particular, the detection of city hotspots is de facto a valuable organization technique for framing detailed knowledge of a metropolitan area, providing high-level summaries for spatial datasets, which are a valuable support for planners, scientists, and policymakers. However, while classic density-based clustering algorithms show to be suitable for discovering hotspots characterized by homogeneous density, their application on multi-density data can produce inaccurate results. In fact, a proper threshold setting is very difficult when clusters in different regions have considerably different densities, or clusters with different density levels are nested. For such a reason, since metropolitan cities are heavily characterized by variable densities, multi-density clustering seems to be more appropriate for discovering city hotspots. Indeed, such algorithms rely on multiple minimum threshold values and are able to detect multiple pattern distributions of different densities, aiming at distinguishing between several density regions, which may or may not be nested and are generally of a non-convex shape. This paper discusses the research issues and challenges for analyzing urban data, aimed at discovering multi-density hotspots in urban areas. In particular, the study compares the four approaches (DBSCAN, OPTICS-xi, HDBSCAN, and CHD) proposed in the literature for clustering urban data and analyzes their performance on both state-of-the-art and real-world datasets. Experimental results show that multi-density clustering algorithms generally achieve better results on urban data than classic density-based algorithms.

Keywords: smart city; density-based clustering; multi-density city hotspots detection; urban data analysis

Citation: Cesario, E.; Lindia, P.; Vinci, A. Detecting Multi-Density Urban Hotspots in a Smart City: Approaches, Challenges and Applications. *Big Data Cogn. Comput.* 2023, 7, 29. https://doi.org/10.3390/bdcc7010029

Academic Editor: Carson K. Leung

Received: 28 December 2022
Revised: 22 January 2023
Accepted: 3 February 2023
Published: 8 February 2023

1. Introduction

Reference Context. Cities worldwide are experiencing significant evolution due to numerous factors, e.g., new forms of communication, new ways of transportation, and fast urbanization. The pervasive and large-scale diffusion of sensing networks, image-scanning devices, and GPS devices is enabling the collection of huge volumes of geo-referenced urban data every day. As more and more data become available, data scientists can analyze such an abundance of urban spatial data to discover predictive and descriptive data-driven models, which can assist city managers in dealing with the major problems that cities face, e.g., human mobility, traffic flows, air pollution, crime forecasts, and virus diffusion [1–9]. In particular, detecting city hotspots is emerging as a frequent task when analyzing urban data. In fact, given the availability of geo-referenced data, it is useful to detect areas where urban events (e.g., crimes, traffic spikes, viral infections, and pollution peaks) occur with a higher density than in other regions of the dataset. Additionally, hotspot detection can serve as a useful organizational technique for elaborating thorough knowledge of an urban area, and their borders and shapes can enable high-level spatial knowledge summaries, which are valuable for policymakers, scientists, and planners [5,10,11]. As an instance, environmental scientists are interested in partitioning a city into uniform regions based on environmental characteristics and pollution density [3,12]. Similarly, during viral emergencies, as recently happened with the COVID-19 pandemic, virologists and epidemiologists are steadily interested in detecting city hotspots in which viruses are spreading with higher densities than other areas of the same city [6,7,13]. Moreover, city administrators can be interested in determining uniform regions of a city with respect to the functions they serve for citizens or visiting people. Additionally, police authorities are interested in detecting crime hotspots (i.e., areas with a high crime density) to ensure public safety in the city territory better [4,5]. Regarding data analysis, the search for intra-hotspot and inter-hotspot models is a hot topic for scientists. For instance, intra-hotspot models can reveal the changes in density within a hotspot over time, and inter-hotspot models can study how the appearance of a given hotspot can affect the generation of other hotspots in a different area [14].

Motivations. In metropolitan cities, the density of events, traffic, or population can differ widely between different areas, making urban regions highly dissimilar regarding density. This issue is made evident in Figure 1, which shows how inter-city and intra-city population densities strongly differ in different metropolitan city areas. Specifically, Figure 1a plots the population density of the 200 densest square kilometer grid cells in six representative cities [15], while the coefficient of variation of the population density of several countries is shown in Figure 1b. Focusing on the first chart (https://garrettdashnelson.github.io/square-density/, accessed on 18 December 2022), we can observe that densities largely vary within the same city, and between several cities. As an instance, New York City represents a classic case of multi-density regions: there are several high-density areas (Manhattan), and many other low-density areas (Queens). Chicago shows similarly top-heavy density pyramids, where the high-density areas (Loop and Near North Side) stand out from the rest of the region [15]. Other cities, such as Boston, San Francisco, and Los Angeles, show similarly multi-density distributions, with a high variation of densities among different city regions. As a second observation, it is worth noting that densities largely vary between several cities. For example, it is worth noting that the lowest-density areas of New York City are even denser than the densest parts of Dallas or Boston, and that even Chicago and Los Angeles' densest areas barely crack into the bottom half of New York City's top 200. On the other side, Figure 1b shows the average, minimum, and maximum values (and the names of the corresponding cities) of the coefficient of variation of the population density for several countries [16]. The coefficient of variation displayed in Figure 1b is defined as the relative standard deviation of urban population density, i.e., $CV = SD/PD$, where given a city, SD is the standard deviation of population density within the city, and PD is the average population density of the same area. Thus, the coefficient of variation is a unit-free measure of the density variation of the population within a city. The higher the coefficient of density variation of a city, the higher the dispersion in the population density of a city. The chart confirms a very high variability of densities within the same country, and between several countries. For example, in Mexico, the coefficient of variation ranges from 1.05 in Mexico City to 14.03 in Navajoa, showing an extremely high dispersion in population density. A similar observation can be made for Korea, the U.S., Canada, and the other listed countries. This aspect must be taken in consideration to properly infer the real hotspots when analyzing urban data. The density of traffic, events, population, etc., in metropolitan cities can largely differ between different areas, making urban regions extremely dissimilar in terms of density. It is worth noting that, in our experience, given an urban area and a set of events

(related to, for example, crimes, COVID infections, and mobility), high-density variations
can be observed in the collected data.

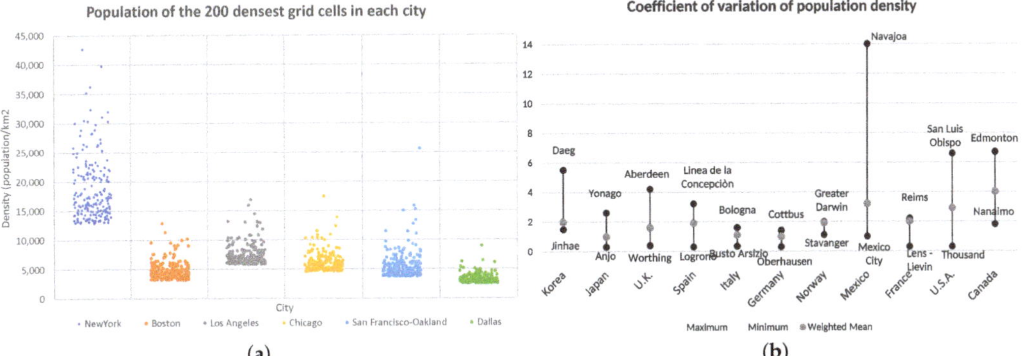

Figure 1. Intra-city and inter-city population densities in metropolitan urban areas. (**a**) Population
densities of the densest 200 cells for a given set of cities. Each cell has a 1 km^2 area [17]. (**b**) Coefficient
of variation of population density across urban areas and countries (2014) [16]. For each country,
the gray dot is the average computed on the coefficient of variation of each city of the country.
The figure also displays, for each country, the minimum and the maximum coefficients of variation,
and the cities where they occur.

Clustering is the most appropriate technique to discover urban hotspots. However, we
can split such algorithms into two groups. The first group includes algorithms that, due to
the adoption of global parameters, define a single minimum threshold value to distinguish
between dense and not-dense areas. Often, a proper threshold setting becomes all the more
difficult when clusters in different regions of the feature space have considerably different
densities, or clusters with different density levels are nested. In such cases, the partitioning
might not be proper with one single-density threshold. In fact, if the chosen threshold is too
high, they can discover several small non-significant clusters that actually do not represent
dense regions; otherwise, if the chosen threshold is too low, they can discover a few large
regions that actually are no longer dense as well. As a matter of fact, the application of
such algorithms to a multi-density dataset, such as urban data, could not achieve good
results. The second group includes algorithms that rely on multiple minimum threshold
values. Such algorithms generally detect multiple pattern distributions of different densities,
aiming at distinguishing between several density regions, which may or may not be nested
and are generally of a non-convex shape. Then, they automatically estimate the number
of threshold values to optimally identify the different density regions, without any prior
knowledge about the data. Such algorithms usually detect better data partitioning than
single-density threshold algorithms, but their drawback is a very high computational cost.

Contributions and plan of the paper. Given the presented context, this paper presents
a study on hotspots detection in urban environments. As the main contribution, the study
compares the most important approaches proposed in the literature for clustering urban
data and analyzes their results on two synthetic datasets and a real-world one, having
in mind two different goals. The experimental evaluation on synthetic state-of-the-art
multi-density datasets is performed to evaluate the clustering quality and the ability of
the algorithms to retrieve proper hotspots. To do that, we exploit two synthetic datasets,
where each point owns a target cluster label, and thus the algorithms could be evaluated
qualitatively and quantitatively by taking advantage of such ground truth information.
The experimental evaluation on real-world data is performed on crime data from the
Chicago Police Department, inherently characterized by points distributed with very
different densities in the city area. Such a concrete scenario is exploited to show the

practical usefulness of density-based clustering algorithms in discovering multi-density urban hotspots in real urban cases.

The remainder of the paper is structured as follows. Section 2 briefly describes the most important density-based approaches in spatial clustering literature, and the most representative projects in that field of research. Section 3 presents a selection of the main density-based clustering algorithms exploited in the literature to analyze urban data, by summarizing how they work. Section 4 provides the comparative experimental evaluation of the different approaches on state-of-the-art datasets. Section 5 shows the algorithm results on a real-world scenario. Finally, Section 6 concludes the paper and plans future research works.

2. Related Works

The analysis of urban data and the detection of urban hotspots from geo-referenced data are very challenging tasks. For this purpose, several approaches have been proposed in the literature, tackling the problem by adopting clustering approaches. In some cases, the discovery of urban hotspots represents one step of a more complex workflow, based on a common inspiring idea of several approaches that first detect geographic hotspots and then extract predictive models of intra-hotspots and/or inter-hotspots. In this section, we briefly review the most representative research work in the area.

The DSPM (density-based sequential pattern mining) approach, aimed at the discovery of mobility patterns from GPS data, is proposed in [2]. The method consists of (i) discovering urban dense regions of interest (more densely passed through ones) and (ii) extracting mobility patterns among those regions. As a case study, the approach is applied to a real-life GPS dataset tracing the movement of taxis in the urban area of Beijing. Additionally, the authors describe a comprehensive validation methodology for assessing the accuracy and quality of detected dense regions and trajectory patterns. The approach relies on the DBSCAN algorithm for detecting dense regions and could be improved by considering multi-density clustering analysis, detecting also lower-dense but homogeneous regions.

An approach to predict ozone concentrations at given target observation stations, based on spatial clustering and multilayer perceptron models, is proposed [18]. In particular, the approach exploits k-means clustering to detect similar stations and then train them together to get a base model for spatial transfer learning. The final models are used to predict the ozone concentration for three-day-ahead prediction horizons. The experimental evaluation, performed using historical data of stations in Germany, has shown higher forecasting accuracy of ozone exceedances with respect to traditional chemical transport models and popular machine learning approaches. Since the work groups sensor stations which are localized on a large area, it could benefit from exploiting multi-density clustering algorithms instead of k-means. Additionally, in a recent paper [19], the application of artificial intelligence (AI) and machine learning (ML) to build air pollution models, aimed at forecasting pollutant concentrations and health risks, is analyzed. The paper depicts how air pollution data can be uploaded into AI-ML models to discover the correlation between exposure to pollution and public health risks, giving a survey of applications and challenges of such a research field. In particular, it is pointed out that explainability is one of the paramount requirements in choosing AI-ML models for analyzing pollution data.

In [20], an approach is proposed to predict high-resolution electric consumption trends at finely resolved spatial and temporal scales. The approach is composed of two steps. First, apartment-level historical electric consumptions data are collected and clustered. Second, the clusters are aggregated based on the consumption profiles of consumers. The clustering analysis is performed by the k-means algorithm, while forecasting models are discovered by two deep learning techniques: long short-term memory unit (LSTM) and gated recurrent unit (GRU). The experimental evaluation was performed on electricity consumption data collected from residential buildings situated in an urban area of South Korea. In particular, a comparative analysis with state-of-the-art machine learning models and deep learning variants showed good performance in terms of building- and floor-level prediction accuracy.

The clustering of the consumption profiles of the consumers does not take into account features related to the location of apartments, buildings and floors. A multi-density hotspot detection can benefit the analysis, as it could group together building in the same city area, maybe constructed in the same years and having similar characteristics.

In [21], the authors designed a workflow composed of five steps, i.e., data pre-processing, feature extraction, machine learning training, performance evaluation, and explainable artificial intelligence, to analyze the effects of changes in land cover, such as deforestation or urbanization, on the local climate. In particular, machine learning models have been trained to learn the relation between land cover changes and temperature changes. Then, explainable artificial intelligence has been further exploited to interpret and analyze the impact of different land cover changes on temperature. Additionally, the experimental results have shown that random forest outperformed other machine learning methods (e.g., linear regression) proposed in the literature for discovering the relation of land cover–temperature changes.

A methodology for discovering behavior rules, correlations, and mobility patterns of visitors attending large-scale public events by analyzing social media posts is proposed in [22]. In particular, the authors describe a multi-step approach based on the detection of hotspots of interest (bounded areas) where the public events are held, collection of the geo-tagged items related to the events, gathering of trajectories of users publishing posts concerning such events, and discovery of touristic mobility patterns. The methodology is tested through two case studies: a mobility pattern analysis on Instagram users who visited EXPO 2015, and behavior modeling of geo-tagged tweets posted by users attending the 2014 FIFA World Cup, showing reasonable predictive accuracy.

A system for geo-localized crime data analysis, named CrimeTracer, is proposed in [23]. The approach is based on a probabilistic framework to discover spatial clusters in urban areas, and it is applied for crime event forecasting. In particular, the algorithm partitions the area of interest in activity spaces, which represent hotspots frequented by known offenders to make their criminal activities. On the bases of such knowledge, spatial crime predictions are performed on each activity space. Another approach for spatial data clustering is proposed in [24], which classifies locations as crime hotposts or no crime hotspots by exploiting one-class support vector machines (SVM). Similarly, in [25] an approach based on recurrent neural network models is designed to analyze spatial information and classify grid-cells as hotspot or not-hotspot.

An approach aiming at detecting crime hotspots in cities and forecasting crime trends in each hotspot is described in [5]. The approach leverages auto-regressive forecasting models and spatial cluster analysis to build a specific crime predictor for each hotspot detected during the spatial clustering analysis. The predictors can estimate crime trends in terms of the number of expected future crime events. The approach is assessed on real-world data, consisting of crime events collected in New York City and Chicago, and is demonstrated effective in terms of forecasting accuracy considering different time horizons. The above reviewed works in crimes analysis [5,23–25] are not capable of considering automatically detected hotspots characterized by different densities.

A predictive approach based on spatial analysis and regressive models is proposed in [13], aiming at discovering spatio-temporal predictive epidemic patterns from infection and mobility data. The algorithm is composed of several steps, starting from the detection of epidemic hotspots (urban areas where infection events occur more densely with respect to others) and mobility hotspots (urban regions more densely visited by mobility traces), to the discovery of epidemic patterns among epidemic hotspots. The approach finally processes each epidemic hotspot and analyzes the infection data of the epidemic hotspots involved in mobility patterns, then it extracts hotspot-specific epidemic forecasting models. The approach has been validated on real-world data regarding mobility and COVID-19 infections in Chicago. The paper focuses only on high-density hotspots in the given analysis and exploits the DBSCAN algorithm for detecting epidemic hotspots. This work can also benefit from the exploitation of other multi-density-based clustering algorithms.

3. Algorithms to Detect Urban Hotspots

This section shortly describes four density-based clustering methods—CHD, DBSCAN, HDBSCAN and OPTICS-Xi—that we selected from the literature as the most used and interesting approaches to analyze urban data.

3.1. DBSCAN

The DBSCAN (density-based spatial clustering of applications with noise) [26] algorithm is the precursor of all density-based clustering algorithms. It was developed to process large datasets with the inherent presence of noise. DBSCAN is capable of discriminating the noise points of a dataset and can detect clusters of any shape with no previous information about the number of expected clusters. Shortly, DBSCAN leverages the concepts of *core points, density-reachability*, and *density-connectivity*. Given two parameters ϵ and *minPts*, a point is a *core point* if there are at least *minPts* points in its neighborhood of radius ϵ (ϵ-neighborhood). A point p is directly density-reachable from a point q if q is a core point and p is in q's ϵ-neighborhood. Two points p and q are *density-reachable* if there exists a chain of directly density-reachable points that connect q and p. Finally, two points p and q are *density-connected* if there exists a core point o such that p and q are density-reachable from o.

DBSCAN builds a cluster of points by iteratively connecting a couple of points that are density-connected, and all the points that are density-reachable from a point of the cluster are in the same cluster. All points that do not belong to any cluster, and thus are not density-connected to any other point, are considered noise points. The DBSCAN can process a dataset of size n in $O(nlogn)$ time if exploiting a proper indexing structure on the data for executing the search for the ϵ-neighborhood. It is worth noting that, given the definitions above, it is clear that DBSCAN can detect clusters having at least a specific predetermined density ($\frac{minPts}{\pi r^2}$), directly determined by the ϵ and *minPts* parameters. For such a reason, it can fail to detect clusters characterized by different densities.

3.2. OPTICS-xi

The OPTICS-xi [27] algorithm is rooted in the concepts of reachability described for the DBSCAN, but it exploits some derived properties to build an ordered structure for the dataset containing information about every ϵ value in a given range, and it uses this structure to generate a proper clustering. The OPTICS indexing structure is based on the assumption that given a constant *min_pts* value, density-based clusters with respect to a higher density (i.e., a lower value for ϵ) are completely contained in density-connected sets with respect to a lower density (i.e., a higher value for ϵ). For each point, the structure stores the *core distance* and the *reachability distance*. Given a parameter *min_pts*, the *core distance* of a point p is the distance ϵ' to its $minPts^{th}$ nearest neighbor (it is undefined whether p has less than *minPts* neighbors). The *reachability distance* of point p with respect to a point o is, intuitively, the smallest distance such that p is directly density-reachable from o if o is a core point. By exploiting these above-introduced concepts, the OPTICS-xi algorithm is capable of generating an indexing structure of the dataset that keeps the cluster hierarchy for a variable neighborhood radius. Now, if a specific value for ϵ is chosen, by exploiting the structure, it is possible to perform a clustering that is very similar to the DBSCAN one. Given the generated values of reachability distance stored in the OPTICS indexing structure, the algorithm first generates the related *reachability plot*, and then it looks at the steep slopes within the graph to find clusters. The ξ ($0 < \xi < 1$) parameter is exploited to define what counts as a steep slope. The results of the *xi* clustering extraction method are very sensitive to the tuning of the ξ parameter. The OPTICS-xi time complexity is $O(nlogn)$.

3.3. HDBSCAN

The HDBSCAN algorithm [28], based on similar concepts defined for OPTICS, computes a complete clustering hierarchy composed of all possible density-based clusters for a large range of density thresholds. Then, it chooses the clustering model that maximizes the overall stability of the extracted clusters. To build such a hierarchy, the HDBSCAN starts from the concepts of *mutual reachability distance* between two core points p and q and given a value for a parameter *min_pts*. The *mutual reachability distance* is defined as the minimum ϵ radius such that p and q are mutually density-reachable. Differently from the above introduced *reachability distance*, the *mutual reachability distance* is symmetric.

HDBSCAN works as follows. First, it builds the clustering hierarchy by computing a *mutual reachability graph*, which is a complete graph where each vertex is a data point, and each edge is weighted with the mutual reachability distance of the linked couple of points. Then, a minimum spanning tree is computed on that graph, integrated by adding (for each vertex) a self-edge, weighted by the *core-distance* of the related data point. The tree is processed by removing the edges in decreasing order with respect to their weight. For each removal, the two involved edges are labeled as roots of a new pair of clusters, or noise if the generated component has not any edge. A variation of the summarized algorithm considers also a given minimum cluster size (*min_cluster_size* parameter), which avoids the generation of clusters having a size lower than *min_cluster_size*. Given the clustering hierarchy, a clustering is extracted which maximizes the overall stability. The notion of stability is derived from the notion of *excess of mass* [29]. HDBSCAN is able to compute the clustering hierarchy and extract the clusters in $O(n^2)$ time, which is in some cases infeasible and represents the main drawback with respect to DBSCAN and OPTICS.

3.4. City Hotspot Detector

The *city hotspot detector* (CHD) algorithm [30] is a multi-density based clustering algorithm that has been purposely designed for processing urban spatial data. The algorithm is composed of several steps, as follows. First, given a fixed *min_pts*, the reachability distance for each point is computed and exploited as an estimator of the density of each data point. Then, the points are sorted with respect to their estimated density, and the density variation between each consecutive couple of points in the ordered list is computed. The obtained density variation list is then smoothed by applying a rolling mean operator considering windows of size s. The points are then partitioned into several *density level sets*, on the basis of the smoothed density variations. Then, a different ϵ value is estimated for each density level set. Finally, each set is analyzed by the DBSCAN algorithm. Specifically, each instance takes in input, a specific ϵ value computed for the analyzed density level set. The set of clusters detected for each partition constitutes the final result of the CHD algorithm. The CHD algorithm runs with $O(nlogn)$ time complexity, where n is the size of the processed dataset. A cluster analysis with the CHD algorithm requires the tuning of more parameters (three) with respect to the previously introduced algorithms.

4. Experimental Evaluation and Results

In this section, we provide a comparative analysis of the four density-based clustering algorithms described in Section 3, namely CHD, DBSCAN, HDBSCAN, and OPTICS-Xi, by assessing the quality of the clusters detected by the algorithms and their ability to process datasets characterized by areas with different densities. The comparison is made on the results gathered by analyzing two datasets provided of the target cluster labels that are considered ground truth during the evaluation process. The experiments were carried out by exploiting the implementations provided by the `scikit-learn` Python library for DBSCAN and OPTICS-xi, the `hdbscan` Python library for HDBSCAN, and the R implementation of the CHD algorithm available at gitlab (CHD R-code: https://gitlab.com/chd3/chd-rcode/, accessed on 18 December 2022).

4.1. Data Description

The datasets chosen for the comparative analysis are *chess* and *compound*, two cluster-labeled datasets available in the literature [31,32], whose data instances and target clusters are shown in Figures 2 and 3. In particular, the two datasets have different characteristics, as reported in the following:

- The *chess* dataset is composed of 618 instances and partitioned in nine target clusters. Each instance is described by X and Y features (Figure 2). Clusters are *very contiguous*, and they have *regular block shapes, different densities and sizes*. In particular, the highest density cluster has a density $\sigma_5^{Chess} = 212.54$ (cluster n. 5, n. of points = 196, area = 0.92), while the lowest density one has a density $\sigma_7^{Chess} = 31.50$ (cluster n. 7, n. of points = 25, area = 0.79).

- The *compound* dataset is composed of 399 instances, described by X and Y features, and partitioned in six target clusters (Figure 3). Clusters are *well separated*, and they have *irregular multi-geometric shapes* (different from the previous dataset), *different densities and sizes*. In this dataset, the highest density cluster has a density $\sigma_6^{Compound} = 6.19$ (cluster n. 6, n. of points = 16, area = 2.58), while the lowest density cluster has a density $\sigma_1^{Compound} = 0.21$ (cluster n. 1, n. of points = 50, area = 236.60).

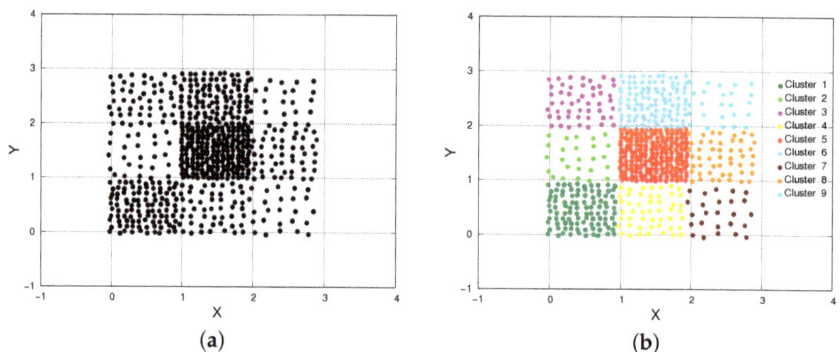

Figure 2. The *Chess* dataset: (**a**) data instances and (**b**) target clusters.

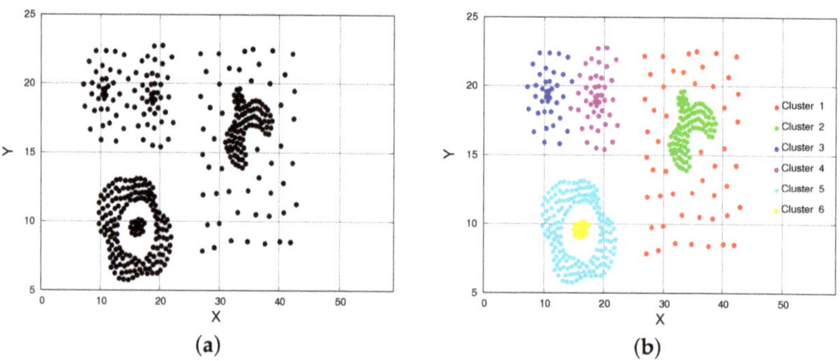

Figure 3. The *Compound* dataset: (**a**) data instances and (**b**) target clusters.

The multi-density distribution of instances, as well as their multi-shape partitions, makes such datasets very appropriate for our analysis because they model different scenarios to test and validate the algorithms on.

4.2. Results on State-of-the-Art Data

In order to evaluate the performance of the selected clustering algorithms over the above-introduced datasets, we compare the results obtained by the cluster analysis, i.e., the *discovered clusters*, to the ground truth labels provided by the datasets, i.e., the *target clusters*. By matching the discovered clusters against the provided target clusters, we can evaluate the effectiveness of the clustering algorithms. To do so, the following set of external metrics, designed to be employed when ground truth labels are available, are here adopted: *Fowlkes, Adjusted Rand, Adjusted Mutual Information (AMI), V-measure, Accuracy, F-*

measure, Jaccard, Γ, Rand and *Homogeneity* (more details about such metrics are reported in [33]).

In general, the listed metrics consider the number of items that are incorrectly allocated, i.e., items not assigned to a cluster of points sharing the same target cluster label. According to an external criterion, the result of a clustering algorithm is more satisfactory when fewer items are incorrectly allocated. All the above-listed metrics can assume values in the range [0, 1], where a value of 1 corresponds to a perfect match between discovered and target clusters, and lower values to the presence of a higher number of incorrectly allocated items. Therefore, such external metrics can be exploited to compare the performance results of clustering algorithms according to objective quantitative criteria.

It is worth noting that, for each clustering algorithm, the choice of the input parameters directly impacts the quality of the results; therefore, in order to make a fair comparison between the clustering algorithms, there is the need to carefully pick the input parameters with respect to the analyzed dataset. Let us recall that CHD receives k, ω and s as input parameters; DBSCAN requires the setting of ϵ and *min_pts*; HDBSCAN receives *min_cluster_size* and *min_pts* [28] as input parameters; and OPTICS-Xi requires the setting of ξ and *min_pts*.

In this paper, we adopted a parameter sweeping methodology for selecting the input parameters. Such a methodology consists in running several instances of each algorithm exploiting different parameter settings. For each algorithm, the parameter settings resulting in the best average performance, computed as the average of the above-listed metrics, are chosen. This process enables the modeler to determine a parameter's "best" value. Table 1 shows some details about the experimental setting adopted during the parameter sweeping. In particular, for each algorithm, the table reports the fixed parameter values, the chosen parameter to be swept and its range of values, the obtained best parameter value, and the corresponding best average performance.

Table 1. Experimental setting for the parameter sweeping for each algorithm.

Dataset	Algorithm	Fixed Parameter	Swept Parameter	Begin	End	Best Average Performance	Best Swept Parameter Value
Chess	CHD	$k = 4, s = 1$	ω	0.1	1.7	0.65	$\omega^* = 1$
	DBSCAN	*min_pts* = 4	ϵ	0.08	0.25	0.47	$\epsilon^* = 0.14$
	HDBSCAN	*min_pts* = 4	*min_cluster_size*	2	18	0.38	*min_cluster_size* = 3
	OPTICS-Xi	*min_pts* = 4	ξ	0.06	0.08	0.13	$\xi^* = 0.066$
Compound	CHD	$k = 4, s = 1$	ω	2.0	2.8	0.86	$\omega^* = 2.5$
	DBSCAN	*min_pts* = 4	ϵ	1.43	1.6	0.83	$\epsilon^* = 1.53$
	HDBSCAN	*min_pts* = 4	*min_cluster_size*	2	18	0.84	*min_cluster_size* = 15
	OPTICS-Xi	*min_pts* = 4	ξ	0.2	0.4	0.82	$\xi^* = 0.33$

Figure 4 reports the first set of experimental results, obtained on the *chess* dataset. The figure shows how quality indices vary versus swept input parameter values. Regarding the CHD algorithm (Figure 4a), it is clear how the trend is strongly affected by the values of the ω parameter, and the best results are obtained by considering $\omega^* = 1.00$. The DBSCAN algorithm is evaluated by varying the ϵ parameter from 0.08 to 0.22 (*minPts* = 4), and the best result is achieved for $\epsilon^* = 0.14$ (see Figure 4b). Similarly, we evaluate different input parameters settings for HDBSCAN (Figure 4c) and OPTICS-xi (Figure 4d). Even in these cases, little variations of the input parameters strongly affect the quality of the results. The best results are achieved considering *min_cluster_size* = 3 for HDBSCAN and $\xi^* = 0.066$ for OPTICS-xi.

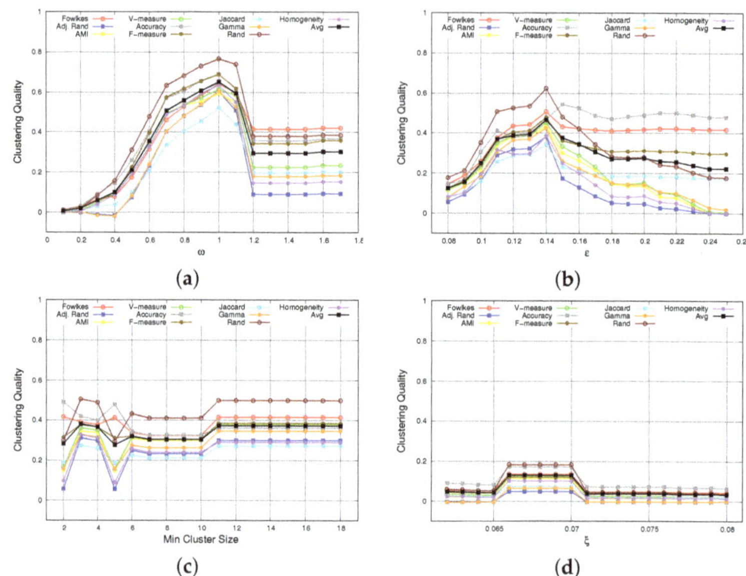

Figure 4. The *Chess* dataset: clustering quality indices vs. different input parameter values. (**a**) CHD. (**b**) DBSCAN. (**c**) HDBSCAN. (**d**) OPTICS-Xi.

Similarly, we run several tests on the *compound* dataset, whose results are reported in Figure 5. In particular, the figure shows how quality indices vary versus input parameter values. We can observe that, even for this dataset, input parameter values strongly affect the clustering quality and performance index values. As a result, we find that CHD achieves the best result for $\omega^* = 2.50$, DBSCAN for $\epsilon^* = 1.53$, HDBSCAN for $min\_cluster\_size^* = 15$ and OPTICS-Xi for $\xi^* = 0.33$.

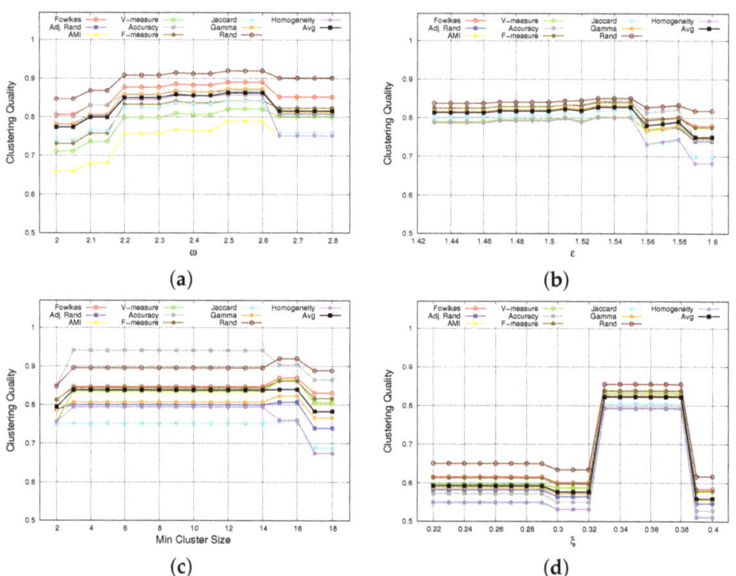

Figure 5. The *Compound* dataset: clustering quality indices vs. different input parameter values. (**a**) CHD. (**b**) DBSCAN. (**c**) HDBSCAN. (**d**) OPTICS-Xi.

A quantitative performance comparison among the considered algorithms is presented in Figure 6, where the values of the clustering indexes are shown for *chess* and *compound* datasets, by only referring to the run with the best combination of input parameters. In addition, Figure 7 plots the number of noise points and the number of detected clusters for both datasets. From the presented results, we can make the following considerations:

- *CHD detects higher quality clusters than DBSCAN, HDBSCAN and OPTICS-Xi.* For both datasets, in fact, Figure 6 shows that CHD achieves better performance than the other three algorithms, for all indices. Specifically, on *chess*, considering the best parameter setting case for each algorithm, CHD achieves an average clustering quality (computed over all indices) equal to 0.65, while DBSCAN, HDBSCAN, and OPTICS-Xi achieve 0.47, 0.38 and 0.13, respectively. Similarly, on *compound*, CHD slightly outperforms the other three algorithms, assessing on an average clustering quality equal to 0.86, while DBSCAN, HDBSCAN, and OPTICS-Xi achieve 0.83, 0.84, and 0.82, respectively. This is an interesting result since it shows that a multi-density approach, applied over such datasets, overtakes the other algorithms in terms of accuracy, compactness, and separability. In addition, the higher the closeness among clusters (*chess* dataset), the more evident the clustering quality improvement.

- *CHD and HDBSCAN detect a lower number of noise points than DBSCAN, and OPTICS-Xi.* Figure 7 shows the number of noise points and the number of clusters detected by the two algorithms. Specifically, Figure 7a shows that CHD, on the *Chess* dataset, is the algorithm detecting the lowest number of noise points (17%). On the *compound* dataset, HDBSCAN detects no noise points, while CHD detects the 5.3% of the total number of instances, which is a very low number as well. The other two algorithms detect a higher number of noise points.

- *CHD largely outperforms the other algorithms when detecting not-well-separated clusters.* Observing Figures 2 and 3, we can observe that the *chess* dataset shows clusters that are very contiguous and not-well-separated, while in the *compound* dataset, the separation among clusters is more evident. Generally, the low separation between clusters is a crucial issue for density-based algorithms to detect proper clusters. Considering the results of our tests performed on both datasets, it is worth noting that, in particular on the *chess* dataset, CHD outperforms the other three algorithms, for all indices (see Figure 6). This means that its application results in being more effective than the other approaches when clusters are very close, which is a classic urban case scenario. On the *compound* dataset (see Figure 6), characterized by well-separated clusters, all four algorithms achieve good results, and the difference in their performance is less evident than in the first dataset.

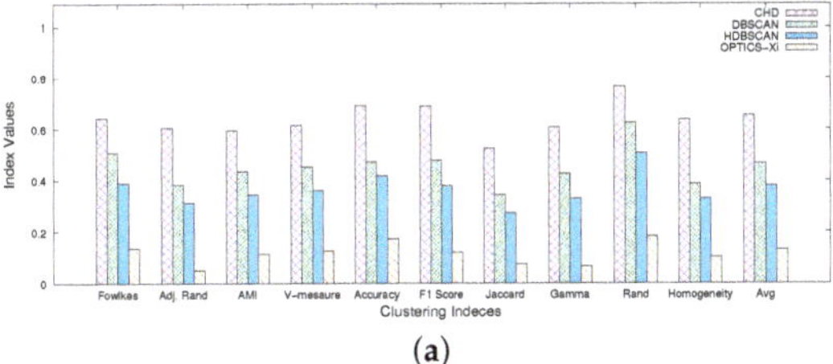

(a)

Figure 6. *Cont.*

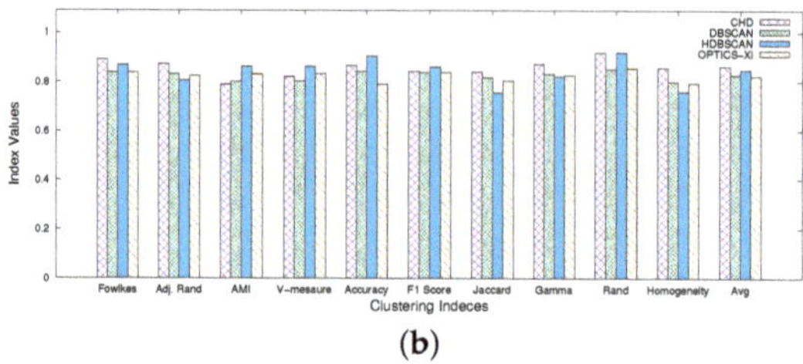

(b)

Figure 6. Best clustering results for the four algorithms on the two datasets: *chess* (**a**) and *compound* (**b**) datasets.

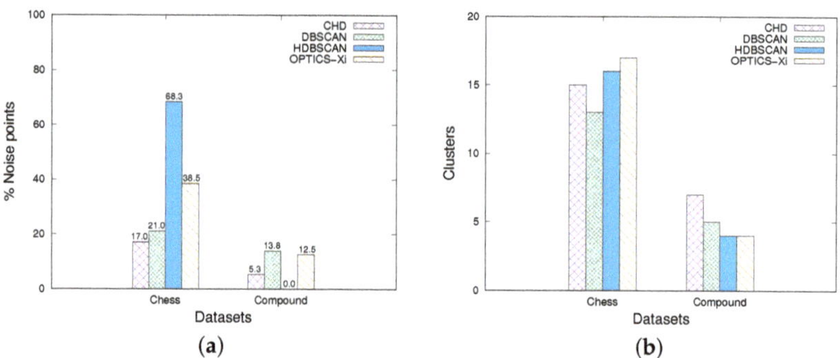

(a)   **(b)**

Figure 7. Number of noise points (**a**) and number of clusters (**b**) detected by the four algorithms on the two datasets.

Finally, Figures 8 and 9 show a qualitative comparison among the clustering models detected by the four algorithms on the two datasets. In particular, by observing Figure 8 (*chess* dataset) we can see that CHD detects 15 clusters, separability is quite good, and the number of noise points (in black) is very low with respect to the other algorithms. On the other side, DBSCAN and HDBSCAN detect a lower number of clusters than CHD, but a high number of noise points. Finally, OPTICS-Xi labels many instances as noise points, which makes the clustering quality very low. On the other side, by observing Figure 9 (*compound* dataset), we can see that the CHD and DBSCAN achieve a good separability among all clusters, while HDBSCAN and OPTICS-Xi are not able to separate the two clusters on the upper left side (cluster 1). It is worth noting that DBSCAN, OPTICS-Xi, and HDBSCAN could not detect the large low-density cluster on the right (cluster 1 in Figure 3b), labeling it as noise. That cluster is detected only by CHD.

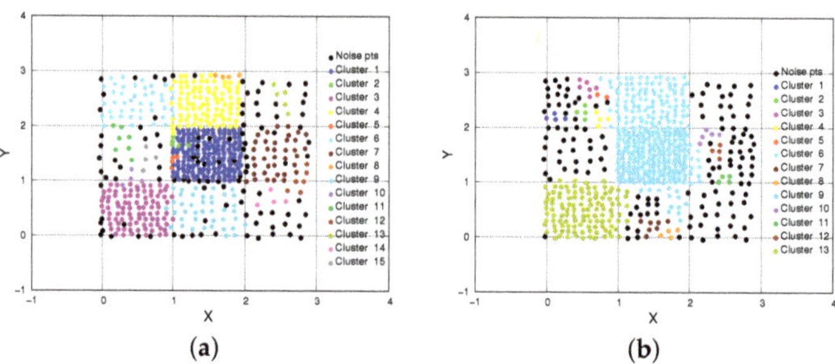

(a)   **(b)**

Figure 8. *Cont.*

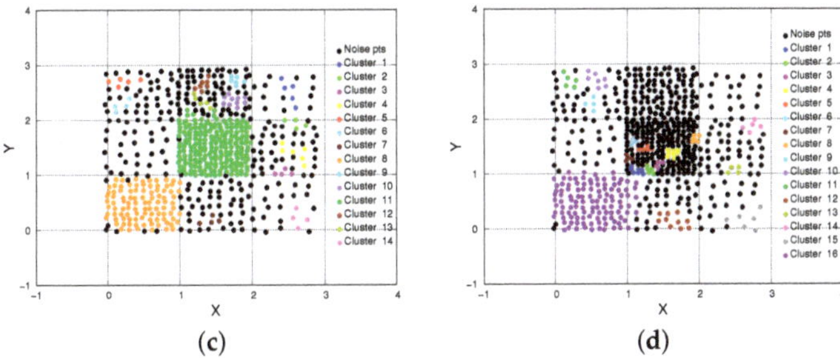

Figure 8. The *Chess* dataset: detected clusters. (**a**) CHD. (**b**) DBSCAN. (**c**) HDBSCAN. (**d**) OPTICS-Xi.

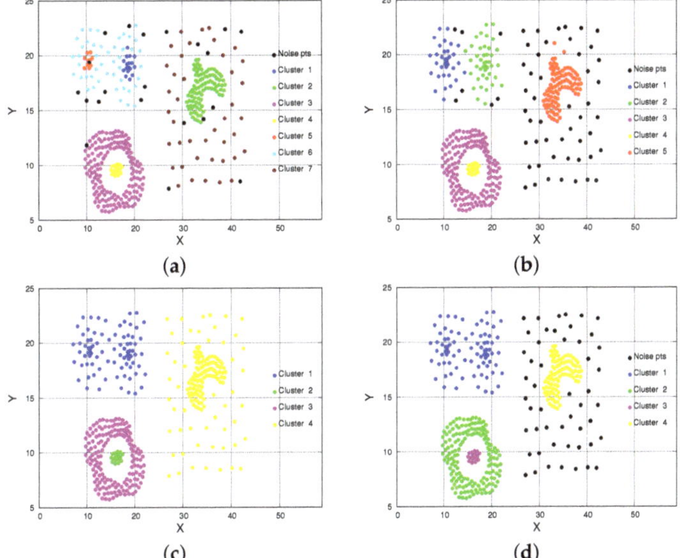

Figure 9. The *Compound* dataset: detected clusters. (**a**) CHD. (**b**) DBSCAN. (**c**) HDBSCAN. (**d**) OPTICS-Xi.

5. A Real-Case Study: Detecting Multi-Density Crime Hotspots in Chicago

To evaluate the performance and assess the effectiveness of the approaches described in Section 3 to discover city hotspots in a real-world scenario, we perform a comparative evaluation on geo-referenced crime events collected over a large area of Chicago. In particular, such tests aim at showing a concrete use case on which density-based clustering analysis can be exploited and the practical usefulness of the selected clustering algorithms to discover city hotspots in real urban cases.

5.1. Data Description

The experimental evaluation presented in this section is performed on the 'Crimes—2001 to present' dataset, consisting of a collection of crime events that occurred in Chicago from January 2001 to the present. The dataset is publicly available on the Chicago Data Portal (https://data.cityofchicago.org/, accessed on 18 December 2022), which also collects and provides open data about various aspects and events of Chicago, e.g., food inspection, traffic crashes, and COVID-19 vaccine diffusion. Each crime in the dataset is both geo-localized (with latitude and longitude) and time-stamped. Furthermore, it includes attributes describing other characteristics of each crime event, e.g., the FBI code and the crime type.

For the sake of our experimental evaluation, we consider only the latitude and longitude of crime events that occurred in 2012 and localized inside the boundary box shown in Figure 10a,b. The area has a perimeter of about 52 km and extends on approximately 135 km. The total number of crime instances is 100,219. The area includes different zones of the city, such as residential, commercial, tourist, and cultural zones, each one characterized by different crime densities. Given such a property, detecting urban hotspots in the area is a good benchmark to compare the performance results of the selected algorithms.

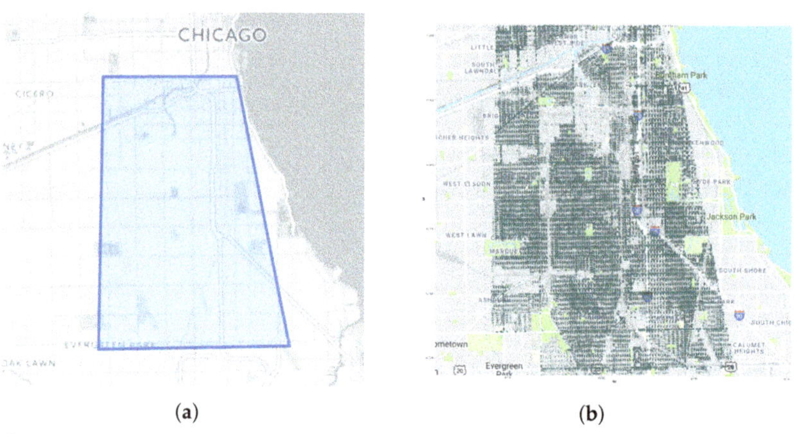

(**a**)   (**b**)

Figure 10. Selected area of Chicago and geo-localized crime events. (**a**) Polygon of the area; (**b**) geo-localized crime events.

5.2. Results

Similarly to the experimental evaluation performed on state-of-art datasets, we first assessed the best parameter settings for a fair comparison between CHD, DBSCAN, HDBSCAN, and OPTICS-Xi. We run several experimental tests to find the parameter settings capable of detecting the highest-quality city hotspots in terms of significance, compactness, and separability. Table 2 shows, for each algorithm, the selected input parameters and some statistics related to the achieved results. In particular, for each algorithm, the table reports the input parameter setting, the number of detected hotspots, the percentage of noise points, and the achieved Silhouette index values. In particular, Silhouette is an internal criterion to compute and evaluate clustering quality, and it is a measure of how similar an object is to its own cluster (cohesion) compared to other clusters (separation). The silhouette ranges from -1 to $+1$, where high values indicate that instances are well-matched to their own cluster and poorly matched to neighboring clusters. Thus, the higher the Silhouette value, the better the clustering quality (a more detailed description of this metric is reported in [33]). The hotspots detected by the considered algorithms are depicted in Figure 11, where they are highlighted through different colors, while noise points are black-colored.

Table 2. Overview of the results obtained by CHD, DBSCAN, HDBSCAN, and OPTICS-Xi.

	Input Parameters	# Hotspots	# Noise Points	Silhouette Index
CHD	$\omega = -0.27, k = 64,$ $s = 5000$	181	5.7%	-0.23
DBSCAN	$\epsilon = 500, minPoints = 60$	78	12.6%	-0.28
HDBSCAN	$min\_cluster\_size = 200,$ $minPoints = 60$	61	34.6%	-0.19
OPTICS-Xi	$\xi = 0.05, minPoints = 60$	279	71.9%	-0.46

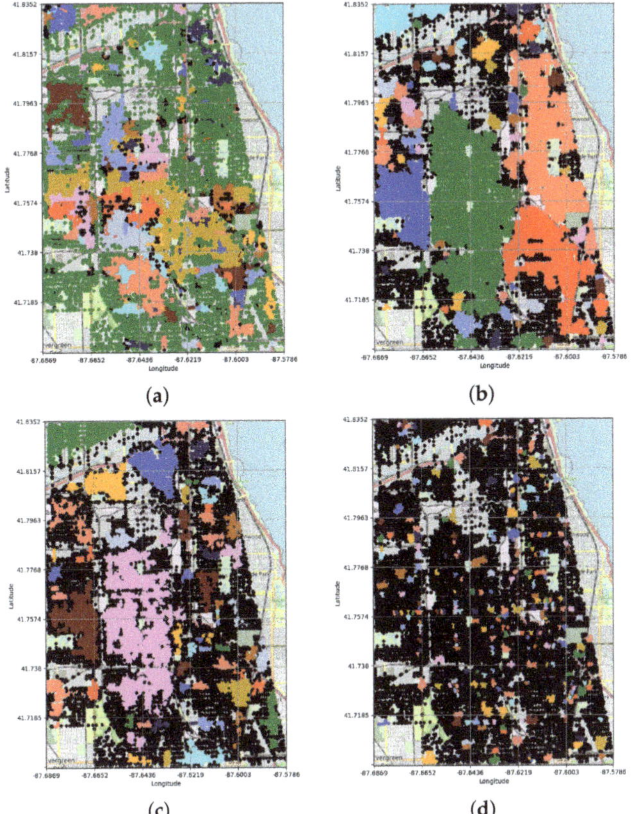

Figure 11. The *Crime* dataset: detected clusters. (**a**) CHD. (**b**) DBSCAN. (**c**) HDBSCAN. (**d**) OPTICS-Xi.

Now, by observing the hotspots detected by the algorithms and shown in Figure 11, and the values reported in Table 2, we can make some considerations:

- *CHD detects a higher number of significant hotspots than DBSCAN, HDBSCAN and OPTICS-Xi.* After a preliminary split in several density level sets, CHD partitions each one by exploiting specific ϵ values (as described in Section 3), finally detecting 181 hotspots; on the other side, DBSCAN and HDBSCAN detect a lower number of clusters, i.e., 78 and 61 hotspots, respectively. Finally, OPTICS-Xi detects 279 (very small) hotspots, which are not very significant.
- *CHD performs higher separation among the hotspots than DBSCAN, HDBSCAN and OPTICS-Xi.* The results depicted in Figure 11 highlight that CHD is able to achieve a more refined spatial partitioning than DBSCAN and HDBSCAN, splitting some areas of the city. Contrariwise, OPTICS-Xi detected a large number of noise points and a lot of very small hotspots. In particular, CHD detects several hotspots in the central area (colored in red, orange, violet, and blue in Figure 11a, whereas DBSCAN and HDB-SCAN labeled such points as only a single hotspot (the large green area in Figure 11b and the large violet area in Figure 11c). Similarly, CHD detects different hotspots in the left-middle part of the analyzed area, while DBSCAN and HDBSCAN label those as only one hotspot (colored in blue and red). OPTICS-Xi fails in a reasonable clustering of points, by detecting only some small hotspots sparsely distributed in the whole area. This shows that CHD is able to perform higher separation than the other algorithms among the city hotspots, by creating clusters having different densities.

- *CHD labels a lower number of noise points than DBSCAN, HDBSCAN, and OPTICS-Xi.* The noise points, which are those points that could not be assigned to a hotspot since they do not satisfy the density requirements of a given algorithm, are colored in black in Figure 11. Table 2 reports that CHD, DBSCAN, and HDBSCAN classify 5.7%, 12.6%, and 34.6% of data instances as noise points, respectively. On the other side, OPTICS-Xi labels almost 72% of total points as noise, showing de facto low-quality results. Considering the first three algorithms, it seems that CHD, in several cases, is able to better detect hotspots characterized by distinct densities, labeling a low percentage of instances as noise points. This is clearly evident by comparing Figure 11a–c. In particular, we can notice that large regions located in the top part and bottom part of the analyzed area are labeled as noise by DBSCAN and HDBSCAN (black-colored blows in Figure 11b,c), while CHD is able to detect several clusters from it (several hotspots colored in green and blue in Figure 11a). Finally, the presence of noise points in Figure 11d is pervasive and diffused, showing low-quality results achieved by OPTICS-Xi.

- *HDBSCAN and CHD achieve higher clustering quality than DBSCAN and OPTICS-Xi.* Table 2 shows that HDBSCAN and CHD assess on silhouette values equal to -0.19 and -0.23, respectively. Indeed, they achieve better results than DBSCAN and OPTICS-xi, whose clustering quality assess on -0.28 and -0.46. Such results show that multi-density clustering (i.e., HDBASCN and CHD) is able to distinguish several density regions and identify proper hotspots in urban environments better than DBSCAN and OPTICS-xi.

6. Conclusions

Detecting urban hotspots in smart cities is a challenging task, due to the fact that geo-spatial urban data, e.g., traffic, crimes, mobility, and events, are generally characterized by multiple densities that can differ widely from one area to another. This paper discussed research issues, challenges and approaches to discover multi-density hotspots in urban areas. Then, it compared the performance of four approaches (i.e., DBSCAN, OPTICS-xi, HDBSCAN, and CHD) available in the literature, and analyzed their performance on synthetic and real-world data. The evaluation on synthetic datasets was performed considering the best parameter setting for each algorithm, selected by a parameter sweeping methodology taking into account several quantitative clustering indexes. Similarly, a qualitative comparison of the different algorithms was performed on real urban data. Overall, the results showed that multi-density clustering algorithms (CHD and HDBSCAN) outperform classic density-based algorithms (DBSCAN and OPTICS-xi) when analyzing data characterized by multiple densities. Therefore, multi-density approaches are more appropriate for urban hotspot detection.

Author Contributions: Conceptualization, E.C. and A.V.; methodology, E.C. and A.V.; software, P.L. and A.V.; validation, E.C. and P.L.; formal analysis, E.C., P.L. and A.V.; investigation, P.L. and A.V.; resources, E.C. and P.L.; data curation, E.C., P.L. and A.V.; writing—original draft preparation, E.C. and A.V.; writing—review and editing, E.C., P.L. and A.V.; visualization, E.C., P.L. and A.V.; supervision, E.C. and A.V.; funding acquisition, E.C. and A.V.; All authors have read and agreed to the published version of the manuscript.

Funding: This work has been partially supported by the "ICSC National Centre for HPC, Big Data and Quantum Computing" (CN00000013) within the NextGenerationEU program, and by European Union—NextGenerationEU—National Recovery and Resilience Plan (Piano Nazionale di Ripresa e Resilienza, PNRR)—Project: "SoBigData.it—Strengthening the Italian RI for Social Mining and Big Data Analytics"—Prot. IR0000013—Avviso n. 3264 del 28/12/2021.

Data Availability Statement: The analyzed datasets are available as follows. The chess dataset is available at https://gitlab.com/chd3/datasets, accessed on 28 December 2022. The compound dataset is available at http://cs.joensuu.fi/sipu/datasets/, accessed on 18 December 2022. The

Chicago "Crimes—2001 to present" dataset is available at https://data.cityofchicago.org/Public-Safety/Crimes-2001-to-Present/ijzp-q8t2, accessed on 18 December 2022.

Conflicts of Interest: The authors declare no conflict of interest.

References

1. Li, L.; Jiang, R.; He, Z.; Chen, X.; Zhou, X. Trajectory data-based traffic flow studies: A revisit. *Transp. Res. Part C Emerg. Technol.* **2021**, *114*, 225–240.
2. Cesario, E.; Comito, C.; Talia, D. An approach for the discovery and validation of urban mobility patterns. *Pervasive Mob. Comput.* **2017**, *42*, 77–92.
3. Ali, M.E.; Hasan, M.F.; Siddiqa, S.; Molla, M.M.; Nasrin Akhter, M. FVM-RANS Modeling of Air Pollutants Dispersion and Traffic Emission in Dhaka City on a Suburb Scale. *Sustainability* **2022**, *15*, 673 . [CrossRef]
4. Wang, Q.; Jin, G.; Zhao, X.; Feng, Y.; Huang, J. CSAN: A neural network benchmark model for crime forecasting in spatio-temporal scale. *Knowl.-Based Syst.* **2020**, *189*, 105–120. [CrossRef]
5. Catlett, C.; Cesario, E.; Talia, D.; Vinci, A. Spatio-temporal crime predictions in smart cities: A data-driven approach and experiments. *Pervasive Mob. Comput.* **2019**, *53*, 62–74.
6. Chintalapudi, N.; Battineni, G.; Amenta, F. COVID-19 virus outbreak forecasting of registered and recovered cases after sixty day lockdown in Italy: A data driven model approach. *J. Microbiol. Immunol. Infect.* **2020**, *53*, 396–403. [PubMed]
7. Ghosh, S.; Bhattacharya, S. A data-driven understanding of COVID-19 dynamics using sequential genetic algorithm based probabilistic cellular automata. *Appl. Soft Comput.* **2020**, *96*, 106692. [CrossRef] [PubMed]
8. Hu, S.; Xiong, C.; Yang, M.; Younes, H.; Luo, W.; Zhang, L. A big-data driven approach to analyzing and modeling human mobility trend under non-pharmaceutical interventions during COVID-19 pandemic. *Transp. Res. Part C Emerg. Technol.* **2021**, *124*, 102955. [CrossRef] [PubMed]
9. Cicirelli, F.; Guerrieri, A.; Mastroianni, C.; Spezzano, G.; Vinci, A. *The Internet of Things for Smart Urban Ecosystems*; Springer: Cham, Switzerland, 2019.
10. Liu, P.; Zhou, D.; Wu, N. VDBSCAN: Varied density based spatial clustering of applications with noise. In Proceedings of the 2007 International Conference on Service Systems and Service Management, Chengdu, China, 9–11 June 2007; pp. 1–4.
11. Mitra, S.; Nandy, J. KDDclus: A simple method for multi-density clustering. In Proceedings of the International Workshop on Soft Computing Applications and Knowledge Discovery (SCAKD 2011), Moscow, Russia, 24 June 2011; pp. 72–76.
12. Cesario, E. Big Data Analysis for Smart City Applications. In *Encyclopedia of Big Data Technologies*; Sakr, S., Zomaya, A.Y., Eds.; Springer: Cham, Switzerland, 2019. [CrossRef]
13. Canino, M.P.; Cesario, E.; Vinci, A.; Zarin, S. Epidemic forecasting based on mobility patterns: An approach and experimental evaluation on COVID-19 Data. *Soc. Networks Anal. Min.* **2022**, *12*, 116.
14. Mastroianni, C.; Cesario, E.; Giordano, A. Efficient and scalable execution of smart city parallel applications. *Concurr. Comput. Pract. Exp.* **2018**, *30*, e4258. [CrossRef]
15. Garrett Dash Nelson. What Micro-Mapping a City's Density Reveals. 9 May 2021. Available online: https://www.bloomberg.com/news/articles/2019-07-09/what-micro-mapping-a-city-s-density-reveals (accessed on 18 December 2022).
16. Organisation for Economic Cooperation and Development (OECD). *Rethinking Urban Sprawl*; OECD: Paris, France, 2018; p. 168. [CrossRef]
17. Center for International Earth Science Information Network—CIESIN—Columbia University. Gridded Population of the World, Version 4 (GPWv4): Population Count, Revision 11, NASA Socioeconomic Data and Applications Center (SEDAC), 2021. Available online: https://sedac.ciesin.columbia.edu/data/set/gpw-v4-population-count-rev11 (accessed on 18 December 2022). [CrossRef]
18. Deng, T.; Manders, A.; Jin, J.; Lin, H.X. Clustering-based spatial transfer learning for short-term ozone forecasting. *J. Hazard. Mater. Adv.* **2022**, *8*, 100168.
19. Krupnova, T.G.; Rakova, O.V.; Bondarenko, K.A.; Tretyakova, V.D. Environmental Justice and the Use of Artificial Intelligence in Urban Air Pollution Monitoring. *Big Data Cogn. Comput.* **2022**, *6*, 75. [CrossRef]
20. Khan, A.N.; Iqbal, N.; Rizwan, A.; Ahmad, R.; Kim, D.H. An Ensemble Energy Consumption Forecasting Model Based on Spatial-Temporal Clustering Analysis in Residential Buildings. *Energies* **2021**, *14*, 3020. [CrossRef]
21. Kolevatova, A.; Riegler, M.A.; Cherubini, F.; Hu, X.; Hammer, H.L. Unraveling the Impact of Land Cover Changes on Climate Using Machine Learning and Explainable Artificial Intelligence. *Big Data Cogn. Comput.* **2021**, *5*, 55. [CrossRef]
22. Cesario, E.; Marozzo, F.; Talia, D.; Trunfio, P. SMA4TD: A social media analysis methodology for trajectory discovery in large-scale events. *Online Soc. Netw. Media* **2017**, *3–4*, 49–62.
23. Tayebi, M.; Ester, M.; Glasser, U.; Brantingham, P. CRIMETRACER: Activity space based crime location prediction. In Proceedings of the Advances in Social Networks Analysis and Mining (ASONAM), 2014 IEEE/ACM International Conference, Beijing, China, 17–20 August 2014; pp. 472–480.
24. Kianmehr, K.; Alhajj, R. Crime Hot-Spots Prediction Using Support Vector Machine. In Proceedings of the Computer Systems and Applications, IEEE International Conference, Dubai, United Arab Emirates, 8 March 2006; pp. 952–959.

25. Zhuang, Y.; Almeida, M.; Morabito, M.; Ding, W. Crime Hot Spot Forecasting: A Recurrent Model with Spatial and Temporal Information. In Proceedings of the 2017 IEEE International Conference on Big Knowledge (ICBK), Hefei, China, 9–10 August 2017.
26. Ester, M.; Kriegel, H.P.; Sander, J.; Xu, X. A density-based algorithm for discovering clusters in large spatial databases with noise. In Proceedings of the Second International Conference on Knowledge Discovery and Data Mining, Portland, OR, USA, 2–4 August 1996; Volume 96, pp. 226–231.
27. Ankerst, M.; Breunig, M.M.; Kriegel, H.P.; Sander, J. OPTICS: Ordering points to identify the clustering structure. In Proceedings of the ACM Sigmod Record, Philadelphia, PA, USA, 1–3 June 1999; Volume 28, pp. 49–60.
28. Campello, R.J.; Moulavi, D.; Zimek, A.; Sander, J. Hierarchical density estimates for data clustering, visualization, and outlier detection. *ACM Trans. Knowl. Discov. Data (TKDD)* **2015**, *10*, 1–51. [CrossRef]
29. Müller, D.W.; Sawitzki, G. Excess mass estimates and tests for multimodality. *J. Am. Stat. Assoc.* **1991**, *86*, 738–746.
30. Cesario, E.; Uchubilo, P.I.; Vinci, A.; Zhu, X. Multi-density urban hotspots detection in smart cities: A data-driven approach and experiments. *Pervasive Mob. Comput.* **2022**, *86*, 101687. [CrossRef]
31. Fränti, P.; Sieranoja, S. K-Means Properties on Six Clustering Benchmark Datasets. 2018. Available online: http://cs.uef.fi/sipu/datasets/ (accessed on 18 December 2022).
32. Zahn, C. Graph-theoretical methods for detecting and describing gestalt clusters. *IEEE Trans. Comput.* **1971**, *100*, 68–86.
33. Jain, A.; Dubes, R. *Algorithms for Clustering Data*; Prentice-Hall: Hoboken, NJ, USA, 1988.

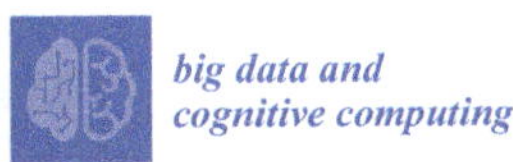
big data and cognitive computing

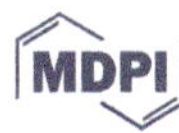

Systematic Review

Disclosing Edge Intelligence: A Systematic Meta-Survey

Vincenzo Barbuto [1], Claudio Savaglio [1,*], Min Chen [2] and Giancarlo Fortino [1]

1   Department of Computer Science, Modeling, Electronics and Systems Engineering (DIMES), Università della Calabria, Via P. Bucci, 87036 Rende, Italy
2   School of Computer Science and Engineering, South China University of Technology, Guangzhou 510641, China
*   Correspondence: csavaglio@dimes.unical.it

Abstract: The Edge Intelligence (EI) paradigm has recently emerged as a promising solution to overcome the inherent limitations of cloud computing (latency, autonomy, cost, etc.) in the development and provision of next-generation Internet of Things (IoT) services. Therefore, motivated by its increasing popularity, relevant research effort was expended in order to explore, from different perspectives and at different degrees of detail, the many facets of EI. In such a context, the aim of this paper was to analyze the wide landscape on EI by providing a systematic analysis of the state-of-the-art manuscripts in the form of a tertiary study (i.e., a review of literature reviews, surveys, and mapping studies) and according to the guidelines of the PRISMA methodology. A comparison framework is, hence, provided and sound research questions outlined, aimed at exploring (for the benefit of both experts and beginners) the past, present, and future directions of the EI paradigm and its relationships with the IoT and the cloud computing worlds.

Keywords: edge intelligence; Internet of Things; edge–cloud continuum; artificial intelligence

1. Introduction

The International Data Corporation (IDC) forecasts that, by 2025, over 150 billion devices will be connected across the globe [1], with the majority of them generating data in real-time. In the same year, the source forecasts also that Internet of Things (IoT) devices located at the network edge will generate over 90 Zettabytes of data, namely more than the half of the Global Datasphere (i.e., the amount of data created, captured, and replicated in any given year across the world).

This shift in the digital landscape, from centralized data centers to a network of dispersed ubiquitous devices, requires a reassessment of the current methods of data analysis and processing to keep pace with the burgeoning volume and velocity of data. Currently, cloud-based data analysis and learning systems enable organizations to store and process vast amounts of data, making them readily accessible from any location at any time [2]. This enables organizations to make rapid and informed decisions, optimize operations, and reduce costs. However, with the increasing volume of data being generated and the high-expectations of IoT services' QoS/QoE [3], there is a growing need for more efficient methods for data processing/analysis and for system management, to be implemented closer to the source of data collection. This is where Edge Intelligence (EI) comes in, as it allows for the processing and analysis of data as much as possible at the network's edge, instead of solely relying on centralized data centers. This truly distributed and pervasive computing approach not only reduces latency and data traffic, but it also enables real-time decision-making, improves scalability, privacy, and reliability, and ultimately, leads to more efficient and effective data analysis.

Being recognized as an extremely promising enabler for many next-generation IoT services in different smart-* domains, in a few years, the EI has become the centerpiece of a wide literature, spanning from very narrow technical contributions to comprehensive

Citation: Barbuto, V.; Savaglio, C.; Chen, M.; Fortino, G. Disclosing Edge Intelligence: A Systematic Meta-Survey. *Big Data Cogn. Comput.* **2023**, *7*, 44. https://doi.org/10.3390/bdcc7010044

Academic Editor: Moulay A. Akhloufi

Received: 31 January 2023
Revised: 21 February 2023
Accepted: 27 February 2023
Published: 2 March 2023

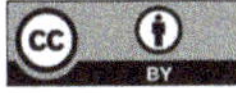

studies and informative analysis. As a result, currently, EI looks like a container of so many entangled concepts (astride IoT, AI, edge and cloud computing, data science) that are complex to approach and even more challenge to productively apply. Therefore, in order to offer an extensive and in-depth understanding of the theoretical basis, architectures, technologies, and application scenarios of the novel and multidisciplinary field of EI, this survey provides an overview of the research efforts made so far, by exploring the literature in accordance with two key principles:

- Comprehensiveness: The research methodology we applied to perform our systematic EI literature review followed the *PRISMA* guidelines [4], a formal protocol consisting of well-defined and reproducible steps centered on clear criteria for the selection of the target articles, aiming at high level of homogeneity and quality [5];
- Effectiveness: Given the infeasibility of an exhaustive study of the whole EI literature, we opted for a systematic review performed in the form of a *tertiary study*, a well-established approach, also known as *meta-analysis* [6], which has the purpose of aggregating and generalizing the main results from large collections of thematically related secondary studies (reviews, surveys, roadmaps, white papers, etc.).

The joint exploitation of these two distinct, but highly compatible, approaches to the research synthesis is a novelty in the EI literature (precisely, only [7] provided a systematic review) but as demonstrated in many other fields [8], it allows summarizing wide bodies of knowledge, quantifying the size, strength, and trend of research directions, and generating new valuable insights. Ultimately, this survey sets out to serve as a valid resource for anyone looking to stay current in this rapidly evolving field and to gain insights into the potential future developments in EI.

This manuscript is organized as follows. In Section 2, we introduce the main concepts to approach the EI paradigm, its diffusion in the IoT scenario, and its relationships with other mainstream paradigms such as edge and cloud computing, AI, etc. In Section 3, we provide a detailed report of the research objectives we pursued and of the search methodology we adopted, thus reviewing the obtained literature in Section 4. Final remarks conclude the manuscript in Section 5.

2. Background

EI has witnessed a significant surge in growth lately, being intrinsically tied to the progression of edge computing. However, at the beginning of the ubiquitous and pervasive computing era, there was a significant deficiency of intelligence at the network's edge in favor of a "remote" intelligence. For example, the primary function of Wireless Sensor Networks (WSNs) [9] was to gather and transmit data according to the "sense-and-forward" paradigm, by means of dumb sensors that were relatively simplistic and resource limited. Therefore, cloud computing emerged as a prevalent enabler for supporting WSNs due to its ability to provide scalable data storage and management, remote monitoring and control, and ease of use. Both WSNs and cloud computing have started, hence, to take advantage of one another: the former found the necessary computing power for implementing intelligent solutions to be fed with a huge amount of real-time data provided by the latter.

As the IoT has gained traction [10], a plethora of more sophisticated devices, known as "smart objects", emerged at the periphery of the network. These devices, such as smart thermostats, security cameras, and connected appliances, promised to make our lives easier by automating daily tasks and providing valuable insights. However, despite their improved capabilities, these devices continued to be heavily reliant on cloud-based infrastructure [11]: indeed, devices still remained unable to take actions without the assistance of the cloud since both the volume and the heterogeneity of the data increased dramatically, and consequently, only simple processing tasks and limited storage operations could be performed locally.

Only in the last decade, a number of issues about the IoT–cloud duo has emerged and pushed for a paradigm shift: indeed, while cloud-based infrastructure does provide the necessary scalability and flexibility for IoT devices, it also introduces a number of challenges. One major concern is the potential for data breaches and privacy violations, as sensitive information is transmitted to and stored on remote servers. Additionally, the reliance on cloud-based infrastructure can also result in unacceptably high latency in field-to-cloud and back transmissions, as well as exorbitant energy and bandwidth consumption. To address these issues, new computing paradigms such as edge and fog computing have emerged, with the intent to carry not only data processing, but more broadly, intelligence (intended as "Interacting, Interoperate, Cooperation, Communicating and Perception" capabilities [12]) as close as possible to the data sources, in the place of remote servers accessed over the Internet.

In this direction, more recently, EI has emerged in order to support the new and ambitious services and scenarios of the IoT. It incorporates both emerging and well-established approaches from edge and cloud computing, AI, data science, and networking to bring intelligence outside the boundaries of the cloud. This approach, also referred to as "Edge AI", pushes as much as possible for local operations, even better if directly on edge devices, such as smartphones, IoT devices, and industrial equipment, rather than in the cloud or a centralized data center. As illustrated in Figure 1, this strategy effectively reduces the amount of data transmitted from the device monitoring a target phenomenon to a remote server, thus reducing the time and the communication that pass between the operations of sensing and actuation. However, the challenge of EI involves not only embedding the characteristics of massive computing systems into tiny, restricted devices, as if trying "to fit an elephant into a small box" [13], but indeed, a full-fledged infrastructure to allow EI, at its extreme, to transform Big Data into intelligent data and to enable real-time device management, system performance, decision-making, and operation monitoring, thus improving overall responsiveness, privacy, effectiveness, and productivity [12,14–16]. Although EI holds the potential to rival the cloud, it cannot maximize its capabilities when employed alone. EI and cloud computing can complement each other seamlessly, with the optimum approach being a synergistic relationship, exemplified by the IoT–edge–cloud continuum [17]. This harmonious connection is crucial in today's technological arena, resulting in enhanced resource utilization, heightened efficiency, and the best outcomes.

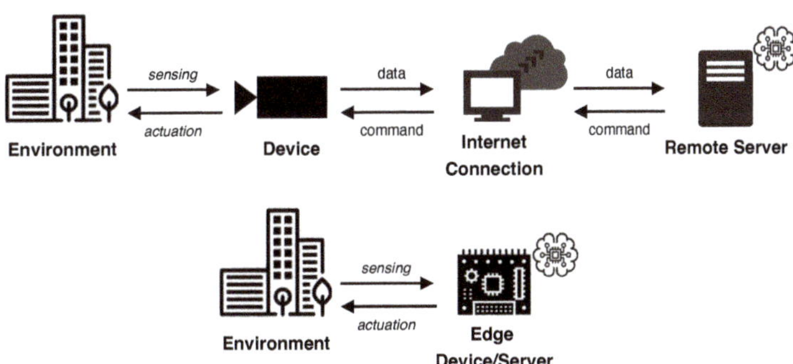

Figure 1. From remote (e.g., cloud-based) to local (e.g., EI) data processing.

3. Research Methodology

We undertook an initial informal search, which, together with personal knowledge, confirmed that there exist a relevant number of contributions on the EI topic and that a systematic review would be appropriate. It also provided the information needed to guide the manual search process. Accordingly, a survey of articles regarding EI spanning 13 years (from January 2011 to February 2023) was conducted in accordance with the guidelines of the PRISMA statement. After the record screening and the report selection processing, we analyzed a total of 50 works. However, they refer to specific domains (e.g., robotics [18] or cyber-security [19]) or technology (e.g., embedded intelligence for

FPGA [20]), to narrow contributions (e.g., a novel version of an algorithm or an optimized model [21,22]), and to broader surveys/review papers outlining definitions, goals, and roadmaps for EI. We decided to focus specifically on the latter and performed a further hand-made selection, which produced a systematic analysis literature in the form of a tertiary study of 14 publications. The undertaken *search plan* is summarized in Table 1, while Figure 2 depicts the flow-chart of the PRISMA-based selection process, detailed in the following subsections.

3.1. Objectives

This review aimed to identify the state-of-the-art on EI, at the confluence of AI, cloud, and edge computing, to bring intelligence as close as possible to the data sources. The survey was conducted to identify the current research trend and research challenges related to EI and to answer the following **Research Questions (RQs):**

- **(RQ1)** What are current definitions or interpretations of EI?
- **(RQ2)** Are there specific reference architectures that help to enable intelligence at the edge?
- **(RQ3)** What are the main topics (intended as broad subjects or themes) addressed by EI?
- **(RQ4)** What are the key techniques (intended as enabling, implementation methods) of EI?
- **(RQ5)** What are the pursued goals, the on-going efforts, and the future challenges for EI?

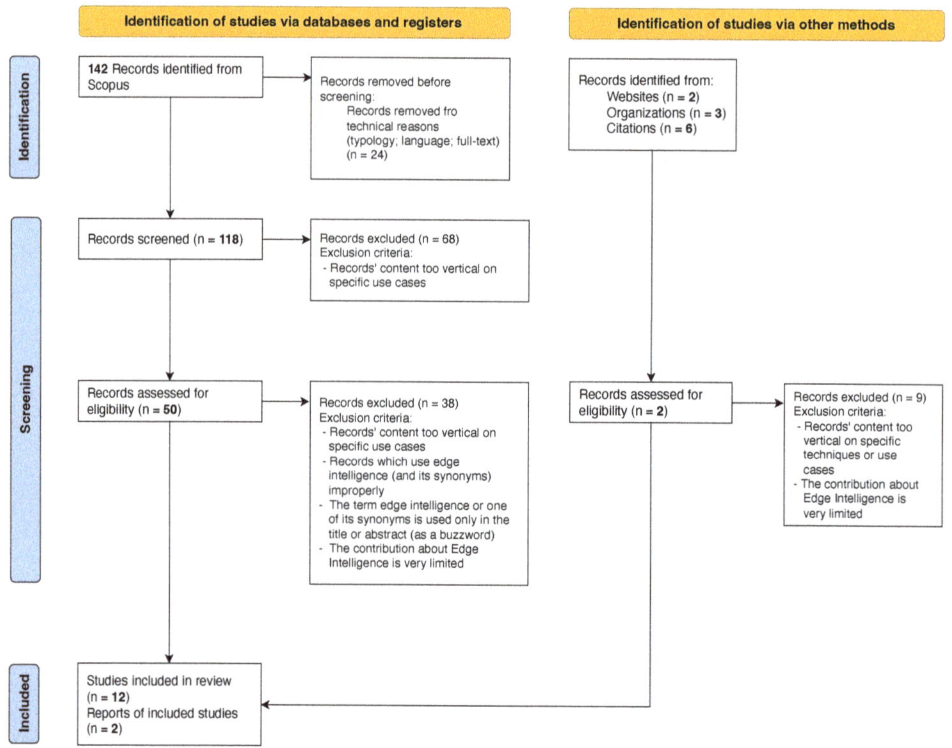

Figure 2. Flow-chart of the literature review selection process according to the PRISMA guidelines.

Table 1. Search plan.

Source	Criteria
Database	ScienceDirect, Scopus, IEEEXplore, ACM Digital Library, Web of Science
Date of publication	2011–2023
Keywords	- Edge intelligence/AI - Embedded intelligence/AI - On-device intelligence/AI
Language	English
Type of Publication	Article, conference paper, book chapter, review, survey
Inclusion Criteria	- Secondary studies on EI - Formal definitions, models, and perspectives of EI - Relevant EI architectures and techniques - EI as the main element of the proposed solution
Exclusion Criteria	- Too vertical contributions on use-cases or single techniques - The EI term used as a buzzword or improperly - The EI-related contribution is very limited

3.2. Search Strategy

An exhaustive search of the articles regarding EI was performed in February 2023 by two of the authors on the following digital libraries: ScienceDirect, Scopus, IEEEXplore, ACM Digital Library, and Web of Science. The search focused on retrieving scientific publications proposing solutions (i.e., models, techniques, approaches, architectures) that aim to understand how to bring intelligence as close as possible to the data sources. The keyword search string was defined according to three key concepts: (i) edge intelligence; (ii) embedded intelligence; (iii) on-device intelligence. Considering such key terms and their synonyms, the following search string was identified:

$$(\text{``edge'' OR ``embedded'' OR ``on-device''}) \text{ AND } (\text{``intelligence'' OR ``AI''}) \tag{1}$$

To find relevant results, we applied the search string to articles' titles, and we forced a distance of a maximum of two words between the key terms. Later on, since the object of our work was specifically on EI's secondary studies, we applied the following search string to manuscripts' abstracts:

$$(\text{survey* OR review* OR literature OR roadmap OR discuss*}) \tag{2}$$

It is worth noting that the search string (2) incorporates the wildcard symbol "*", and this allows for the stemming task over key terms such as "survey", "review", and "discussion".

3.3. Eligibility Criteria

The articles were eligible for selection if they met all of the following inclusion criteria:

- The work is a literature review, survey, or mapping study that specifically delves into the EI realm;
- A model or at least a formal definition of EI is proposed or adopted;
- The work uses EI as the main element of the proposed solution;
- Either EI-based or EI-enabling architectures or techniques are presented.

The articles were excluded from the selection if they met one of the following exclusion criteria:

- The work is too vertical on use cases (ranging from individual domains such as autonomous vehicles [23] and the smart grid [24] to general IoT-based applications [25]), techniques (e.g., information fusion for EI [26], neural-network-based self-learning architecture [27]), algorithm customization (e.g., combination of blockchain and k-means algorithm [28]), or model/platform optimization [20,29];
- The terms "edge intelligence" and "embedded intelligence" or one of their synonyms are contained only in the title, abstract, or keywords and are missing in the main body of the article [21,30,31];
- The concept of EI or one of its synonyms is either defined or used improperly [32,33];
- The work is a pre-print and/or its extension has been already included (as for [34] with respect to [35]).

3.4. Study Selection

Figure 2 depicts the flow-chart of the approach adopted to select the articles according to the PRISMA guidelines [4]. The search in the digital libraries using the search string provided a total of **142** articles. In order to discard studies not relevant to our review, we removed the papers due to the following technical criteria, based on: (1) the type of publication, by eliminating materials such as editorials, short papers, posters, theses, dissertations, brief communications, commentaries, and unpublished works; (2) articles partially or wholly not written in English; (3) papers with text unavailable in full. In this step, a total of 24 papers were removed, obtaining 118 publications. To select the appropriate studies for this review, in the first screening task, only the records (title, abstract, and keyword) of each article were analyzed independently by two of the authors. Each researcher evaluated the title and the abstract according to the eligibility criteria to decide if that paper should be included in the next screening phase. A paper included by one of the researchers resulted in a full-text assessment in the next phase, so 50 papers were selected by the reviewers in this phase. In the last phase, all the researchers read the full papers and decided whether to include the work in the review based on the eligibility criteria and on criteria of relevance, rigorousness, credibility, and quality. Most of the papers were excluded in this phase because EI was used only in the title or abstract (as a buzzword) [36–39] or only in the related works Section [40], and therefore, it did not represent a fundamental element of the solution proposed in the manuscript [41,42]. To guarantee the high quality of the selected studies, final inclusion of a paper in the review was reached by consensus among the researchers (i.e., only if the majority of the researchers evaluated it as suitable for the review, or in case of parity, a discussion between the researchers took place to decide about the inclusion). In this phase, the researchers selected and analyzed a total of 20 papers. In parallel, we performed also an extensive *snowballing* search to identify other eligible studies (relevant, but not found by our query) according to the references' lists (*back-in-time search*) and citations (*forward-in-time search*) of the included studies. In particular, we repeated our query by including the term "intelligence continuum", which is sometimes used to refer to smart solutions distributed across all the architectural levels, hence including the edge. Finally, for the sake of maximum comprehensiveness, we also attempted to search for *gray literature*, thus covering relevant documents, unlisted in electronic databases since they are usually provided by both government and professional organizations, such as technical reports, Ph.D. theses, patents, company's white papers, etc. Lastly, **14** secondary studies specifically related to EI were analyzed in more detail, and they are reported and compared in the framework of Table 2.

4. Literature Review

Already from an initial screening of our search results, we observed that the literature related to EI is not well consolidated. Although the term EI occasionally appears in older EI-related works such as [16,41], only in the last decade has the research established clearer boundaries of the domain, and only in the last four years (2019–2023) have more systematic studies been published in conference proceedings and journals, mostly. From a deep study of all the analyzed works, indeed, we were able to identify a clear classification of the studies under the general umbrella of EI: the majority of them are truly narrowed on specific techniques and domains (e.g., [18,19,43–45]), while few horizontal studies seek to explore the fundamentals, perspectives, and trends of EI (whereas with coarse-grained [42,46] or fine-tuned [12,14,35] analysis). However, as previously pointed out, the specific aim of this survey was to methodically shed light on the state-of-the-art of EI by performing a systematic analysis (interesting and somewhat surprisingly, there is only a systematic literature review [7] and a systematic classification [35]) in the form of a tertiary study, thus centering our analysis on comprehensive reviews, surveys, roadmaps, etc. In this direction, given the time of writing, milestone works are [12,35,47], which provide key contributions by discussing core components and concepts, designing theoretical frameworks, and analyzing technology drivers, exploring capabilities, benefits, opportunities, gaps, and use cases for current EI scenarios, as well as for the next decade. These three manuscripts are the most-cited ones (with more than 200+ citations in a short period of time), but obviously, many other interesting and relevant findings came from the other works identified adopting the research methodology discussed in Section 3 and whose comparative analysis is summarized in Table 2. Therefore, driven by the Research Questions (RQs) outlined in Section 3.1, we carried out an accurate literature analysis, whose research directions and main findings (enclosed in dotted boxes) are concisely presented in Figure 3.

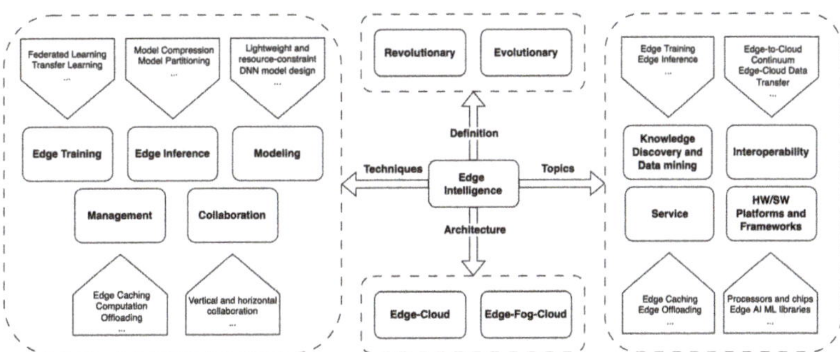

Figure 3. Directions and main findings (enclosed in dotted boxes) of the performed study on EI.

Table 2. Comparison framework for the analyzed literature.

Title	Year	Cit. #	SLR	EI Definition	Ref. Architecture	Topics Addressed	Key Techniques	Hardware Tools	Software Tools	Use Cases
Distributed intelligence on the Edge-to-Cloud Continuum: A systematic literature review [7]	2022	8	Yes	No	No	- KDD - Interoperability - Platforms/ Frameworks	- Edge Training - Edge Inference - Modeling - Collaboration - (indirect contributions)	- Edge devices - Processors	- ML on the continuum - Data Analytics on the continuum - Simulation and Emulation systems	- Healthcare - Smart Factory - Smart Agriculture - Smart Cities - Automotive
Edge Intelligence: Paving the Last Mile of Artificial Intelligence With Edge Computing [12]	2019	703	No	Revolutionary: "The marriage of edge computing and AI"	2-layer	- KDD - Platforms/ Frameworks	- Edge Training - Edge Inference	Edge devices	- Systems and Frameworks on EI Model Training, Inference	- Smart Factory - Smart City - Smart Home - Entertainment
The Many Faces of Edge Intelligence [14]	2022	0	No	Evolutionary: "An emerging computing paradigm that enables AI functionalities at the network edge"	3-layer	Outlook	No	No	No	- Smart City - Automotive
Edge Intelligence [15]	2019	0	No	Revolutionary: "Edge computing with machine learning and advanced networking capabilities"	2-layer	Standardization	No	Edge devices	No	- Smart Factory - Smart City - Public Safety
Edge Intelligence: Empowering Intelligence to the Edge of Network [35]	2021	19	No	Revolutionary: "A set of connected systems and devices for data collection, caching, processing and analysis proximity to where data are captured based on AI."	2-layer	- KDD - Service	- Edge Training - Edge Inference - Modeling - Management	No	No	- Smart Factory - Smart City - Healthcare

Table 2. *Cont.*

Title	Year	Cit. #	SLR	EI Definition	Ref. Architecture	Topics Addressed	Key Techniques	Hardware Tools	Software Tools	Use Cases
Edge Intelligence: The Confluence of Edge Computing and Artificial Intelligence [47]	2020	239	No	Revolutionary: "The integration of edge computing and AI"	No	- KDD - Service	- Edge Inference - Management	No	No	- Automotive - Smart Home - Smart City
OpenEI: An open framework for edge intelligence [48]	2019	47	No	Evolutionary: "The capability to enable edges to execute AI algorithms"	No	- Platforms/Frameworks - Interoperability	- Edge Training - Edge Inference - Modeling	Hardware modules	- Running environments - Edge-based deep learning packages	- Automotive - Smart Home - Healthcare - Public Safety
Edge Intelligence: Challenges and Opportunities [49]	2020	1	No	Evolutionary: "The next stage of edge computing, which allows to run AI applications at the edge of the network"	3-layer	- KDD - Platforms/Frameworks - Service	- Edge Training - Edge Inference - Modeling	- Edge AI chips - Edge Computing Platforms	- Edge AI programming libraries	- Automotive - Smart factory - Smart city - Healthcare
Artificial Intelligence in the IoT Era: A Review of Edge AI Hardware and Software [50]	2022	2	No	Evolutionary: "The modern trend of moving artificial intelligence computation near to the origin of data sources"	No	- Platforms/Frameworks - Outlook	Edge Inference	- Hardware devices - NVIDIA Jetson devices	- ML Frameworks - Mobile SDK - Software for MCU - Model conversion lib. for MCU	No
Convergence of Edge Computing and Deep Learning: A Comprehensive Survey [51]	2020	486	No	Revolutionary: "The combination of edge computing and AI"	2-layer	- KDD - Platforms/Frameworks - Service - Outlook	- Edge Training - Edge Inference - Management - Collaboration	AI hardware for Edge Computing	Edge frameworks for DL	- Smart city - Automotive - Smart home - Smart factory
Edge Intelligence: A Robust Reinforcement of Edge Computing and Artificial Intelligence [52]	2021	0	No	Revolutionary: "The combination of edge computing and AI"	No	- KDD - Service	No	No	No	- Automotive - Military

Table 2. *Cont.*

Title	Year	Cit. #	SLR	EI Definition	Ref. Architecture	Topics Addressed	Key Techniques	Hardware Tools	Software Tools	Use Cases
Roadmap for edge AI: A Dagstuhl Perspective [53]	2022	8	No	Revolutionary: "A fast evolving domain that merges edge computing and AI"	No	Outlook	No	No	No	- Automotive - Entertainment - Smart Factory - Healthcare
Edge Intelligence: Concepts, Architectures, Applications, and Future Directions [54]	2022	4	No	Revolutionary: "The confluence of edge computing with machine learning, or artificial intelligence in the broad sense"	2-layer	- KDD - Platforms/ Frameworks - Outlook	Edge training	Edge devices	Edge intelligence frameworks	- Automotive - Entertainment - Smart home - Smart city - Smart factory
Edge Intelligence: The Convergence of Humans, Things, and AI [55]	2019	25	No	Revolutionary: "A new paradigm in which intelligence is gradually be pushed from the cloud closer to the edge"	No	- Outlook - Platforms/ Frameworks	No	Edge AI chips and modules	- Sw for AI lifecycle managing - Edge Computing platforms	- Smart City - Automotive - Healthcare - Corporate

Referring to **RQ1**, albeit almost twelve years have passed since the first appearance of the term [16] (also referred to as "Edge AI" in [41]), there is still not a formal definition of EI. All the surveyed works promote similar definitions of EI in which the terms edge computing and AI appear, naturally side-by-side. With a deeper look, however, these definitions can be classified into two groups:

- *Evolutionary EI definitions*, which "simply" mean EI as the next stage of current edge computing [14,48–50], where edge nodes self-process their own data, being empowered through lightened AI algorithms (individually measured in terms of <accuracy, latency, energy, memory footprint> [48]) or pre-trained models (intended as "pluggable AI capabilities for edge computers" [51]);
- *Revolutionary EI definitions*, which propose EI as a new paradigm combining ("the amalgam", "the marriage", "the confluence") both novel and existing approaches, techniques, and tools from different areas (mainly from edge computing and AI, but also approximate computing, cognitive science, etc.) and realizing a fully distributed intelligence among end devices, edge nodes, and cloud servers [12,15,35,47,51–54].

The definitions of the first groups aim to stress the achieved independence of edge nodes from the cloud, but, in this way, they definitively narrow down the scope of EI; the EI definition of the second group, instead, exposes a holistic perspective (not centered on the algorithmic capabilities of single edge nodes), reasoning in terms of a seamless edge–cloud ecosystem [35], promoting a continuum between the two domains and all their actors, technology enablers, etc. [53]. Indeed, for example, in [12], six EI levels are defined, and they form a collaborative hierarchy to be integrated for the design of efficient EI solutions. Far from providing the umpteenth EI definition, we adhered to the latter definition, and we believe that the "evolutionary" one limits the potential of EI: indeed, in order to enable novel IoT services or to optimize the overall system performance, all the available system's data and resources should be fully and opportunistically exploited. Just in the direction of such a full-fledged EI vision, Refs. [47,51] provide an interesting interpretation, by identifying two complementary contributions, namely *"AI for Edge"* (or Intelligent Edge) and *"AI on Edge"*, also referred to in [55] as *"AI for Operations"* and *"Operations for AI"*. The former focuses on providing optimal solutions to solve key problems in edge computing (e.g., data offloading, energy management, nodes coordination) with the help of popular AI techniques, while the latter studies how (i.e., which hardware platforms, programming framework, methods, and tools) to perform the whole process of AI model building, i.e., training, inference, and optimization, on edge devices despite their intrinsic resource limitations.

Referring to **RQ2**, it was found that a reference architecture purposely designed for EI is still missing. Indeed, even if the international community is actively working towards the development of a comprehensive edge computing reference architecture [56–59] with a relevant portion of "intelligence" located on edge devices, the full development of an "Edge-native AI system" is currently far away, being only sketched in [27,35]. With respect to the analyzed works, half of them (7 out of 14 [7,47,48,50,52,53,55]) do not deal with such a point, while the remaining ones discuss a multi-level architecture, which is, implicitly or explicitly, strongly influenced by the IoT and by the ETSI MEC reference architecture [14,60]; indeed, these edge computing architectures look tailored to conform and mirror the IoT's layered structure, which generally consists of various and closely intertwined layers that manage different system functionalities, such as data collection, processing, and management [61]. Notably, the majority of surveyed works (5 out of 7 [12,15,35,51,54]) expose *two-layer architectures* (i.e., edge and cloud layers), while only [14,49] include a third, intermediate layer, which is mainly responsible for networking (from LAN to WAN) and interoperability (protocol conversion) tasks. Therefore, it emerges that the fog computing layer is losing attractiveness, being embedded in the so-called "thick Edge" (including, exactly, gateways and other specific-purpose devices), except for some industrial use cases demanding particular requirements. This can be due to the ever-increasing power and miniaturization and lowering cost of IoT boards and microcomputers, which, most of the time, can perform typical fog computing duties (caching, pre-processing, etc.). Such a trend is especially noticeable in [51], whose authors define an "Edge Computing network" layer by distinguishing, from one side, devices such as base stations and gateways and, from the other side, tablets, smartphones, smartwatches, etc. Interestingly, only [55] and, primarily, [7] markedly stress the importance of a seamless interaction between the architectures, by presenting ad hoc methods, libraries, and frameworks for machine learning and data analytics on the *edge-to-cloud continuum*, in the spotlight today thanks to the recent initiative "European Cloud, Edge and IoT Continuum" led by the European Commission [62].

Referring to **RQ3**, an examination of the selected works revealed a common focus on EI's general objectives, applications, and use cases (especially [14,50,51,53–55]), while key technical topics can be grouped primarily into four categories we purposely grounded:

1. Knowledge Discovery and Data mining (KDD), which encompasses all aspects pertaining to the extraction of valuable insights and patterns from the vast data generated by end devices;
2. Hardware platforms and software frameworks, namely those commercial devices and software tools that concretely allow enabling intelligence at the network edge;
3. Service, which encompasses all non-functional aspects (from service placement, composition, and orchestration to mobility, offloading, caching, etc.) related to the support and maintenance of IoT services at the edge layer;
4. Interoperability, which focuses on those methods and mechanisms enabling different devices, systems, and networks to be readily connected and exchange information.

A preponderance of the reviewed literature (8 out of 14 [7,12,35,47,49,51,52,54]) concentrated on the category *KDD*, thereby shedding light on techniques pertaining to data cleaning and preprocessing, feature selection and extraction, and model building and evaluation. Notably, within this category, the subjects of edge training and edge inference have garnered significant interest among researchers, as they pertain to the key methods and techniques that address the challenges of implementing intelligent systems at the edge of the network. Additionally, over half of the works (8 out of 14, [7,12,48–51,54]) also address topics related to *HW platforms and SW frameworks*, enumerating the mainstream legacy of EI software and hardware tools. One of the key findings was the prevalent use of GPU, FPGA, and ASIC hardware chips in supporting intelligence at the edge of the network. These chips are favored for their ability to provide the necessary computational power and flexibility for real-time data processing and analysis, leading to the development of various hardware platforms based on them that are widely used in current Edge AI applications. Examples include the Nvidia Jetson family (GPU-based), the Google Coral Edge TPU (ASIC-based), and the Horizon Sunrise (FPGA-based), all of which are known for their high performance and energy efficiency. Additionally, the machine learning libraries that are most-frequently referenced in the analyzed works include TensorFlow Lite, Core ML, and Pytorch Mobile. These libraries are widely used for developing and deploying models on edge devices, and some of them, such as TensorFlow Lite, have been specifically optimized to run natively on hardware configurations such as the Google Coral family. An intriguing discovery is the introduction of an open framework for EI, also known as OpenEI, presented in the paper [48]. This lightweight software platform imbues the edge with sophisticated processing and data-sharing capabilities. OpenEI comprises a deep learning package that is specifically optimized for resource-constrained edge devices, including a plethora of refined AI models, providing a streamlined solution for the deployment of EI applications. Then, we found that approximately half of the examined literature (5 out of 14 [35,47,49,51,52]) focuses on the primary techniques that seek to sustain and preserve the added value of IoT *services*. Within this category, edge caching and edge offloading have been the most-extensively researched [35,51,52], as they address the critical need for efficient data management and processing at the edge of the network, followed by ever-green (well-explored in the past, yet still crucial) topics such as service placements, user mobility, topology management, etc. [47,49]. Finally, an intriguing discovery is that only a minority of the reviewed papers (4 out of 14 [7,14,15,48]) reserves an adequate discussion on the *interoperability* topic, whereas its centrality has been widely recognized in the IoT ecosystem: these works agree that a rapid adoption of EI technologies by vendors and industry go through IoT gateways and unified interfaces for the system life-cycle (e.g., cross-platform software and RESTful AP for requirements assessment, authentication, resource discovery, system configuration, and deployment), but additionally, they focus on different aspects. For example, Ref. [48] delves into the transfer of data between edge nodes and cloud servers, emphasizing the importance of seamless collaboration; instead, Ref. [7] conducts an in-depth analysis of the collaborative aspect of the edge-to-cloud continuum, while, finally, Ref. [15] primarily concentrates on standardization, but from an industry perspective (by shedding light on requirements, potentials, and gaps in multiple use cases and domains, such as manufacturing, smart cities, and smart buildings). Conversely, there is no reference (if not as an open point in [12,35]) about semantic technologies.

Referring to **RQ4**, a noteworthy outcome is that 5 papers [14,15,52,53,55] out of the 14 did not provide insights on any specific enabling techniques for EI, but rather, focused on imparting a general overview of their principal contribution. As for the remaining nine works [7,12,35,47–51,54], a thorough analysis resulted in the classification of EI's key technologies into the following categories:

1. Edge inference, which covers all techniques for near-real-time inference, i.e., as close as possible to the data sources;
2. Edge training, which encompasses all techniques that aid in training complex ML models on constrained and resource-limited devices;
3. Modeling, which encompasses all techniques that aid in designing ML models' architectures suitable for resource-limited devices;
4. Management, which encompasses all techniques that aid in managing the vast amount of real-time data at the edge layer;
5. Collaboration, which includes techniques that aim to improve the interoperability between nodes across the edge-to-cloud continuum.

The categories that the majority of the analyzed works center on are edge inference [7,12,35,47–51] and edge training [7,12,35,49,51,54] (respectively, 8 and 6 out of 9). This is indicative of ongoing research efforts aimed at understanding the most-efficient ways to train ML models and provide timely predictions and analyses as close as possible to both end-devices and end-users. *Edge inference* pertains to the utilization of a pre-trained model or algorithm to make predictions or classify new data on edge devices or servers. The majority of current AI models are optimized for deployment on devices with ample computational resources, making them unsuitable for edge environments. The reviewed literature, however, identifies two main challenges in enabling efficient edge inference [12,35,48,51]: designing models that are suitable for deployment on resource-constrained edge devices or servers and accelerating inference to provide real-time responses. One widely discussed approach to addressing these challenges is model compression (for reducing the size and computational requirements of existing models without affecting their accuracy) and, especially, its techniques of network pruning and parameter quantization. Another prominent approach discussed in the literature is model partitioning, which involves transferring the computationally intensive portions of a model to an edge server or neighboring mobile device, thus reducing the workload on the endpoint device and significantly enhancing inference performance: in this regard, the technique of model early exit has garnered much attention, as it enables the use of output data from early layers of a DNN to achieve a classification result, thus enabling the inference process to be completed using only a subset of the full DNN model. Unlike traditional centralized training methods that are executed on powerful servers or computing clusters, *edge training* is typically performed in a decentralized manner by using a training dataset located on devices with less computational power at the network's edge. This poses several challenges such as selecting the appropriate training architecture, increasing the training speed, and optimizing performance. The surveyed works propose various techniques to address these issues. The most-commonly used architectures in the literature are "solo training" [35,51], where tasks are performed on a single device, and "collaborative training" [35,49,51], where multiple devices work together to train a shared model or algorithm. It is noteworthy that solo training has higher hardware requirements, which are often unavailable, and as consequence, several works focus on collaborative training architectures and techniques such as Federated Learning (FL) (which has been proposed in several variations such as communication-efficient FL, resource-optimized FL, security-enhanced FL and hierarchical FL [35,51]) and knowledge transfer learning. The latter method involves training a primary network (referred to as the "teacher network") on a base dataset and then transferring the acquired knowledge, in the form of learned features, to a secondary network (referred to as the "student network") for further training on a target dataset. This technique promises to drastically reduce the energy costs of model training on both end devices and edge servers. Approximately half of the papers (4 out of 9 [7,35,48,49]) also deal with *modeling* techniques for the design of ML models aimed at fully leveraging the limited resources of edge devices. According to the literature reviewed [7,12,35,47,49,51,54], it was noticed that deep learning outperformed other machine learning methods in a variety of tasks, including image classification, object detection, and face recognition. These deep learning models are commonly referred to as Deep Neural Networks (DNNs) due to their layered architecture. Despite the fact that DNNs can take on a variety of structures [12,49,51], such as Multilayer Perceptrons (MLPs), Convolutional Neural Networks (CNNs), and Recurrent Neural Networks (RNNs), the surveyed works primarily focus on the general DNN architecture. The increasing complexity and computational demands of modern DNN models make it challenging to run them on edge devices with limited resources, such as mobile devices, IoT terminals, and embedded devices. To address this challenge, recent works such as [7,35,48,49] focus on designing lightweight and resource-constraint DNN models that are more suitable for edge environments. According to [35], this approach can significantly improve the performance of training and inference tasks on edge devices. The categories of management and collaboration received relatively less attention in the analyzed works, with only 3 [35,47,51] and 2 [7,51] papers, respectively, out of 9 addressing these topics. The *management* techniques primarily focus on optimizing data retrieval and processing speed and on minimizing power consumption and thermal stress on the edge device. Edge caching and computation offloading are widely used techniques to achieve these goals [35,51,52]: the former involves storing frequently accessed data on edge devices, reduces latency, and increases data retrieval speed; the latter, on the other hand, distributes the computational workload among a group of edge devices and encompasses various strategies such as Device-to-Cloud (D2C), Device-to-Edge (D2E), Device-to-Device (D2D), and hybrid offloading [35,52]. The *collaboration* category delves into methods for fostering cooperation and coordination among edge devices and other network entities such as vertical and horizontal collaboration and integral and partial task offloading [51]. It is particularly notable to observe the survey [7] through its extensive citation and analysis of a plethora of works, making a significant, albeit indirect, contribution to all the categories outlined, except for "management".

Finally, answering **RQ5**, the most-frequently mentioned application use cases in the reviewed literature pertain to the domains of smart cities [12,15], smart homes [48,51], smart factories [7,35], healthcare [49,50], entertainment [52,54], and automotive [47,51]. Notably, healthcare applications related to disease prediction [63,64], automotive applications exploiting connected and autonomous vehicles [65,66], as well as smart factory applications for the Industrial IoT [49,67] have been receiving significant attention from both industry professionals and researchers. The benefits of EI, such as low-latency communication, crucial in life-or-death situations, reduced bandwidth consumption, essential for energy efficiency in resource-limited devices, and enhanced privacy through the local storage of sensitive information, render these areas particularly appealing. Then, most of the surveyed works report some well-known, yet still unaddressed challenges typical of distributed computing and, hence, of the IoT [61], such as scalability [53,55], security and privacy [12,50,52], ethical issues [7,53], pervasiveness and ubiquity [7,14], resource optimization [48,52,54], heterogeneity [14,15,50,54], data scarcity and consistency [35,47,54], etc. However, these issues generally refer to the edge computing scenario rather than EI, whose main specific open challenges (and related future directions), instead, focus on:

- Understanding the performance of EI applications and finding a balance between effectiveness and efficacy [47,52], thanks to a targeted exploitation of HW/SW co-design techniques [48,68] and the development of novel, full-fledged simulators [69] specifically tailored to EI;
- Designing comprehensive architecture for EI [51], natively provided with the continuum concept and, possibly, with a standardized API, data model, workflow, and notations [14,15,50];
- Developing pervasive intelligent infrastructures that already consider the integration with 5G and 6G technology to facilitate EI solutions [15,27,29,35];
- Outlining engineering methodologies for resource-friendly EI models and situation-aware networking techniques [12,14,47–49], drawing from different computing, networking, and data science paradigms;
- Promoting programming and software platforms for EI [12,48], as well as lightweight OS for the edge devices [48]; with respect to the former, the most well-known are IoT Edge Microsoft Azure https://azure.microsoft.com/it-it/products/iot-edge/, accessed on 30 January 2023, Cisco Edge Intelligence https://www.cisco.com/c/en/us/solutions/internet-of-things/edge-intelligence.html, accessed on 30 January 2023, AWS IoT Greengrass https://aws.amazon.com/greengrass/, accessed on 30 January 2023, IoT Core https://cloud.google.com/iot-core?hl=it, accessed on 30 January 2023, Google Coral https://coral.ai/, accessed on 30 January 2023, NVIDIA Jetson https://www.nvidia.com/it-it/autonomous-machines/embedded-systems/, accessed on 30 January 2023, and Open VINO https://docs.openvino.ai/latest/index.html, accessed on 30 January 2023, while obvious OS candidates for edge devices are open-source and Linux-based such as Wind River, Android Things, or RedHat (whereas there are others as well such as Azure RTOS, VxWorks, FreeRtos, etc.);
- Conceiving of innovative incentive and business models along with cutting-edge applications to promote the combination of theory and practice [35,49,51].

Although they all are relevant, some of the identified gaps in the EI literature are particularly challenging. For example, particular emphasis should be given to the preliminary evaluation of EI solutions under development; indeed, while there exist some simulators conceived for IoT and edge computing scenarios, only [70,71] specifically focus on EI and on the many orthogonal issues it leads across the edge–cloud continuum [72]. Then, open (horizontal, vertical, and specialty) standards [12,50], robust platform abstractions [51], and flexible programming approaches that are deployment-transparent [73,74] are also key to deal with the inherent heterogeneity, scalability, and dynamicity of EI scenarios. In particular, even if standardization processes are typically burdensome efforts of indefinite duration and results (as taught by the IoT), commonly accepted practices should be established, possibly integrating the existing de jure and de facto standards and operating frameworks. Finally, themes such as equal accessibility [53] and governance [29,55], trustworthiness, and explainability [27,75], which already have gained attention in conventional AI systems, are carefully observed by institutions, and therefore, they deserve further research efforts from both industry and academia.

5. Conclusions

IoT systems and related services need to be truly supported by a pervasive, reliable, and effective intelligence to unleash their disruptive potential in our daily lives. Cloud-ification has so far helped, but the latest candidate to burst onto the scene is EI, whose rich, though fresh, recent literature reflects its broad appeal and usefulness. This survey provided both a quantitative and qualitative analysis of the large body of knowledge related to EI and rapidly accumulated in the last decade by means of a systematic literature review of secondary study according to the well-known PRISMA guidelines.

As a final takeaway of this survey, we recognize that the ETSI MEC reference architecture provides a solid base for EI system engineering; however, the realization of AI functionalities is open, and intelligence has not yet been considered as a built-in capability of the edge system [14]. As result, it is still not completely clear how and where the EI capabilities should be built into the edge systems to achieve its maximum yield, while further specifications (mainly for standardized APIs, software constructs, interoperability mechanisms, supporting infrastructures) need to be developed. In particular, the latest concept of the edge–cloud continuum, at its extreme, may lead to isomorphic EI architectures, allowing the identical service provision among edge devices, gateways, and servers [14,76]; from such a perspective, data and computation can be transferred dynamically and performed on any level of the cloud–edge architecture that provides the optimal QoS/QoE, thus ultimately diluting or even dissolving the boundaries between the cloud and edge.

To conclude, we attempted to disclose the wide research area of EI, and we hope that this survey can supply basic knowledge to enable new researchers to enter the area, current researchers to continue developments, and practitioners to apply the results, being confident that huge research efforts will be carried out to completely realize EI in the incoming years.

Author Contributions: All authors contributed equally to this paper. All authors have read and agreed to the published version of the manuscript.

Funding: The research leading to this work was carried out under the Italian MIUR, PRIN 2017 Project "Fluidware" (CUP H24I17000070001), and under the "MLSysOps Project" (Grant Agreement 101092912) funded by the European Community's Horizon Europe Programme.

Data Availability Statement: Data sharing not applicable.

Conflicts of Interest: The authors declare no conflict of interest.

References

1. Reinsel, D.; Gantz, J.; Rydning, J. The Digitization of the World from Edge to Core. 2018. Available online: https://www.seagate.com/files/www-content/our-story/trends/files/idc-seagate-dataage-whitepaper.pdf?Tag=Sponsorships (accessed on 30 January 2023).
2. Biswas, A.R.; Giaffreda, R. IoT and cloud convergence: Opportunities and challenges. In Proceedings of the 2014 IEEE World Forum on Internet of Things (WF-IoT), Seoul, Republic of Korea, 6–8 March 2014 ; IEEE: Piscataway, NJ, USA, 2014; pp. 375–376.
3. Fizza, K.; Banerjee, A.; Mitra, K.; Jayaraman, P.P.; Ranjan, R.; Patel, P.; Georgakopoulos, D. QoE in IoT: A vision, survey and future directions. *Discov. Internet Things* **2021**, *1*, 4. [CrossRef]
4. Page, M.J.; McKenzie, J.E.; Bossuyt, P.M.; Boutron, I.; Hoffmann, T.C.; Mulrow, C.D.; Shamseer, L.; Tetzlaff, J.M.; Moher, D. Updating guidance for reporting systematic reviews: Development of the PRISMA 2020 statement. *J. Clin. Epidemiol.* **2021**, *134*, 103–112. [CrossRef] [PubMed]
5. Bramer, W.M.; De Jonge, G.B.; Rethlefsen, M.L.; Mast, F.; Kleijnen, J. A systematic approach to searching: An efficient and complete method to develop literature searches. *J. Med Libr. Assoc. JMLA* **2018**, *106*, 531. [CrossRef] [PubMed]
6. Čehovin, G.; Bosnjak, M.; Lozar Manfreda, K. Meta-analyses in survey methodology: A systematic review. *Public Opin. Q.* **2018**, *82*, 641–660. [CrossRef]
7. Rosendo, D.; Costan, A.; Valduriez, P.; Antoniu, G. Distributed intelligence on the Edge-to-Cloud Continuum: A systematic literature review. *J. Parallel Distrib. Comput.* **2022**, *166*, 71–94. [CrossRef]
8. Littell, J.H.; Corcoran, J.; Pillai, V. *Systematic Reviews and Meta-Analysis*; Oxford University Press: Oxford, UK, 2008.
9. Lewis, F.L. Wireless sensor networks. In *Smart Environments: Technologies, Protocols, and Applications*; John Wiley & Sons: New York, NY, USA, 2004; pp. 11–46.
10. Atzori, L.; Iera, A.; Morabito, G. The internet of things: A survey. *Comput. Netw.* **2010**, *54*, 2787–2805. [CrossRef]
11. Fortino, G.; Guerrieri, A.; Russo, W.; Savaglio, C. Integration of agent-based and cloud computing for the smart objects-oriented IoT. In Proceedings of the 2014 IEEE 18th International Conference on Computer Supported Cooperative Work in Design (CSCWD), Hsinchu, Taiwan, 21–23 May 2014; IEEE: Piscataway, NJ, USA, 2014; pp. 493–498.
12. Zhou, Z.; Chen, X.; Li, E.; Zeng, L.; Luo, K.; Zhang, J. Edge intelligence: Paving the last mile of artificial intelligence with edge computing. *Proc. IEEE* **2019**, *107*, 1738–1762. [CrossRef]

13. Nayak, S.; Patgiri, R.; Waikhom, L.; Ahmed, A. A review on edge analytics: Issues, challenges, opportunities, promises, future directions, and applications. *Digit. Commun. Netw.* **2022**. [CrossRef]
14. Peltonen, E.; Ahmad, I.; Aral, A.; Capobianco, M.; Ding, A.Y.; Gil-Castineira, F.; Gilman, E.; Harjula, E.; Jurmu, M.; Karvonen, T.; et al. The Many Faces of Edge Intelligence. *IEEE Access* **2022**, *10*, 104769–104782. [CrossRef]
15. Edge Intelligence. 2019. Available online: https://www.iec.ch/system/files/2019-09/content/media/files/iec_wp_edge_intelligence_en_lr.pdf (accessed on 30 January 2023).
16. Guo, B.; Zhang, D.; Wang, Z. Living with internet of things: The emergence of embedded intelligence. In Proceedings of the 2011 International Conference on Internet of Things and 4th International Conference on Cyber, Physical and Social Computing, Dalian, China, 19–22 October 2011; IEEE: Piscataway, NJ, USA, 2011; pp. 297–304.
17. Bittencourt, L.; Immich, R.; Sakellariou, R.; Fonseca, N.; Madeira, E.; Curado, M.; Villas, L.; DaSilva, L.; Lee, C.; Rana, O. The internet of things, fog and cloud continuum: Integration and challenges. *Internet Things* **2018**, *3*, 134–155. [CrossRef]
18. Feng, R.; Feng, X. Robot, Edge Intelligence and Data Survey. In Proceedings of the 2021 IEEE Intl Conf on Dependable, Autonomic and Secure Computing, Intl Conf on Pervasive Intelligence and Computing, Intl Conf on Cloud and Big Data Computing, Intl Conf on Cyber Science and Technology Congress (DASC/PiCom/CBDCom/CyberSciTech), AB, Canada, 25–28 October 2021; IEEE: Piscataway, NJ, USA, 2021; pp. 843–848.
19. Xu, S.; Qian, Y.; Hu, R.Q. Edge intelligence assisted gateway defense in cyber security. *IEEE Netw.* **2020**, *34*, 14–19. [CrossRef]
20. Seng, K.P.; Lee, P.J.; Ang, L.M. Embedded intelligence on FPGA: Survey, applications and challenges. *Electronics* **2021**, *10*, 895. [CrossRef]
21. Lalapura, V.S.; Amudha, J.; Satheesh, H.S. Recurrent neural networks for edge intelligence: A survey. *ACM Comput. Surv. (CSUR)* **2021**, *54*, 1–38. [CrossRef]
22. Liu, X. Model Optimization Techniques for Embedded Artificial Intelligence. In Proceedings of the 2021 2nd International Conference on Computing and Data Science (CDS), Stanford, CA, USA, 28–29 January 2021; IEEE: Piscataway, NJ, USA, 2021; pp. 1–6.
23. Cunneen, M.; Mullins, M.; Murphy, F. Autonomous vehicles and embedded artificial intelligence: The challenges of framing machine driving decisions. *Appl. Artif. Intell.* **2019**, *33*, 706–731. [CrossRef]
24. Molokomme, D.N.; Onumanyi, A.J.; Abu-Mahfouz, A.M. Edge intelligence in Smart Grids: A survey on architectures, offloading models, cyber security measures, and challenges. *J. Sens. Actuator Netw.* **2022**, *11*, 47. [CrossRef]
25. Bourechak, A.; Zedadra, O.; Kouahla, M.N.; Guerrieri, A.; Seridi, H.; Fortino, G. At the Confluence of Artificial Intelligence and Edge Computing in IoT-Based Applications: A Review and New Perspectives. *Sensors* **2023**, *23*, 1639. [CrossRef]
26. Zhang, Y.; Jiang, C.; Yue, B.; Wan, J.; Guizani, M. Information fusion for edge intelligence: A survey. *Inf. Fusion* **2022**, *81*, 171–186. [CrossRef]
27. Xiao, Y.; Shi, G.; Li, Y.; Saad, W.; Poor, H.V. Toward self-learning edge intelligence in 6G. *IEEE Commun. Mag.* **2020**, *58*, 34–40. [CrossRef]
28. Qiu, X.; Yao, D.; Kang, X.; Abulizi, A. Blockchain and K-means algorithm for edge AI computing. *Comput. Intell. Neurosci.* **2022**, *2022*, 1153208. [CrossRef]
29. Raith, P.; Dustdar, S. Edge Intelligence as a Service. In Proceedings of the 2021 IEEE International Conference on Services Computing (SCC), Chicago, IL, USA, 5–10 September 2021; IEEE: Piscataway, NJ, USA, 2021; pp. 252–262.
30. Ciampi, L.; Gennaro, C.; Carrara, F.; Falchi, F.; Vairo, C.; Amato, G. Multi-camera vehicle counting using edge-AI. *Expert Syst. Appl.* **2022**, *207*, 117929. [CrossRef]
31. Feng, H.; Mu, G.; Zhong, S.; Zhang, P.; Yuan, T. Benchmark analysis of yolo performance on edge intelligence devices. *Cryptography* **2022**, *6*, 16. [CrossRef]
32. Bellas, F.; Guerreiro-Santalla, S.; Naya, M.; Duro, R.J. AI Curriculum for European High Schools: An Embedded Intelligence Approach. *Int. J. Artif. Intell. Educ.* **2022**, 1–28. [CrossRef]
33. Grandinetti, J. Examining embedded apparatuses of AI in Facebook and TikTok. *AI Soc.* **2021**, 1–14. [CrossRef] [PubMed]
34. Xu, D.; Li, T.; Li, Y.; Su, X.; Tarkoma, S.; Jiang, T.; Crowcroft, J.; Hui, P. Edge intelligence: Architectures, challenges, and applications. *arXiv* **2020**, arXiv:2003.12172.
35. Xu, D.; Li, T.; Li, Y.; Su, X.; Tarkoma, S.; Jiang, T.; Crowcroft, J.; Hui, P. Edge intelligence: Empowering intelligence to the edge of network. *Proc. IEEE* **2021**, *109*, 1778–1837. [CrossRef]
36. Welagedara, L.; Harischandra, J.; Jayawardene, N. Edge Intelligence Based Collaborative Learning System for IoT Edge. In Proceedings of the 2021 IEEE 12th Annual Information Technology, Electronics and Mobile Communication Conference (IEMCON), Vancouver, BC, Canada, 27–30 October 2021; IEEE: Piscataway, NJ, USA, 2021; pp. 0667–0672.
37. Lee, M.; She, X.; Chakraborty, B.; Dash, S.; Mudassar, B.; Mukhopadhyay, S. Reliable edge intelligence in unreliable environment. In Proceedings of the 2021 Design, Automation & Test in Europe Conference & Exhibition (DATE), Grenoble, France, 1–5 February 2021; IEEE: Piscataway, NJ, USA, 2021; pp. 896–901.
38. Cui, Q.; Zhu, Z.; Ni, W.; Tao, X.; Zhang, P. Edge-intelligence-empowered, unified authentication and trust evaluation for heterogeneous beyond 5G systems. *IEEE Wirel. Commun.* **2021**, *28*, 78–85. [CrossRef]
39. Hafeez, T.; Xu, L.; Mcardle, G. Edge intelligence for data handling and predictive maintenance in IIOT. *IEEE Access* **2021**, *9*, 49355–49371. [CrossRef]

40. Shaeri, M.; Afzal, A.; Shoaran, M. Challenges and opportunities of edge ai for next-generation implantable BMIs. In Proceedings of the 2022 IEEE 4th International Conference on Artificial Intelligence Circuits and Systems (AICAS), Incheon, Republic of Korea, 13–15 June 2022; IEEE: Piscataway, NJ, USA, 2022; pp. 190–193.

41. Xiao, P. *Artificial Intelligence Programming with Python*, 1st ed.; Wiley: New York, NY, USA, 2011.

42. Ramya, R.; Ramamoorthy, S. Survey on Edge Intelligence in IoT-Based Computing Platform. In *Ambient Communications and Computer Systems: Proceedings of RACCCS 2021*; Springer: Berlin, Germany, 2022; pp. 549–561.

43. Leroux, S.; Simoens, P.; Lootus, M.; Thakore, K.; Sharma, A. TinyMLOps: Operational Challenges for Widespread Edge AI Adoption. In Proceedings of the 2022 IEEE International Parallel and Distributed Processing Symposium Workshops (IPDPSW), Lyon, France, 30 May–3 June 2022; IEEE: Piscataway, NJ, USA, 2022; pp. 1003–1010.

44. Seng, K.P.; Ang, L.M. Embedded intelligence: State-of-the-art and research challenges. *IEEE Access* **2022**, *10*, 59236–59258. [CrossRef]

45. Zhang, J.; Letaief, K.B. Mobile edge intelligence and computing for the internet of vehicles. *Proc. IEEE* **2019**, *108*, 246–261. [CrossRef]

46. Joshi, K.; Anandaram, H.; Khanduja, M.; Kumar, R.; Saini, V.; Mohialden, Y.M. Recent Challenges on Edge AI with Its Application: A Brief Introduction. In *Explainable Edge AI: A Futuristic Computing Perspective*; Springer: Berlin, Germany, 2022; pp. 73–88.

47. Deng, S.; Zhao, H.; Fang, W.; Yin, J.; Dustdar, S.; Zomaya, A.Y. Edge intelligence: The confluence of edge computing and artificial intelligence. *IEEE Internet Things J.* **2020**, *7*, 7457–7469. [CrossRef]

48. Zhang, X.; Wang, Y.; Lu, S.; Liu, L.; Shi, W. OpenEI: An open framework for edge intelligence. In Proceedings of the 2019 IEEE 39th International Conference on Distributed Computing Systems (ICDCS), Dallas, TX, USA, 7–10 July 2019; IEEE: Piscataway, NJ, USA, 2019; pp. 1840–1851.

49. Hu, H.; Jiang, C. Edge intelligence: Challenges and opportunities. In Proceedings of the 2020 International Conference on Computer, Information and Telecommunication Systems (CITS), Hangzhou, China, 5–7 October 2020; IEEE: Piscataway, NJ, USA, 2020; pp. 1–5.

50. Sipola, T.; Alatalo, J.; Kokkonen, T.; Rantonen, M. Artificial Intelligence in the IoT Era: A Review of Edge AI Hardware and Software. In Proceedings of the 2022 31st Conference of Open Innovations Association (FRUCT), Helsinki, Finland, 27–29 April 2022; IEEE: Piscataway, NJ, USA, 2022; pp. 320–331.

51. Wang, X.; Han, Y.; Leung, V.C.; Niyato, D.; Yan, X.; Chen, X. Convergence of edge computing and deep learning: A comprehensive survey. *IEEE Commun. Surv. Tutor.* **2020**, *22*, 869–904. [CrossRef]

52. Parekh, B.; Amin, K. Edge Intelligence: A Robust Reinforcement of Edge Computing and Artificial Intelligence. In *Innovations in Information and Communication Technologies (IICT-2020)*; Springer: Berlin, Germany, 2021; pp. 461–468.

53. Ding, A.Y.; Peltonen, E.; Meuser, T.; Aral, A.; Becker, C.; Dustdar, S.; Hiessl, T.; Kranzlmüller, D.; Liyanage, M.; Maghsudi, S.; et al. Roadmap for edge AI: A Dagstuhl perspective. *arXiv* **2022**, arXiv:2112.00616.

54. Mendez, J.; Bierzynski, K.; Cuéllar, M.; Morales, D.P. Edge Intelligence: Concepts, architectures, applications and future directions. *ACM Trans. Embed. Comput. Syst. (TECS)* **2022**, *21*, 1–14. [CrossRef]

55. Rausch, T.; Dustdar, S. Edge intelligence: The convergence of humans, things, and Ai. In Proceedings of the 2019 IEEE International Conference on Cloud Engineering (IC2E), Prague, Czech Republic, 24–27 June 2019; IEEE: Piscataway, NJ, USA, 2019; pp. 86–96.

56. Iyengar, A.; Ouyang, C. Edge Computing Architecture. Available online: https://www.ibm.com/cloud/architecture/architectures/edge-computing/reference-architecture/ (accessed on 30 January 2023).

57. Hallsten, J.; Viorel, P.; Petterson, S. IIC: Industrial IOT Reference Architecture. 2022. Available online: https://www.iiot-world.com/industrial-iot/connected-industry/iic-industrial-iot-reference-architecture/ (accessed on 30 January 2023).

58. Isaja, M. Reference Architecture for Factory Automation using Edge Computing and Blockchain Technologies. In *The Digital Shopfloor-Industrial Automation in the Industry 4.0 Era*; River Publishers: Aalborg, Denmark, 2022; pp. 71–101.

59. Edge Computing Reference Architecture 2.0. Available online: http://en.ecconsortium.net/Lists/show/id/82.html (accessed on 30 January 2023).

60. Sabella, D.; Vaillant, A.; Kuure, P.; Rauschenbach, U.; Giust, F. Mobile-edge computing architecture: The role of MEC in the Internet of Things. *IEEE Consum. Electron. Mag.* **2016**, *5*, 84–91. [CrossRef]

61. Fortino, G.; Guerrieri, A.; Savaglio, C.; Spezzano, G. A Review of Internet of Things Platforms through the IoT-A Reference Architecture. In Proceedings of the International Symposium on Intelligent and Distributed Computing, Bhubaneswar, India, 19–23 January 2022; Springer: Berlin, Germany, 2022; pp. 25–34.

62. De Majo, C.; Giuffrida, M. Understanding Cloud-Edge-IoT: Challenges and Opportunities—Webinar Highlights. 2022. Available online: https://zenodo.org/record/7185383#.Y_7TRh9ByUl (accessed on 30 January 2023). [CrossRef]

63. Ooko, S.O.; Mukanyiligira, D.; Munyampundu, J.P.; Nsenga, J. Edge AI-based respiratory disease recognition from exhaled breath signatures. In Proceedings of the 2021 IEEE Jordan International Joint Conference on Electrical Engineering and Information Technology (JEEIT), Amman, Jordan, 16–18 November 2021; IEEE: Piscataway, NJ, USA, 2021; pp. 89–94.

64. Ooko, S.O.; Mukanyiligira, D.; Munyampundu, J.P.; Nsenga, J. Synthetic Exhaled Breath Data-Based Edge AI Model for the Prediction of Chronic Obstructive Pulmonary Disease. In Proceedings of the 2021 International Conference on Computing and Communications Applications and Technologies (I3CAT), Ipswich, UK, 15 September 2021; IEEE: Piscataway, NJ, USA, 2021; pp. 1–6.

65. Liu, S.; Liu, L.; Tang, J.; Yu, B.; Wang, Y.; Shi, W. Edge computing for autonomous driving: Opportunities and challenges. *Proc. IEEE* **2019**, *107*, 1697–1716. [CrossRef]
66. He, Y.; Zhao, N.; Yin, H. Integrated networking, caching, and computing for connected vehicles: A deep reinforcement learning approach. *IEEE Trans. Veh. Technol.* **2017**, *67*, 44–55. [CrossRef]
67. Li, L.; Ota, K.; Dong, M. Deep learning for smart industry: Efficient manufacture inspection system with fog computing. *IEEE Trans. Ind. Inform.* **2018**, *14*, 4665–4673. [CrossRef]
68. Bringmann, O.; Ecker, W.; Feldner, I.; Frischknecht, A.; Gerum, C.; Hämäläinen, T.; Hanif, M.A.; Klaiber, M.J.; Mueller-Gritschneder, D.; Bernardo, P.P.; et al. Automated HW/SW co-design for edge ai: State, challenges and steps ahead: Special session paper. In Proceedings of the 2021 International Conference on Hardware/Software Codesign and System Synthesis (CODES+ ISSS), Austin, TX, USA, 10–15 October 2021; IEEE: Piscataway, NJ, USA, 2021; pp. 11–20.
69. Savaglio, C.; Campisano, G.; Di Fatta, G.; Fortino, G. IoT services deployment over edge vs cloud systems: A simulation-based analysis. In Proceedings of the IEEE INFOCOM 2019-IEEE Conference on Computer Communications Workshops (INFOCOM WKSHPS), Paris, France, 29 April–2 May 2019; IEEE: Piscataway, NJ, USA, 2019; pp. 554–559.
70. Wang, C.; Li, R.; Li, W.; Qiu, C.; Wang, X. SimEdgeIntel: A open-source simulation platform for resource management in edge intelligence. *J. Syst. Archit.* **2021**, *115*, 102016. [CrossRef]
71. Savaglio, C.; Fortino, G. A simulation-driven methodology for IoT data mining based on edge computing. *ACM Trans. Internet Technol. (TOIT)* **2021**, *21*, 1–22. [CrossRef]
72. Abreu, D.P.; Velasquez, K.; Curado, M.; Monteiro, E. A comparative analysis of simulators for the cloud to fog continuum. *Simul. Model. Pract. Theory* **2020**, *101*, 102029. [CrossRef]
73. Casadei, R.; Pianini, D.; Placuzzi, A.; Viroli, M.; Weyns, D. Pulverization in cyber-physical systems: Engineering the self-organizing logic separated from deployment. *Future Internet* **2020**, *12*, 203. [CrossRef]
74. Casadei, R.; Fortino, G.; Pianini, D.; Placuzzi, A.; Savaglio, C.; Viroli, M. A Methodology and Simulation-based Toolchain for Estimating Deployment Performance of Smart Collective Services at the Edge. *IEEE Internet Things J.* **2022**, *9*, 20136–20148. [CrossRef]
75. Corchado, J.M.; Ossowski, S.; Rodríguez-González, S.; De la Prieta, F. Advances in explainable artificial intelligence and edge computing applications. *Electronics* **2022**, *11*, 3111. [CrossRef]
76. Taivalsaari, A.; Mikkonen, T. A taxonomy of IoT client architectures. *IEEE Softw.* **2018**, *35*, 83–88. [CrossRef]

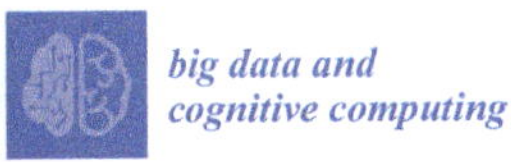
big data and cognitive computing

MDPI

Review

Enhancing Digital Health Services with Big Data Analytics

Nisrine Berros [1,*], Fatna El Mendili [2], Youness Filaly [1] and Younes El Bouzekri El Idrissi [1]

1   Engineering Sciences Laboratory, National School of Applied Sciences, Ibn Tofail University, Kenitra 14000, Morocco

2   Image Laboratory, School of Technology, Moulay Ismail University, Meknes 50050, Morocco

*   Correspondence: nisrine.berros@uit.ac.ma

Abstract: Medicine is constantly generating new imaging data, including data from basic research, clinical research, and epidemiology, from health administration and insurance organizations, public health services, and non-conventional data sources such as social media, Internet applications, etc. Healthcare professionals have gained from the integration of big data in many ways, including new tools for decision support, improved clinical research methodologies, treatment efficacy, and personalized care. Finally, there are significant advantages in saving resources and reallocating them to increase productivity and rationalization. In this paper, we will explore how big data can be applied to the field of digital health. We will explain the features of health data, its particularities, and the tools available to use it. In addition, a particular focus is placed on the latest research work that addresses big data analysis in the health domain, as well as the technical and organizational challenges that have been discussed. Finally, we propose a general strategy for medical organizations looking to adopt or leverage big data analytics. Through this study, healthcare organizations and institutions considering the use of big data analytics technology, as well as those already using it, can gain a thorough and comprehensive understanding of the potential use, effective targeting, and expected impact.

Keywords: big health data; electronic health records; analytics; machine learning; NoSQL database

Citation: Berros, N.; El Mendili, F.; Filaly, Y.; El Bouzekri El Idrissi, Y. Enhancing Digital Health Services with Big Data Analytics. *Big Data Cogn. Comput.* **2023**, *7*, 64. https://doi.org/10.3390/bdcc7020064

Academic Editors: Domenico Talia and Fabrizio Marozzo

Received: 13 February 2023
Revised: 9 March 2023
Accepted: 16 March 2023
Published: 30 March 2023

1. Introduction

The health sector has always generated a large amount of data due to the increased record-keeping needs in the context of patient care [1]. Much of this available and particularly valuable data are in a semi-structured or unstructured form. Further, its diverse and dynamic nature makes it challenging to extract valuable insights through the use of traditional analytical methods [2]. Thus, big data in the field of health is an important issue, not only because of its enormous volume but also because of its diversity and how quickly it can be managed [3]. The human capacity to process this data is limited, making effective decision support necessary. Due to this, big data analytics must be integrated into the health industry. Big data analytics has the capability to examine a diverse set of intricate data and generate valuable information that would otherwise be unobtainable. In the healthcare field, it can not only detect emerging trends but also enhance the quality of healthcare, decrease costs, and facilitate prompt decision-making [4]. As stated in the McKinsey International Institute report, if big data are harnessed and used effectively, the U.S. healthcare system value will be saved more than $300 billion annually, with approximately two-thirds of that amount coming from a reduction in healthcare costs of around 8%. By making use of big data technology and the automated analysis of the results, it is possible for useful information to emerge that until recently has remained in obscurity. The ability of big data analytics to recognize the heterogeneity of diseases allows not only a timely diagnosis but also for the evaluation of existing treatments [5,6]. Big data analytics can turn large amounts of continuous data into actionable insights by analyzing and connecting information from multiple sources. This capability to provide this kind of insight is especially crucial, particularly in emergency medical situations, as it can greatly determine the outcome of a patient's life or death [7]. We have seen during the coronavirus pandemic the usefulness of medical data and how such information can be helpful in the management of health crises during a pandemic. Health organizations must seriously consider integrating the technological tools required to treat this massive amount of data that has the potential to save lives. The digitization of clinical examinations and medical records in healthcare systems has become a widespread and accepted norm since the development of computer systems and their potential [8].

1.1. Motivation

The main contribution of this article is to give an analytical insight into the use of big data analytics in medical institutions. This paper aims to understand how big data are applied in the field of digital health services, to present the available tools and applications, describe the most important actions and research work, as well as the technical and organizational challenges that arise. Healthcare organizations and institutions considering implementing big data analytics technology, as well as those already using it, have the opportunity through this study to gain a comprehensive and detailed understanding of its potential for use, effective targeting, expected impact, and the challenges they will face.

1.2. Research Methodology

For this review, we focused on exploring major questions related to big data analytics in healthcare. We conducted a thorough search of the literature articles indexed in Scopus, Web of Science, Science Direct, and other reputable databases. We used a combination of keywords and Boolean operators to refine our search, including terms related to big data analytics, healthcare, and data analysis. We selected articles based on their relevance to our research question, as well as their citation count and impact factor. Using Zotero, a reference management tool, we organized the selected articles and made notes on their content and findings. We also reviewed relevant conference proceedings to ensure the comprehensive coverage of the topic. By conducting a thorough review of the literature, we aimed to provide a comprehensive overview of the current state of knowledge on big data analytics in healthcare. Figure 1 presents the research methodology used.

1.3. Paper Organization

This review paper will be organized as follows: first, in the introduction, we present our motivations and work related to the topic. Then, the concept of using big data in health will be discussed. The second part focuses specifically on the features and sources most commonly used for big data analysis in healthcare. Additionally, instances of the classification of analytics in medicine are provided. Then, in Part 3, an overview of machine learning techniques and their uses in medicine are presented. The big data technology stack in healthcare is presented in Part 4. In Part 5, different technical and organizational challenges in healthcare are discussed and analyzed.In part 6 a Proposed Strategy for Implementing Big Data Analytics in Healthcare is presented.The final part of the paper is the conclusion, where will summarize and draw final insights (Figure 2).

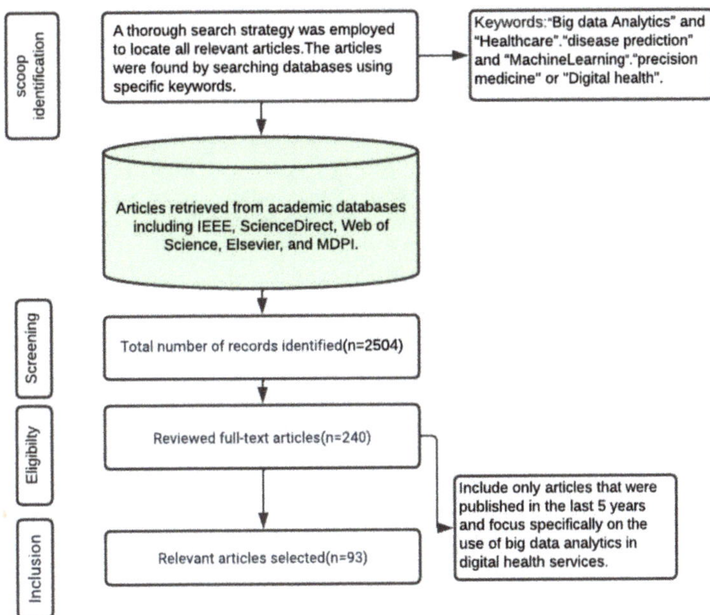

Figure 1. Research methodology followed.

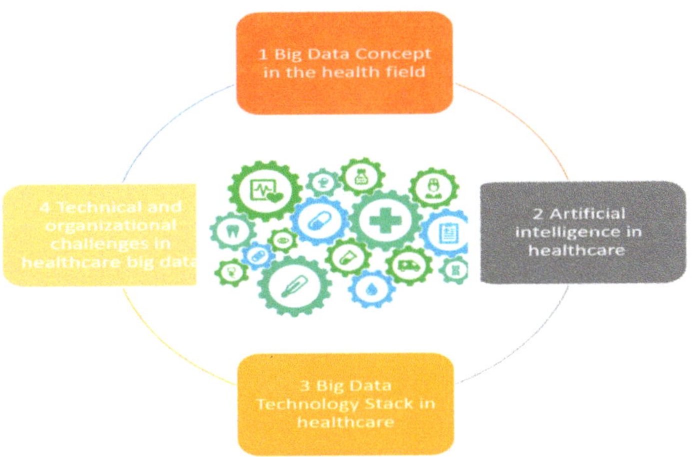

Figure 2. Topics covered in this article.

1.4. Existing Surveys

There are many studies in the literature that show the potential big data analytics can offer to medical organizations and what type of data can be analyzed. However, very few studies have shown how data analysis technology is performed in the healthcare sector and what the major organizational challenges are that an organization willing to integrate big data into their system may face. Table 1 presents a summary of the key related reviews, including a description of each review's contribution and the topic covered. A comparison of our work to the others is provided at the bottom of the table.

Table 1. An overview of the related work.

ID	Reference	Year	Overview
1	[9]	2015	This survey examines the utilization of big data in healthcare and explores the benefits it can bring to the healthcare industry. It delves into the various data sources that should be utilized and brought together for analysis. Numerous difficulties with big healthcare data are also addressed.
2	[10]	2016	This paper addresses both the difficulties and potential of big data in the medical industry, including the pipeline for processing it. It also presents a variety of machine-learning techniques for mining and analyzing data.
3	[11]	2018	This paper gives an in-depth look at the technologies and techniques used to create analytical applications in healthcare. It examines the progression of healthcare big data and the data mining algorithms used, including their general usage and specific applications in healthcare. Additionally, it covers the essential platforms and technologies needed for a successful health analytics solution.
4	[12]	2019	This paper discusses the significant impacts of big data on various medical actors and healthcare providers, as well as the difficulties in utilizing all of this big data and the applications that are already accessible.
5	[13]	2019	In this article, the authors investigate the various technologies, tools, and applications used for data integration in healthcare. They also address the current difficulties encountered when integrating large amounts of healthcare data and explore potential future research opportunities in this field.
6	[14]	2020	This paper covers technological advances and advancements in big data analytics in healthcare as well as infrastructure, artificial intelligence (AI), and cloud computing. In addition, it also explores the primary techniques, frameworks, and resources for big healthcare data analytics in medical engineering.
7	[15]	2020	This paper provides an overview of big data analytics systems used in healthcare and highlights the various algorithms, techniques, and tools that can be implemented in cloud, wireless, and internet of things environments. The authors propose the concept of SmartHealth as a way to bring all these platforms together and have a unified standard learning healthcare system for the future.
8	[16]	2021	This study places particular emphasis on applications of big data analytics for the healthcare field, especially NoSQL databases. The authors also propose a BDA architecture dubbed Med-BDA for the healthcare industry to address BDA's issues in this field. They also present strategies to make their proposals successful, and the authors in this article also make a comparison with the literature to justify the importance of their work.
9	[17]	2021	This article discusses the use of ML, big data, and blockchain technology in medicine, healthcare, public health surveillance, and case prediction during the COVID-19 pandemic and other epidemics. It also covers potential challenges for medical professionals and health technologists in creating future-oriented models to enhance human life.
10	[5]	2022	This paper examines the fundamental concepts of big data, its management, analysis, and potential applications, specifically in the field of health.
11	[8]	2022	The primary objective of this paper is to gather and categorize the utilization of big data from various perspectives and to provide a comprehensive analysis of the application of big data analytics within medical institutions in Poland.
12	[18]	2022	This study examines the literature on big data applications in the context of the COVID-19 pandemic, specifically focusing on their use in four key industries, including healthcare. By comparing the utilization of big data applications before and during the pandemic, the paper provides an overview of the current significance of big data in the COVID-19 era and how these applications align with relevant big data analytics models.
13	[4]	2022	This survey explores the utilization of big data (BD) in the fields of pharmacy, pharmacology, and toxicology. It examines how researchers have employed BD to address issues and discover solutions. The survey uses a comparative analysis to examine the application of big data in these three domains.

1.5. Current Survey

Our study provides a comprehensive and in-depth examination of the utilization of big data analytics in medical institutions. Unlike other surveys on the subject, we not only present a summary of the available tools and applications but also delve deeper into the key actions and research efforts being undertaken in this field. Additionally, we address the technical and organizational challenges that arise when implementing big data analytics in digital health services. In the end, we offer a simple strategy that can be adopted by organizations that want to integrate big data analytics based on the best practice in the field of healthcare. The goal of this study was to provide healthcare organizations and institutions with a clear understanding of the potential use, effective targeting, and expected impact of big data analytics technology, thus helping them make informed decisions about its implementation.

2. Big Data Concepts in the Health Field

Big data are generally viewed as a set of data that are too large or too heterogeneous and complex in structure to be handled by traditional data processing software. Big data challenges include collecting, storing, analyzing, transferring, sharing, and visualizing the information it contains. Scientists, entrepreneurs, and medical professionals are often required to use data from a range of sources, including big data from the international literature, the Internet, medical records, patient registries, and even 'smart' devices.

2.1. Features of Big Data in Healthcare

- Volume

In digital health, the increase in the amount of data is a result of both the digitization of already available data and the creation of new data formats. The volume of data available consists of personal medical records, radiology and fluoroscopy images, clinical trials, surveys, demographic data, human genomes, genetic sequences, etc. The exponential rise in data in the healthcare industry is due to the integration of new types of big data, including three-dimensional images, biological data, and data from sensor technologies. To handle the large volumes of healthcare data, for example, authors in [19] have used natural language processing (NLP) techniques to extract meaningful information from clinical notes in EHRs for complementary and integrative health (CIH). By automating the extraction of CIH information, this research can address the challenge of dealing with the volume of unstructured data in EHRs.

- Variety

Traditionally, the vast majority of data available in healthcare have been unstructured data, such as medical records and handwritten notes from medical and nursing staff describing symptoms, indications, behavior, medical images, etc. Of course, there has been an upsurge in structured data in recent years, such as electronic drug prescribing information, quantitative data on an instrument and test measurements, and general data that are attempted to be recorded in a single structure so that they can be used as a basis for data analysis. In addition to the data that are obviously recorded, data from new sources, such as wellness devices that record patients' pulse or sleep time, social networks, and genomic research, the use of different data sources allows for the obtaining of faster and more reliable results. In the study [20], the authors demonstrate how monitoring social media conversations related to vaccines can address the various problems of big data by providing a way to organize and make sense of a large amount of unstructured social media data.

- Velocity

In healthcare, most data traditionally come from static sources, such as X-rays, hospital documents, patient records, health logs, etc. In some applications, however, it is necessary to process and use the data in real-time, for example, to monitor blood pressure and heart function during surgery [21]. There are also cases where data processing is necessary at a relatively slower pace, such as the daily determination of glucose levels in diabetics [22]. Another example is information about a known disease, which develops at a much slower rate in terms of percentage compared to a new epidemic that is developing. In the latter case, the data arrive at a high rate and are "new" information. It is imperative to quickly process this information in order to resolve the matter in a timely manner. To analyze healthcare data in real-time or near real-time, researchers have proposed the use of big data analytics to develop predictive models that can detect and respond to health emergencies. For example, using machine learning algorithms to predict the outbreak of infectious disease and monitor the spread of the disease in real-time [23].

- Veracity

There are several similarities between the study of data reliability in financial transactions and healthcare: the accuracy of patient data, correctly filling in hospital or clinic fields, patient insurance, linkage to bank accounts, the recording of payment amounts, etc. [3]. Of course, in the health sector, there are data that are not observed in other sectors, such as information about a diagnosis, treatment, administration of medication, care, and any other information deemed necessary to be recorded. The validity of these data is, in any case, as important as the data mentioned above. Ensuring the accuracy of big data is critical in healthcare to prevent medical errors, incorrect diagnoses, and treatment decisions. To address this issue, various techniques such as data cleaning, data validation, data integration, and normalization are used to ensure that the data are reliable and consistent.

- Value

The cost of healthcare is unsustainable and constantly rising. However, the multiple benefits offered by the use and exploitation of big data in healthcare are far more numerous. For example, in the study [24], the authors developed machine learning algorithms to predict hospital readmissions and reduce healthcare costs. The algorithms were able to accurately predict readmissions, and healthcare providers were able to intervene early and provide targeted interventions to reduce the risk of readmission.

The following figure, Figure 3, illustrates the 5 Vs of big data in the healthcare sector.

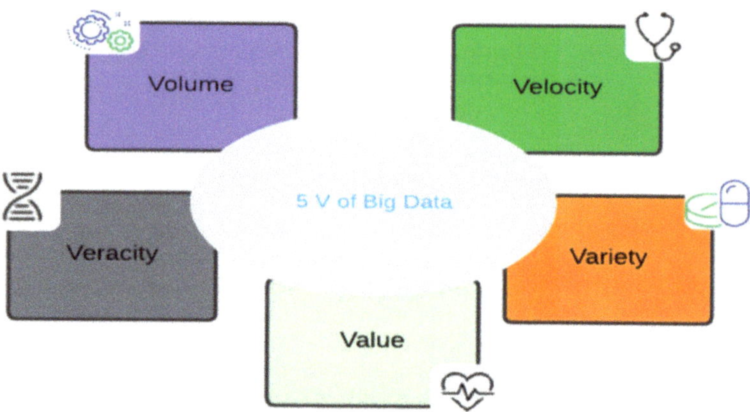

Figure 3. Big data characteristics in the healthcare sector.

2.2. Data Sources

For the healthcare sector, relevant data are needed to build systems that have a positive impact on the health and well-being of individuals. In this section, we introduce three data sources and analyze how each can be leveraged through concrete examples.

- Electronic Health Records

Electronic patient records are a source of an enormous amount of data containing information about the social, demographic, medical, and health aspects of the patient's health. However, without reliable decision support, the human brain can only process a certain amount of information. In order to develop real-time knowledge and support systems that are preventive, predictive, and diagnostic in the healthcare industry, it is important to have an infrastructure that is constantly updated. Computational models are required to assist medical professionals in data organization, pattern recognition, and result interpretation [25]. the following table shows some of the possible data that an electronic medical record may contain, as well as their data type (Table 2).

Table 2. Possible content of an electronic medical record.

Data	Format of Representation
First and Last Name	Text
Gender	Code
Date of birth	Date
Clinical notes	Text
Laboratory tests, X-ray tests	Code/Number
Radiological examinations	Image/Signal
Medications	Number/code/Text
Vaccines	Code

- Social networks

The resurgence of communication via social networks is one of the most important factors in the dramatic evolution of healthcare. According to a recent estimate, approximately one billion tweets have been exchanged, illustrating the depth of communication between organizations, patients, and providers. Social networks now offer researchers new ways to reach out to patients and include them in their research. One such project is TuAnalyze, a collaboration between TuDiabetes1 and Boston Children's Hospital that allows diabetics to track, assess, and share their findings while actively participating in diabetes research [26]. Without a doubt, one of the most intriguing applications of data analytics is its ability to predict and monitor significant epidemics for the benefit of public health. Predictions of major health outcomes, such as an exacerbation of asthma attacks, can be improved by combining social network analysis with environmental data. Specifically, Google searches, Twitter activity, and air quality data can be used to estimate the number of daily emergency room admissions for an asthma event [27]. According to a study published in [28], there was a rise in tweets discussing the situation in Nigeria at least three days before the Ebola outbreak was brought to public attention and seven days before the Centers for Disease Control issued an official alert. As a result, many researchers are now harnessing social media's potential to advance global awareness and improve health.

- Internet of Things

Millions of people use devices to monitor various aspects of their health behavior. These devices can monitor things such as heart rate, mobility, sleep quality, and blood sugar quality. The recorded data can be used to detect any danger and alert a physician, depending on the service offered by the device, all in real-time [29]. Due to advances in technology, particularly sensor technology, there is a growing interest in wearable and implantable sensors. These technological advances have made continuous and multimodal sensing possible. Simultaneously, advances in sensor miniaturization, noise reduction, and microelectronics development have increased the flexibility and reliability of implantable sensors [30].

2.3. Healthcare Big Data Analytics Classification

Several types of big data analytics are used in the healthcare industry (Figure 4), including descriptive analytics, diagnostic analytics, and predictive and prescriptive analytics [18]. In this section, we discuss the specifics of each type of analysis and how it manifests itself in the healthcare field.

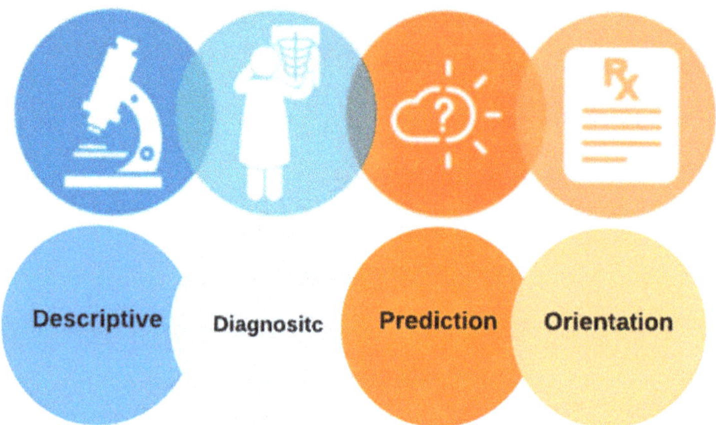

Figure 4. Classification of big data analytics in healthcare.

(a)   Descriptive Analytics

Descriptive analytics consists of the description of the existing situation and helps to outline the picture of past performance on the basis of historical data and through the use of business intelligence and data mining. To perform this level of analysis, various techniques are used [31]. Descriptive analysis, known as unsupervised learning, among other things, summarizes what happens in the management of health services and what effect does a parameter have on the system? Descriptive analysis is the simplest level of understanding and use. It is a simple description of the data, with no further analysis, exploration, or analysis. The descriptive analysis defines, characterizes, aggregates, and classifies data in order to provide health practitioners with useful information for understanding and analyzing decisions, performance, and consequences. For example, this includes discharge rates, the average length of stay, and other relevant metrics for hospitals.

(b)   Diagnostic Analytics

Diagnostic analytics seeks to explain why certain events occurred and what factors contributed to them. For example, diagnostic analytics attempts to understand the reasons behind the frequent readmissions of some patients [32] using various methods such as clustering and decision trees. To find the source of an issue and help people understand its nature and impact, an extensive examination and guided analysis of the existing data utilizing tools such as imaging techniques are required [33]. This may include the ability to understand the effects of system inputs and processes on performance. For instance, there are a number of significant factors, such as patient, provider, or organization-related issues, that may contribute to longer wait times for the provision of some healthcare services [34,35].

(c)   Predictive Analytics

Predictive analytics reflect the ability to predict future events while assisting in the identification of trends and identifying potential uncertain outcomes; for example, it may be asked to predict whether or not a patient will develop complications. Predictive models are often constructed using machine learning techniques. Predictive analytics use massive data sets to improve customer experience, improving results compared to conventional business strategies [7]. They are used to analyze large volumes of data, as well as unstructured data, which produce the results to predict future developments. From an information science perspective, predicting future developments based on current data sets is a difficult issue. Business intelligence programs of this kind help to calculate data streams on a larger scale, including social media content, shopping experiences, users' daily activities, and surveys [36]. For example, a pharmacist may need to know how much of a medicinal preparation to keep in stock in the inventory in anticipation of an outbreak of an epidemic. A doctor may also need to predict certain clinical events, such as the length of a patient's stay, the possibility that a patient will choose to undergo surgery, or the possibility that a patient will have complications or even die [4].

(d)   Prescriptive Analytics

Decisions in the prescriptive analysis must be based on a wide range of practical alternatives, which can enable decision-makers in an organization to diagnose emerging opportunities or problems and recommend the best course of action to capitalize on the analysis provided in time while also taking into account the consequences and expected outcomes of decisions [37]. This analysis method automatically synthesizes Big Data and provides insights into a large number of possible outcomes before an analysis is performed. This information can be used by the decision-maker to support their actions. Prescriptive analytics give advice on what should be performed, what the best outcome will be, and how they can obtain it.

3. Artificial Intelligence in Medical Field

The use of artificial intelligence in medical research has the potential to lead to extremely sophisticated e-Health [38]. Machine learning (ML) is recognized as one of the most important scientific fields that can be integrated into the processes of diagnosis, prognosis, and even the treatment of diseases with the help of clinical decision support systems [39]. Another point about using machine learning techniques in healthcare is the elimination of human involvement to some degree, which reduces the likelihood of human error. This is particularly relevant when processing automation tasks; tedious routine work is where humans make the most errors [17]. In contrast, deep learning is a subfield of machine learning, which is a more sophisticated method that enables computers to automatically extract, analyze, and grasp relevant information from unstructured data by mimicking human thinking and learning [40]. Due to the volume of data generated for each patient, machine learning techniques have enormous potential in the healthcare field. The algorithms listed below are commonly used in health informatics.

- K-Nearest Neighbor Algorithm

We can define the k-nearest neighbor (k-NN) technique as a non-parametric algorithm, which means that the data set determines the model's structure. This is the reason why it is widely used; it does not rely on theoretical mathematical assumptions [41]. It also belongs to so-called "lazy" algorithms, which means that it does not need to learn or train all the data used in the prediction phase, and all the data can be used for the "test" phase. As a result, data learning is faster, and prediction is slower and more expensive and is thus more time and memory-consuming.

- Support Vector Machines (SVM)

Support vector machines, or SVMs, are a group of techniques used in classification and regression. They belong to a family of generalized linear classifiers. SVM is a practical method for classifying data. Typically, training and testing data for a classification task comprise certain data instances. Each instance in the training set includes a goal value and a number of other attributes. SVM classification is an example of fully supervised learning. Known labels aid in determining whether or not a system is on the right track [42]. According to [43], the SVM classifier has superior performance compared to other classifiers based on machine learning. Arrhythmic beat classification is used for anomaly detection in the electrocardiogram. The following figure (Figure 5) depicts a Support Vector Machine (SVM) model in two dimensions.

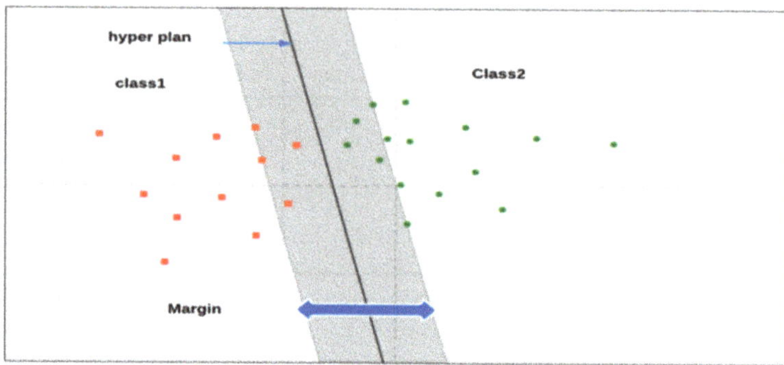

Figure 5. SVM model in two dimensions.

- K-Means Clustering Techniques

It has been demonstrated that data clustering is a useful technique for identifying structures in medical datasets. The k-means partitioning algorithm is one of the most popular and widely used clustering algorithms, and it belongs to a larger class of learning techniques that do not require unsupervised learning [44]. Clustering a dataset using k-means is simple. The fundamental idea is to find k centroids, one for each cluster, and link each element to the closest centroid, as long as the number (k) of clusters (groups) to be formed is predetermined.

- Artificial Neural Networks

Artificial neural networks streamline representations of the brains of living things, particularly humans. Their functions and the structure of biological neural networks are similar to those of biological neurons in the brain. They attempt to combine the function of the human brain with a strictly abstract mathematical way of thinking, thus distinguishing artificial intelligence from biology and the classical function of computers [45]. Figure 6 depicts the fundamental structure of the algorithm.

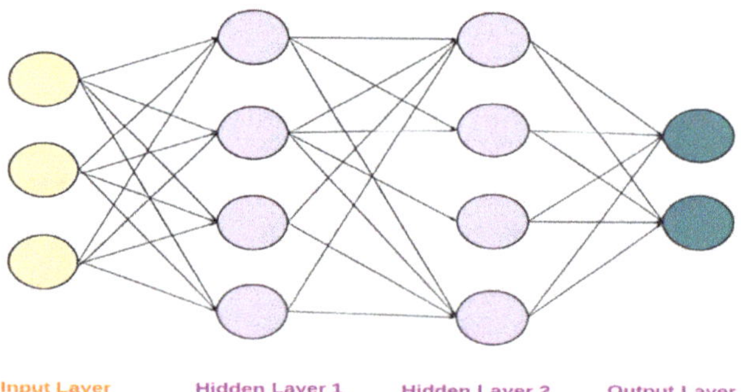

Figure 6. A neural network's basic structure.

However, scientists, with the source inspired by the structure of the biological neuron, have managed to create an equivalent model of the so-called artificial neuron. A biological neuron receives input signals in the form of electrical impulses in its dendrites, processes them, and then transmits them to neighboring neurons via the axis and synapses. The primary goal of using artificial neural networks is to solve specific problems or to work autonomously in certain processes, such as image recognition. The issue of opacity in artificial neural networks is of critical concern, especially in safety-critical applications where the ability to comprehend and interpret decisions is paramount. Due to the black-box nature of neural networks, it can be challenging to identify potential sources of error or bias, hindering our understanding of the underlying mechanisms behind decisions. While generating explanations or using more interpretable models have been proposed to address this issue, they may reduce accuracy or increase complexity. Therefore, it is essential for researchers and practitioners to weigh the trade-offs that are involved in using neural networks in safety-critical contexts and ensure that their use is justifiable and appropriately evaluated.

- Application of Machine Learning in Healthcare

There has been a considerable amount of research in recent publications to diagnose, predict or identify diseases. Nowadays, a variety of diseases are extensively diagnosed using different machine learning (ML) algorithms because of improvements in processing power and substantial studies on the subject [46]. The authors in [47] proposed a computational approach that relies on the SVM algorithm to predict Alzheimer's disease by utilizing gene and protein sequencing information. According to the obtained results in their research, the accuracy of their technique for Alzheimer's disease detection was 85.7%. U. Ahmed et al. [48] designed a framework consisting of two types of models: an SVM model and an ANN model. In order to predict if a patient has diabetes or not, these models examine the dataset to identify if a diabetes diagnosis is positive or negative. The prediction accuracy of their suggested fused technique was 94.87%. S. Thapa et al. [46] suggested a method for detecting Parkinson's disease patients based on feature selection and support vector machines. Based on the experiment's findings, TSVM can be a better classifier for a problem involving binary classifications such as Parkinson's disease delineation. To track the characteristics of brain tumors and improve detection efficiency, the authors in [49] developed a convolutional neural network-based model and MRI detection technology. This research model's main function is to segment and recognize MRIs: it employs a convolutional layer to improve recognition efficiency. Zheng et al. [50] used fusion k-means and SVMs to identify breast cancer. K-means were used in the experiment to identify the different hidden patterns of cancerous and benign tumors. H. K. van der Burgh et al. [51] merged clinical information from individuals with amyotrophic lateral sclerosis (a condition that results in the loss of neurons that regulate voluntary muscles) with MRI pictures. By using deep neural networks and this data, scientists were able to predict survivorship. M. Ghiasi et al. [52] designed a model dubbed the classification and regression tree (CART) model to detect coronary heart disease based on a decision tree learning algorithm. When compared to the reported targets, the results of the CART models showed the highest possible accuracy for coronary heart disease diagnosis (100%). D. Brinati et al. [53] created an interactive decision tree model to help clinicians identify COVID-19-positive patients using blood test analysis and machine learning instead of a PCR test. Their research demonstrated the feasibility and utility of using the latter two tools as an alternative to polymerase chain reaction (PCR) testing. While authors in [54] built a system based on the electronic medical record to help doctors categorize and prioritize patients in the emergency department, their system uses image data transformation as an input and a convolutional neural network algorithm as a classifier, to select patients who should go to the emergency department. The model presents a good performance of 0.86%.

In summary, Table 3 depicts in detail the applications of different machine learning techniques in healthcare analytics.

As shown in Table 3, machine learning methods can be used for a variety of applications, such as disease diagnosis, patient risk stratification, drug discovery, and resource optimization. The choice of algorithm depends on the specific use case and the type of data being analyzed. Some algorithms, such as logistic regression and decision trees, are well-suited for binary classification tasks, while others, such as clustering and neural networks, can be used for unsupervised learning and more complex tasks. While machine learning algorithms can be powerful tools for healthcare analysis, it is important to consider their limitations and potential biases. Machine learning algorithms should be validated and tested to ensure their accuracy and reliability in real-world healthcare settings.

Table 3. Recent uses of machine learning in the healthcare field.

Year	Application of Machine Learning in Medicine Context of Research	Technique Used
2020	Using various data balancing techniques to improve liver disease prediction [55]	
2019	Predicting Opioid Use Disorder [56]	Random Forest
2018	Prediction of osteoarthritis disease [57]	
2022	Prediction of Coronary Artery Disease and Acute Coronary Syndrome [58]	
2020	Neurological disease prediction [59]	Ensemble Learning
2020	Prediction of heart disease risk [60]	
2022	A Gene Prediction Function for Type 2 Diabetes Mellitus [61]	
2020	Prediction of graft dysfunction in pediatric liver transplantation [62]	Logistic regression
2020	Diabetes Progression Index Score Prediction [63]	
2022	Clinical Diagnosis of Alzheimer's Disease [64]	
2021	Classification of MRI images of brain tumors [65]	Support vector Machines
2021	Early Alzheimer's Disease Detection Using Blood Plasma Proteins [66]	
2019	Breast Cancer Detection Using the Decision Tree [67]	
2019	Predicting breast cancer survivability [68]	Decision trees
2020	Liver Diseases Prediction using KNN [69]	
2018	Lower Back Pain Classification [70]	K nearest Neighbors
2018	Heart disease diagnosis [71]	
2021	Prediction of cardiovascular disease via anomaly detection based on grouping [72]	
2021	Estimated number of confirmed COVID-19 cases [73]	K-means
2017	Dengue fever forecast [74]	
2022	Recognizing human activity from sensor data [75]	
2019	Classify lesions in optical tomographic images of breast masses [76]	Neural Networks
2017	Automatic identification of nasopharyngeal carcinoma [77]	

The capacity of researchers is greatly facilitated by open access to epidemiological, management, and clinical data in the health sector, which should help increase the volume of data and improve the quality of scientific research, as well as the scientific reach of institutions and the research community. In fact, the dominant trend in healthcare, which promises the most significant innovations, is that of data-driven patient care. Recording and collating all a patient's information provides a more accurate picture of the care being performed and, in general, of population health management. It can also reduce inappropriate drug prescriptions and, in many cases, save lives.

4. Big Data Technology Stack in Healthcare

Once the fundamental issues regarding the use, collection, and management of big data in healthcare have been understood, it is appropriate to explore the tools provided by technology for data use. As is almost always the case in areas of software use, there is also in the use of big data the possibility of choosing between the use of open-source software and commercial solutions, which require the use of financial resources. The chosen platform must, in any case, manage data entry, processing, storage, and retrieval, as well as provide data analysis capabilities. This section presents the main options available.

4.1. Infrastructure and Virtualization

To be able to store and process huge amounts of health data efficiently, hardware resources ranging from highly scalable storage systems to computing resources for data centers, and HPC systems are required. For this purpose, there are three subareas: cloud and grid solutions, data centers and HPC systems [78]. Cloud solutions provide the user with the illusion of virtually infinite computing and storage resources and thus allow companies and researchers to easily acquire them. Cloud solutions hide the details of the proposed hardware and rely on technologies for implementing large data centers. Data centers are needed for building cloud infrastructures as well as for in-house companies to provide computing and storage resources. For data centers, commodity hardware is primarily used to scale horizontally in a cost-effective manner.

4.1.1. Apache Hadoop

Hadoop [79] is an open framework based on a distributed system that stores and processes very large computational clusters on core architecture and is reinforced by three primary elements, as shown in Figure 7.

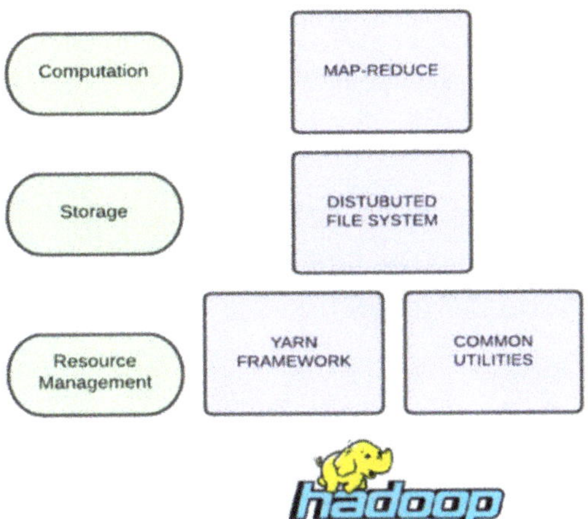

Figure 7. The structure of apache Hadoop.

The core of Hadoop consists of a storage component called HDFS, a distributed file system, a processing component based on the map-reduce model, and a resource manager called YARN, "Yet Another Resource Negotiator" [80]. Hadoop splits the data into large blocks and distributes them among the diverse compute nodes that make up the computing system. It then transfers the code for execution to the nodes so that parallels, i.e., the simultaneous processing of data, can take place on those nodes [81]. In essence, the location property of the data is exploited, and nodes manage the individual data to which they have access. Finally, it should be noted that while the basic structure of Hadoop consists of the elements already mentioned, Apache extensions are often used to enrich Hadoop's capabilities, depending on the situation, with the most important ones being Apache Spark, Apache Storm, Apache Flink, Apache Hive, Apache HBase, Apache Flume, Apache Sqoop, and Apache Pig. Hadoop could potentially be employed to develop medical analytics solutions. However, as previously stated, it is a batch big data platform that fails to fully capitalize on the potential of real-time emergencies [11].

4.1.2. Apache Spark

Spark was created after Hadoop and provides the developer with an interface focused on a data structure known as a "Resilient Distributed Dataset" (RDD) that is intended to be a collection of objects distributed across a set of compute nodes, which provide efficient hardware failure management [82]. On the other hand, Spark provides the capacity to perform computations in shared memory, where the speed is significantly higher than on a disk. In this way, it becomes possible to implement iterative algorithms that access data multiple times on each iteration, without this coming at the expense of computational time, since the data access time in memory is faster and "closer" to the processor of the compute nodes. Apache Spark, in addition to the way it handles big data, offers the following key extensions [83]:

- Spark SQL: allows queries to be performed on data using SQL in conjunction with the Java, Scala, Python, and R programming languages.
- Spark Streaming: allows for the processing of streaming data, i.e., data that enters the system while calculations are already underway on the previous data. This

feature is very important because in Hadoop, new data cannot be preprocessed during processing, but the entire data set must be available when a MapReduce process is started. Java, Scala, and Python programming languages are supported.

- MLlib: This is a machine learning library that allows this type of algorithm to run up to 100 times faster than Hadoop.
- GraphX: Provides an API (application programming interface) for graphical data, allowing for productive computations using iterative algorithms.

Figure 8 shows the components of Apache Spark.

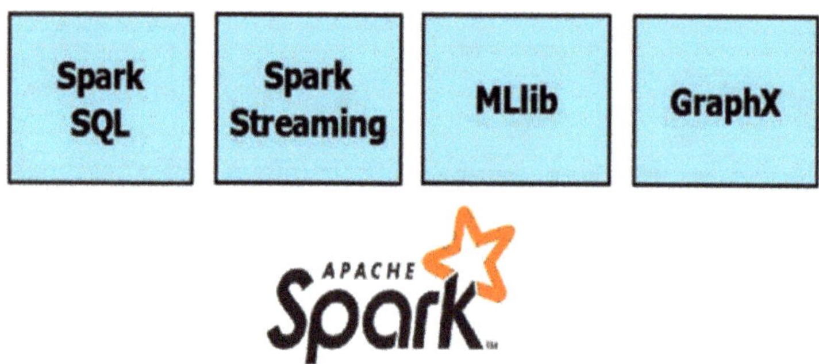

Figure 8. Apache Spark components.

Apache Spark can collect data from a variety of health data sources. It can handle large amounts of structured, semi-structured, and unstructured healthcare data, such as electronic health records (EHRs), diagnostic images, and genetic information. It can also preprocess, clean, and transform the data into a format suitable for analysis. Spark streaming components such as MLib can be employed to analyze healthcare data in real time, which is produced by wearable health devices [84]. The data consists of crucial health metrics such as weight, blood pressure, respiratory rate, ECG, and blood glucose levels. By utilizing machine learning algorithms, the analysis can detect any potential critical health conditions before they manifest. For example, the authors in [85] created a health status prediction system in real-time for breast cancer by utilizing Spark streaming and machine learning. The system was designed to predict health status using machine learning models applied to streaming data. In the same context, the authors in [86] have suggested a heart disease monitoring system that utilizes the Spark framework for continuous and real-time monitoring. The system also employs the random forest algorithm with MLlib to build a prediction model for heart disease.

In summary, Apache Spark's ability to process, analyze, and integrate large amounts of healthcare data, combined with its machine learning and real-time capabilities, make it a valuable tool for addressing big data healthcare problems.

4.2. The Use of NoSQL Databases

Relational databases, structured on the basis of the SQL language, have been the most popular data management method for many years among organizations and technology professionals. With the advent of big medical data, which are characterized by both its large size and diverse structure, there is a need to be able to process data on a large scale in order to draw consistent conclusions [87]. SQL-based systems cannot provide a stand-alone solution to the problem of managing these data. This problem can be solved by using NoSQL databases, which offer dynamic data management, flexibility, and scalability over relational databases. Their characteristics make them ideal for managing large, non-homogeneous data that are frequently updated and have frequently changed data field formats, in addition to the data itself [82]. The main NoSQL database options are MongoDB, Neo4j, CouchBase, Dynamo DB, HBase, and Cassandra. For healthcare companies, the use of MongoDB has dominated over others. MongoDB is provided by 10Gen and can be effectively combined with the use of JSON (JavaScript Object Notation), XML, etc. According to the company itself, MongoDB is flexible, easy to use, and offers high performance, availability, and automatic scaling. Among other important features, it has the ability to perform text searches and connect to Hadoop. According to the official solution website, some indicative examples of solutions provided by MongoDB in the healthcare industry include:

- The creation of a complete patient profile that includes all tests performed on the patient and extracts useful relationships between them using data mining techniques. It is easy to modify and add new test data to the profile and compare old and new data.
- Early detection and containment of epidemics: big data has the potential to save human lives in situations where no other method can. Collecting data on emerging diseases, which have the potential to spread, widely, could be leveraged by applications that could serve as a tool for medical personnel and the extraction of risk indicators, such as the speed of spread, the number of people affected, symptoms, comparisons with data from previous epidemics, and suggesting the possibility of rapidly implementing population containment measures if necessary.
- The early diagnosis of rare diseases: it is possible to identify rare diseases that may have a common set of symptoms, but each of them or a subset of them is not a formidable indication. This observation is especially important because medical practitioners make their diagnoses primarily based on the experience and history of the patients they have examined in the past, which makes the process of early diagnosis of rare diseases extremely difficult, given the nature of human reasoning. Applications that have a large statistical dataset make it very easy to extract indicators to identify a disease and are an extremely useful tool for medical staff.
- Immediate consultation in real-time: in the case of laboratory data from patient tests, it is possible for medical personnel to draw immediate quantitative conclusions. As measurements from all types and sources of data can be visually displayed in single tables via graphs, there is no need for an independent review of individual tests by attending physicians.

4.3. Commercial Platforms for Healthcare Data Analytics

A large number of databases that are available in the field of drug development create the need to identify priorities and methods for selecting appropriate information from a vast universe of big data. In this context, the Open PHACTS initiative implements the semantic weight-based search of research questions conducted in the context of pharmaceutical research [88]. The Open PHACTS program has a clear impact in several ways. The most important contribution is the use of the system in scientific research. Several scientific publications have resulted from the extensive use of this system, which allows for data analysis that has been very difficult to achieve in the past. Many pharmaceutical companies have integrated their internal data into Open PHACTS so that they can easily query all the information they have, whether public or private. Another contribution comes from the realization that large amounts of diverse semantic pharmaceutical data can be analyzed efficiently, thus improving data quality. The success of the Open PHACTS project has demonstrated the practicality of using data in biomedical research. Indeed, the fact that providers have chosen to offer their data reinforces the value of the action and helps sustain the Open PHACTS system.

Another very interesting project is the Artemis project. This project uses mining techniques, patented by McGregor, that are designed for non-trivial and possibly meaningful abstract information from huge datasets, where the digital data are generated by monitoring devices [89]. The analysis system employs abstraction techniques on the input data to identify recurrent patterns. It subsequently evaluates whether individuals with various health conditions, including infections, respiratory distress syndrome, and different forms of sleep apnea, exhibit similar data patterns in their normal state. The Artemis project leverages three medical connectivity systems provided by Capsule Tech, ExcelMedical, and True Process clinical centers to continuously feed real-time data into a cloud-based database and analytics platform powered by IBM's InfoSphere and DB2 relational database [90].

IBM Watson is a complex computer system capable of answering questions in natural language. Medical personnel express in natural language the problem they are facing, describing symptoms and other relevant factors. Watson then performs an analysis and compiles a list of possible causes [91]. The sources of big data that Watson refers to can be physician and nurse notes and records, the electronic medical records of patients, clinical trials and research, scientific articles, as well as the information provided by patients themselves. Although it was developed and advertised as a diagnostic and treatment consultant, in reality, Watson was primarily used to treat patients who had already been diagnosed with a disease by suggesting ways to treat it [92].

The subsequent table presents a comparative analysis of various big data technologies applied in the context of healthcare.

The right technology for healthcare data analytics is determined by several factors, including the complexity and volume of the data, the system's required speed and scalability, the resources available, expert knowledge, and the defined targets and use cases. In general, open-source tools such as Hadoop and Spark provide a cost-effective and flexible solution for handling huge and varied healthcare datasets, as well as supporting various machine learning algorithms and techniques. They may, however, necessitate more technical skills and maintenance efforts than commercial tools. Commercial tools such as IBM Watson, Artemis, and Open PHACTS, on the other hand, often come with pre-built models and features that can accelerate the development and deployment of healthcare analytics applications, as well as provide more user-friendly interfaces and support services. They may, however, be more expensive and have fewer customization options. When selecting a technology for healthcare data analytics, healthcare professionals should carefully evaluate their specific needs and constraints, as well as factors such as data security, regulatory compliance, interoperability, and ethical considerations. It is also important to remember that technology selection is a continuous process that may necessitate continuous evaluation and optimization in response to changing needs and advances in the field. Table 4 represents a comparative analysis of various big data technologies in healthcare.

Table 4. Comparative analysis of various big data technologies in healthcare.

	Hadoop	**Spark**	**IBM Watson**	**Artemis**	**Open PHACTS**
Data Storage	HDFS (Hadoop Distributed File System)	RDDs (Resilient Distributed Datasets)	IBM Cloud Object Storage	MySQL, PostgreSQL, Oracle	Virtuoso Universal Server
Data Processing	Map Reduce, Hadoop Ecosystem (Pig, Hive, HBase, etc.)	Spark Core, Spark SQL, Spark Streaming, GraphX, MLlib	Watson Studio, SPSS Modeler	Cypher Query Language, RDF triplestores	SPARQL, RDF triplestores
Data Integration	Apache Nifi, Talend, Pentaho	Apache Nifi, Talend, Pentaho	IBM InfoSphere DataStage, Talend	ETL tools, REST APIs	ETL tools, REST APIs
Healthcare Applications	Clinical Decision Support, Drug Discovery, Genomics, Imaging Analytics	Predictive Analytics, Electronic Health Records Analysis, Clinical Decision Support	Drug Discovery, Genomics, Precision Medicine	Clinical Trials, Patient Data Management	Drug Discovery, Pharmacovigilance, Disease Networks

5. Technical and Organizational Challenges in Healthcare Big Data

The challenges that arise when using big data analytics technology are numerous and are particularly important to make the effort effective. The challenges are heterogeneous and diverse. The key points that a healthcare provider must consider in each case in this context are as follows:

(a)   Data repositories

Although it has already been reported that the available health data are growing exponentially, the majority of it is in individual repositories: a phenomenon that has been called "data silos" [93]. These are essentially data repositories that are kept within an organization or even individual parts of organizations and are not accessible to the outside world. The lack of a common spirit of collaboration between organizations and internally between different departments inevitably hinder data sharing. It is, therefore, up to the institution concerned to ensure that this risk is avoided by developing the right spirit among employees, which is usually not a standard procedure.

(b)   Data quality

Data quality refers to all the key characteristics that describe big data, as presented in detail in the previous section. In particular, there are four categories (4 vs.), and the following challenges are encountered:

- Volume: For efficient exploitation of data, the ability to manage and store the volume of data as well as determine their size must be ensured. Scalability is almost always required, as needs are constantly increasing, as is the volume to be exploited.
- Velocity: Any organization must consider the speed with which it can store, process, and use available data and continuously improve its performance, especially when the rate of data arrival is fast.
- Validity: Ensuring the validity of the data is critical to the project's needs and is a demanding process.
- Variety: Identifying all data sources, the technical challenges that each source imposes, and managing them effectively is an integral part of any big data analysis effort and is a major challenge.

(c)   Periodic data refresh

This is a purely technical issue, but one that can create difficulties if it is not respected. It is essentially about data management. In some cases, it is necessary to periodically delete or update data, and the systems available have specific capabilities. Therefore, there is a need to ensure that dynamic data management can be performed.

(d)   Analytics challenges

Beyond the technical requirements, it is extremely important to "decrypt" the data, to understand it, and to develop analytical thinking and methods to create value. It is common for data to be misinterpreted by humans, leading to results that are not desired.

(e)   Application of expertise

The needs of the health sector are constantly increasing through new research, observations, scientific articles, etc. However, at the same time, the technological capabilities that can help meet the needs are also increasing. Therefore, it is essential to be aware of technological developments and to intervene, if necessary, to overcome the inherent difficulties and extend the system's functionality.

(f)   Prediction models

A key area of big data analytics is the generation of models that estimate and predict various situations. Specifically, in the healthcare industry, there is a need for the continuous study of data and the estimation of expected events to maximize the benefits and value of the data.

(g)   Legal issues

There is a wide range of legal issues that need to be addressed, and it is necessary to keep abreast of developments in this area. System security must be ensured against unauthorized access to data by unauthorized persons. In this context, the challenges are the same as in the area of security systems, which require a lot of time and effort. On the other hand, health information is extremely sensitive and should never be used to directly or indirectly identify individuals: a concept that is known as patient privacy. The challenge is even greater, especially in the absence of a stable and universally accepted framework.

The following figure, Figure 9, illustrates the key challenges in the healthcare sector regarding the use of big data.

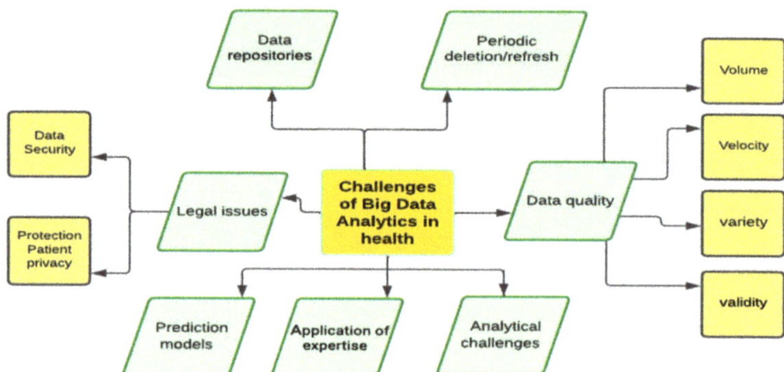

Figure 9. Key challenges in the healthcare sector regarding the use of big data.

The need to develop tools and methods to meet all the issues raised by the use of big data in healthcare organizations requires a collective, organized, and rigorously defined effort.

6. Proposed Strategies for Implementing Big Data Analytics in Healthcare for Smart City

In the context of the Smart City concept, the integration of big data analytics in healthcare can play a critical role in improving the overall quality of life. Healthcare providers can gain a more comprehensive understanding of the community's health needs by leveraging the vast amounts of data that are generated by various sources such as wearable devices, electronic health records, and social media platforms. This can lead to more effective and targeted interventions in addressing health issues, as well as the development of proactive healthcare strategies to avoid illnesses in the first place. Furthermore, the use of big data analytics can aid in the optimization of healthcare resource allocation, lowering costs and increasing efficiency. As such, it is crucial for healthcare organizations and institutions to consider the Smart City context when developing and implementing big data analytics strategies in healthcare.

Based on the best practices in the field of big data analytics in healthcare, we provide a general framework for healthcare organizations to follow; by applying this simple strategy, health professionals can effectively leverage the potential of big data analytics to improve patient outcomes in their medical institutions.

- ✓ Define the goals and objectives: Clearly define the goals and objectives of the big data analytics initiative, such as improving patient outcomes, reducing healthcare costs, or enhancing the quality of care.
- ✓ Develop a comprehensive data strategy: Develop a comprehensive data strategy that outlines how the data will be collected, stored, processed, and analyzed to support the big data analytics initiative.
- ✓ The identification of tools and applications to be used: Invest in the right technology and infrastructure to support big data analytics, such as cloud computing, data warehouses, and data analytics tools. The effective use of big data technologies has many benefits, including the ability to measure the effectiveness and efficiency of interventions in real clinical practice. At the same time, it offers the possibility

of aggregating epidemiological, clinical, economic, and management data that can contribute to the generation of correlation information between the health of humans, economic resources, and health outcomes.

✓ Maximizing the Use of Current Knowledge: It is imperative to adopt a perspective that integrates and uses existing knowledge. This approach will enhance data comprehension, facilitate the systematic generation of novel insights, and foster a data-driven culture within the medical institution.

✓ Create a medical network: Collaborate with patients, healthcare providers, and researchers to ensure that the big data analytics project aligns with their needs and goals.

✓ Establishing a Strong Legal Framework for Personal Data Protection: Data protection, in particular, plays a key role in the successful implementation of big data. Particular attention must be paid to the processing of personal data, and it is important to take into account the legal framework conditions and technological possibilities for its implementation.

✓ Progressive development and continuous monitoring: A progressive integration can help better monitor and continually evaluate the big data analytics initiative to ensure that it is delivering value and positively impacting patient care.

In the following figure (Figure 10), the suggested strategy for implementing big data in the healthcare industry is summarized.

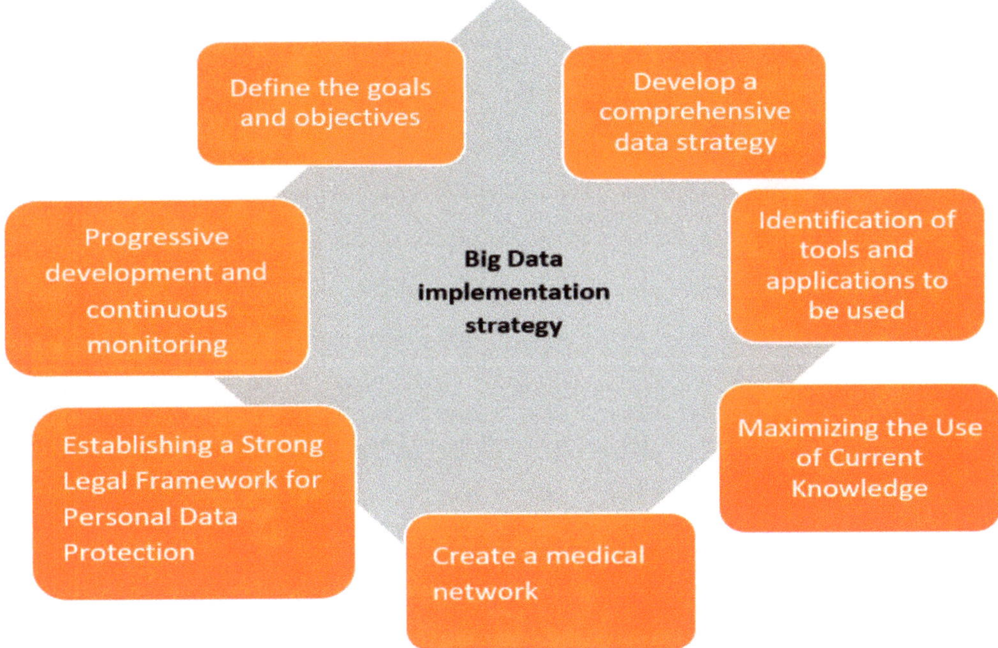

Figure 10. Suggested strategy for implementing big data in the healthcare industry.

7. Conclusions

There is no doubt that financial and human resources will be invested in the near future to improve health services through big data analytics. The number of problems solved through their use is enormous, and at present, there does not seem to be an alternative technology with comparable potential. For this reason, it is certain that the use of data on a large scale will concern not only "large" institutions and organizations in the future but that each clinic and doctor will have to use the technological tools available to them in order to provide health services. This is optimal because large sums of money are wasted unnecessarily, either due to inefficient management resulting from poor handling or incorrect treatment and diagnosis. More importantly, the human factor, i.e., the radical upgrade of health services that can usher in a new era, is the most important reason to dispel any doubts about the proliferation of big data analysis in the future. This paper demonstrates the abundance of opportunities to deliver more targeted, large-scale, and cost-effective healthcare by leveraging the available data and big data analytics. However, the healthcare sector has been shown to have specific characteristics and challenges that require additional research efforts in order to fully benefit from the opportunities. In our next work, we will propose a methodology to develop big data analysis in the health field and design a new flexible architecture that meets the challenges mentioned in this review.

Author Contributions: Methodology and Conceptualization, N.B.; validation and review, F.E.M. and Y.E.B.E.I.; writing—original draft preparation, N.B. and Y.F. All authors have read and agreed to the published version of the manuscript.

Funding: This research received no external funding.

Data Availability Statement: Not applicable.

Conflicts of Interest: The authors declare no conflict of interest.

References

1. Manogaran, G.; Thota, C.; Lopez, D.; Vijayakumar, V.; Abbas, K.M.; Sundarsekar, R. Big Data Knowledge System in Healthcare. In *Internet of Things and Big Data Technologies for Next Generation Healthcare*; Bhatt, C., Dey, N., Ashour, A.S., Eds.; Springer International Publishing: Cham, Switzerland, 2017; pp. 133–157. [CrossRef]
2. Munawar, H.S.; Qayyum, S.; Ullah, F.; Sepasgozar, S. Big Data and Its Applications in Smart Real Estate and the Disaster Management Life Cycle: A Systematic Analysis. *Big Data Cogn. Comput.* **2020**, *4*, 4. [CrossRef]
3. Raghupathi, W.; Raghupathi, V. Big data analytics in healthcare: Promise and potential. *Health Inf. Sci. Syst.* **2014**, *2*, 3. [CrossRef] [PubMed]
4. Bhaskaran, K.L.; Osei, R.S.; Kotei, E.; Agbezuge, E.Y.; Ankora, C.; Ganaa, E.D. A Survey on Big Data in Pharmacology, Toxicology and Pharmaceutics. *Big Data Cogn. Comput.* **2022**, *6*, 161. [CrossRef]
5. Dash, S.; Shakyawar, S.K.; Sharma, M.; Kaushik, S. Big data in healthcare: Management, analysis and future prospects. *J. Big Data* **2019**, *6*, 54. [CrossRef]
6. Strickland, N.H. PACS (picture archiving and communication systems): Filmless radiology. *Arch. Dis. Child.* **2000**, *83*, 82–86. [CrossRef]
7. Janke, A.T.; Overbeek, D.L.; Kocher, K.E.; Levy, P.D. Exploring the Potential of Predictive Analytics and Big Data in Emergency Care. *Ann. Emerg. Med.* **2016**, *67*, 227–236. [CrossRef]
8. Batko, K.; Ślęzak, A. The use of Big Data Analytics in healthcare. *J. Big Data* **2022**, *9*, 3. [CrossRef]
9. Wang, L.; Alexander, C.A. Big Data in Medical Applications and Health Care. *Curr. Res. Med.* **2015**, *6*, 1–8. [CrossRef]
10. Tresp, V.; Overhage, J.M.; Bundschus, M.; Rabizadeh, S.; Fasching, P.A.; Yu, S. Going Digital: A Survey on Digitalization and Large-Scale Data Analytics in Healthcare. *Proc. IEEE* **2016**, *104*, 2180–2206. [CrossRef]
11. Harerimana, G.; Jang, B.; Kim, J.W.; Park, H.K. Health Big Data Analytics: A Technology Survey. *IEEE Access* **2018**, *6*, 65661–65678. [CrossRef]
12. Bahri, S.; Zoghlami, N.; Abed, M.; Tavares, J.M.R.S. BIG DATA for Healthcare: A Survey. *IEEE Access* **2019**, *7*, 7397–7408. [CrossRef]
13. Dhayne, H.; Haque, R.; Kilany, R.; Taher, Y. In Search of Big Medical Data Integration Solutions—A Comprehensive Survey. *IEEE Access* **2019**, *7*, 91265–91290. [CrossRef]
14. Wang, L.; Alexander, C.A. Big data analytics in medical engineering and healthcare: Methods, advances and challenges. *J. Med. Eng. Technol.* **2020**, *44*, 267–283. [CrossRef]
15. Shafqat, S.; Kishwer, S.; Rasool, R.U.; Qadir, J.; Amjad, T.; Ahmad, H.F. Big data analytics enhanced healthcare systems: A review. *J. Supercomput.* **2020**, *76*, 1754–1799. [CrossRef]
16. Imran, S.; Mahmood, T.; Morshed, A.; Sellis, T. Big data analytics in healthcare A systematic literature review and roadmap for practical implementation. *IEEE/CAA J. Autom. Sinica* **2021**, *8*, 1–22. [CrossRef]
17. Chattu, V.K. A Review of Artificial Intelligence, Big Data, and Blockchain Technology Applications in Medicine and Global Health. *Big Data Cogn. Comput.* **2021**, *5*, 41. [CrossRef]
18. Al-Sai, Z.A.; Husin, M.H.; Syed-Mohamad, S.M.; Abdin, R.M.S.; Damer, N.; Abualigah, L.; Gandomi, A.H. Explore Big Data Analytics Applications and Opportunities: A Review. *Big Data Cogn. Comput.* **2022**, *6*, 157. [CrossRef]

19. Zhou, H. Developing Natural Language Processing to Extract Complementary and Integrative Health Information from Electronic Health Record Data. In Proceedings of the 2022 IEEE 10th International Conference on Healthcare Informatics (ICHI), Rochester, MN, USA, 11–14 June 2022; pp. 474–475. [CrossRef]
20. Piedrahita-Valdés, H.; Piedrahita-Castillo, D.; Bermejo-Higuera, J.; Guillem-Saiz, P.; Bermejo-Higuera, J.R.; Guillem-Saiz, J.; Sicilia-Montalvo, J.A.; Machío-Regidor, F. Vaccine Hesitancy on Social Media: Sentiment Analysis from June 2011 to April 2019. *Vaccines* **2021**, *9*, 28. [CrossRef]
21. Khaloufi, H.; Abouelmehdi, K.; Beni-hssane, A.; Saadi, M. Security model for Big Healthcare Data Lifecycle. *Procedia Comput. Sci.* **2018**, *141*, 294–301. [CrossRef]
22. Kumar, D.R.; Rajkumar, K.; Lalitha, K.; Dhanakoti, V. Bigdata in the Management of Diabetes Mellitus Treatment. In *Internet of Things for Healthcare Technologies 73*; Chakraborty, C., Banerjee, A., Kolekar, M.H., Garg, L., Chakraborty, B., Eds.; Springer Singapore: Singapore, 2021; pp. 293–324. [CrossRef]
23. Alfred, R.; Obit, J.H. The roles of machine learning methods in limiting the spread of deadly diseases: A systematic review. *Heliyon* **2021**, *7*, e07371. [CrossRef]
24. Wang, H.; Cui, Z.; Chen, Y.; Avidan, M.; Abdallah, A.B.; Kronzer, A. Predicting Hospital Readmission via Cost-Sensitive Deep Learning. *IEEE/ACM Trans. Comput. Biol. Bioinf.* **2018**, *15*, 1968–1978. [CrossRef] [PubMed]
25. Leff, D.R.; Yang, G.-Z. Big Data for Precision Medicine. *Engineering* **2015**, *1*, 277–279. [CrossRef]
26. Weitzman, E.R.; Kelemen, S.; Mandl, K.D. Surveillance of an Online Social Network to Assess Population-level Diabetes Health Status and Healthcare Quality. *Online J. Public Health Inform.* **2011**, *3*, ojphi.v3i3.3797. [CrossRef] [PubMed]
27. Ram, S.; Zhang, W.; Williams, M.; Pengetnze, Y. Predicting Asthma-Related Emergency Department Visits Using Big Data. *IEEE J. Biomed. Health Inform.* **2015**, *19*, 1216–1223. [CrossRef] [PubMed]
28. Odlum, M.; Yoon, S. What can we learn about the Ebola outbreak from tweets? *Am. J. Infect. Control* **2015**, *43*, 563–571. [CrossRef]
29. Ma, Y.; Wang, Y.; Yang, J.; Miao, Y.; Li, W. Big Health Application System based on Health Internet of Things and Big Data. *IEEE Access* **2017**, *5*, 7885–7897. [CrossRef]
30. Darwish, A.; Sayed, G.I.; Hassanien, A.E. The Impact of Implantable Sensors in Biomedical Technology on the Future of Healthcare Systems. In *Intelligent Pervasive Computing Systems for Smarter Healthcare*, 1st ed.; Sangaiah, A.K., Shantharajah, S., Theagarajan, P., Eds.; Wiley: Hoboken, NJ, USA, 2019; pp. 67–89. [CrossRef]
31. Islam, M.S.; Hasan, M.M.; Wang, X.; Germack, H.D.; Noor-E-Alam, M. A Systematic Review on Healthcare Analytics: Application and Theoretical Perspective of Data Mining. *Healthcare* **2018**, *6*, 54. [CrossRef]
32. Fisahn, C.; Sanders, F.H.; Moisi, M.; Page, J.; Oakes, P.C.; Wingerson, M.; Dettori, J.; Tubbs, R.S.; Chamiraju, P.; Nora, P.; et al. Descriptive analysis of unplanned readmission and reoperation rates after intradural spinal tumor resection. *J. Clin. Neurosci.* **2017**, *38*, 32–36. [CrossRef]
33. Yu, Y.; Li, M.; Liu, L.; Li, Y.; Wang, J. Clinical big data and deep learning: Applications, challenges, and future outlooks. *Big Data Min. Anal.* **2019**, *2*, 288–305. [CrossRef]
34. Simpao, A.F.; Ahumada, L.M.; Gálvez, J.A.; Rehman, M.A. A review of analytics and clinical informatics in health care. *J. Med. Syst.* **2014**, *38*, 45. [CrossRef]
35. Khalifa, M. Health Analytics Types, Functions and Levels: A Review of Literature. *Stud. Health Technol. Inform.* **2018**, *251*, 137–140.
36. Alharthi, H. Healthcare predictive analytics: An overview with a focus on Saudi Arabia. *J. Infect. Public Health* **2018**, *11*, 749–756. [CrossRef]
37. Mosavi, N.S.; Santos, M.F. How Prescriptive Analytics Influences Decision Making in Precision Medicine. *Procedia Comput. Sci.* **2020**, *177*, 528–533. [CrossRef]
38. Dicuonzo, G.; Galeone, G.; Shini, M.; Massari, A. Towards the Use of Big Data in Healthcare: A Literature Review. *Healthcare* **2022**, *10*, 1232. [CrossRef]
39. Khan, P.; Kader, F.; Islam, S.M.R.; Rahman, A.B.; Kamal, S.; Toha, M.U.; Kwak, K.-S. Machine Learning and Deep Learning Approaches for Brain Disease Diagnosis: Principles and Recent Advances. *IEEE Access* **2021**, *9*, 37622–37655. [CrossRef]
40. Chauhan, N.K.; Singh, K. A Review on Conventional Machine Learning vs. Deep Learning. In Proceedings of the 2018 International Conference on Computing, Power and Communication Technologies (GUCON), Greater Noida, India, 28–29 September 2018; pp. 347–352. [CrossRef]
41. Xing, W.; Bei, Y. Medical Health Big Data Classification Based on KNN Classification Algorithm. *IEEE Access* **2020**, *8*, 28808–28819. [CrossRef]
42. Wang, L.; Liu, J.; Zhu, S.; Gao, Y. Prediction of Linear B-Cell Epitopes Using AAT Scale. In Proceedings of the 2009 3rd International Conference on Bioinformatics and Biomedical Engineering, Beijing, China, 11–13 June 2009; pp. 1–4. [CrossRef]
43. Venkatesan, C.; Karthigaikumar, P.; Paul, A.; Satheeskumaran, S.; Kumar, R. ECG Signal Preprocessing and SVM Classifier-Based Abnormality Detection in Remote Healthcare Applications. *IEEE Access* **2018**, *6*, 9767–9773. [CrossRef]
44. Li, Y.; Wu, H. A Clustering Method Based on K-Means Algorithm. *Phys. Procedia* **2012**, *25*, 1104–1109. [CrossRef]
45. Hasson, U.; Nastase, S.A.; Goldstein, A. Direct Fit to Nature: An Evolutionary Perspective on Biological and Artificial Neural Networks. *Neuron* **2020**, *105*, 416–434. [CrossRef]
46. Thapa, S.; Adhikari, S.; Ghimire, A.; Aditya, A. Feature Selection Based Twin-Support Vector Machine for the Diagnosis of Parkinson's Disease. In Proceedings of the 2020 IEEE 8th R10 Humanitarian Technology Conference (R10-HTC), Kuching, Malaysia, 1–3 December 2020; pp. 1–6. [CrossRef]

47. Xu, L.; Liang, G.; Liao, C.; Chen, G.-D.; Chang, C.-C. An Efficient Classifier for Alzheimer's Disease Genes Identification. *Molecules* **2018**, *23*, 3140. [CrossRef]

48. Ahmed, U.; Issa, G.F.; Khan, M.A.; Aftab, S.; Said, R.A.T.; Ghazal, T.M.; Ahmad, M. Prediction of Diabetes Empowered with Fused Machine Learning. *IEEE Access* **2022**, *10*, 8529–8538. [CrossRef]

49. Wang, W.; Bu, F.; Lin, Z.; Zhai, S. Learning Methods of Convolutional Neural Network Combined with Image Feature Extraction in Brain Tumor Detection. *IEEE Access* **2020**, *8*, 152659–152668. [CrossRef]

50. Zheng, B.; Yoon, S.W.; Lam, S.S. Breast cancer diagnosis based on feature extraction using a hybrid of K-means and support vector machine algorithms. *Expert Syst. Appl.* **2014**, *41*, 1476–1482. [CrossRef]

51. van der Burgh, H.K.; Schmidt, R.; Westeneng, H.-J.; de Reus, M.A.; van den Berg, L.H.; van den Heuvel, M.P. Deep learning predictions of survival based on MRI in amyotrophic lateral sclerosis. *Neuroimage Clin.* **2016**, *13*, 361–369. [CrossRef] [PubMed]

52. Ghiasi, M.M.; Zendehboudi, S.; Mohsenipour, A.A. Decision tree-based diagnosis of coronary artery disease: CART model. *Comput. Methods Programs Biomed.* **2020**, *192*, 105400. [CrossRef]

53. Brinati, D.; Campagner, A.; Ferrari, D.; Locatelli, M.; Banfi, G.; Cabitza, F. Detection of COVID-19 Infection from Routine Blood Exams with Machine Learning: A Feasibility Study. *J. Med. Syst.* **2020**, *44*, 135. [CrossRef]

54. Yao, L.-H.; Leung, K.-C.; Hong, J.-H.; Tsai, C.-L.; Fu, L.-C. A System for Predicting Hospital Admission at Emergency Department Based on Electronic Health Record Using Convolution Neural Network. In Proceedings of the 2020 IEEE International Conference on Systems, Man, and Cybernetics (SMC), Toronto, ON, Canada, 11–14 October 2020; pp. 546–551. [CrossRef]

55. Ambesange, S.; Vijayalaxmi, A.; Uppin, R.; Patil, S.; Patil, V. Optimizing Liver disease prediction with Random Forest by various Data balancing Techniques. In Proceedings of the 2020 IEEE International Conference on Cloud Computing in Emerging Markets (CCEM), Bengaluru, India, 6–7 November 2020; pp. 98–102. [CrossRef]

56. Wadekar, A. Predicting Opioid Use Disorder (OUD) Using A Random Forest. In Proceedings of the 2019 IEEE 43rd Annual Computer Software and Applications Conference (COMPSAC), Milwaukee, WI, USA, 15–19 July 2019; Volume 1, pp. 960–961. [CrossRef]

57. Aprilliani, U.; Rustam, Z. Osteoarthritis Disease Prediction Based on Random Forest. In Proceedings of the 2018 International Conference on Advanced Computer Science and Information Systems (ICACSIS), Yogyakarta, Indonesia, 27–28 October 2018; pp. 237–240. [CrossRef]

58. Jamthikar, A.D.; Gupta, D.; Mantella, L.E.; Saba, L.; Johri, A.M.; Suri, J.S. Ensemble Machine Learning and Its Validation for Prediction of Coronary Artery Disease and Acute Coronary Syndrome Using Focused Carotid Ultrasound. *IEEE Trans. Instrum. Meas.* **2022**, *71*, 2503810. [CrossRef]

59. Kaur, S.; Aggarwal, H.; Rani, R. Neurological disease prediction using ensembled Machine Learning Model. In Proceedings of the 2020 Sixth International Conference on Parallel, Distributed and Grid Computing (PDGC), Waknaghat, India, 6–8 November 2020; pp. 410–414. [CrossRef]

60. Mienye, I.D.; Sun, Y.; Wang, Z. An improved ensemble learning approach for the prediction of heart disease risk. *Inform. Med. Unlocked* **2020**, *20*, 100402. [CrossRef]

61. Alshamlan, H.; Taleb, H.B.; Al Sahow, A. A Gene Prediction Function for Type 2 Diabetes Mellitus using Logistic Regression. In Proceedings of the 2020 11th International Conference on Information and Communication Systems (ICICS), Irbid, Jordan, 7–9 April 2020; pp. 1–4. [CrossRef]

62. Prodanova, K.; Uzunova, Y. Prediction of Graft Dysfunction in Pediatric Liver Transplantation by Logistic Regression. In Proceedings of the 2020 International Conference on Mathematics and Computers in Science and Engineering (MACISE), Madrid, Spain, 14–16 January 2020; pp. 260–263. [CrossRef]

63. Lei, L. Prediction of Score of Diabetes Progression Index Based on Logistic Regression Algorithm. In Proceedings of the 2020 International Conference on Virtual Reality and Intelligent Systems (ICVRIS), Zhangjiajie, China, 18–19 July 2020; pp. 954–956. [CrossRef]

64. Bhagyashree, S.R. Clinical Diagnosis of Alzheimer's Disease Employing Support Vector Machine. In Proceedings of the 2022 IEEE International Conference on Distributed Computing and Electrical Circuits and Electronics (ICDCECE), Ballari, India, 23–24 April 2022; pp. 1–5. [CrossRef]

65. Shahajad, M.; Gambhir, D.; Gandhi, R. Features extraction for classification of brain tumor MRI images using support vector machine. In Proceedings of the 2021 11th International Conference on Cloud Computing, Data Science & Engineering (Confluence), Noida, India, 28–29 January 2021; pp. 767–772. [CrossRef]

66. Eke, C.S.; Jammeh, E.; Li, X.; Carroll, C.; Pearson, S.; Ifeachor, E. Early Detection of Alzheimer's Disease with Blood Plasma Proteins Using Support Vector Machines. *IEEE J. Biomed. Health Inform.* **2021**, *25*, 218–226. [CrossRef]

67. Sathiyanarayanan, P.; Pavithra, S.; Saranya, M.S.A.; Makeswari, M. Identification of Breast Cancer Using The Decision Tree Algorithm. In Proceedings of the 2019 IEEE International Conference on System, Computation, Automation and Networking (ICSCAN), Pondicherry, India, 29–30 March 2019; pp. 1–6. [CrossRef]

68. Fu, B.; Liu, P.; Lin, J.; Deng, L.; Hu, K.; Zheng, H. Predicting Invasive Disease-Free Survival for Early Stage Breast Cancer Patients Using Follow-Up Clinical Data. *IEEE Trans. Biomed. Eng.* **2019**, *66*, 2053–2064. [CrossRef]

69. Ambesange, S.; Nadagoudar, R.; Uppin, R.; Patil, V.; Patil, S.; Patil, S. Liver Diseases Prediction using KNN with Hyper Parameter Tuning Techniques. In Proceedings of the 2020 IEEE Bangalore Humanitarian Technology Conference (B-HTC), Vijiyapur, India, 8–10 October 2020; pp. 1–6. [CrossRef]

70. Sandag, G.A.; Tedry, N.E.; Lolong, S. Classification of Lower Back Pain Using K-Nearest Neighbor Algorithm. In Proceedings of the 2018 6th International Conference on Cyber and IT Service Management (CITSM), Parapat, Indonesia, 7–9 August 2018; pp. 1–5. [CrossRef]
71. Pawlovsky, A.P. An Ensemble Based on Distances for a kNN Method for Heart Disease Diagnosis. In Proceedings of the 2018 International Conference on Electronics, Information, and Communication (ICEIC), Honolulu, HI, USA, 24–27 January 2018; pp. 1–4. [CrossRef]
72. Ripan, R.C.; Sarker, I.H.; Hossain, S.M.M.; Anwar, M.; Nowrozy, R.; Hoque, M.M.; Furhad, H. A Data-Driven Heart Disease Prediction Model Through K-Means Clustering-Based Anomaly Detection. *SN Comput. Sci.* **2021**, *2*, 112. [CrossRef]
73. Vadyala, S.R.; Betgeri, S.N.; Sherer, E.A.; Amritphale, A. Prediction of the number of COVID-19 confirmed cases based on K-means-LSTM. *Array* **2021**, *11*, 100085. [CrossRef]
74. Manivannan, P.; Devi, P.I. Dengue Fever Prediction Using K-Means Clustering Algorithm. In Proceedings of the 2017 IEEE International Conference on Intelligent Techniques in Control, Optimization and Signal Processing (INCOS), Srivilliputtur, India, 23–25 March 2017; pp. 1–5. [CrossRef]
75. Sarkar, A.; Hossain, S.K.S.; Sarkar, R. Human activity recognition from sensor data using spatial attention-aided CNN with genetic algorithm. *Neural Comput. Appl.* **2022**, *35*, 5165–5191. [CrossRef]
76. Xu, Q.; Wang, X.; Jiang, H. Convolutional neural network for breast cancer diagnosis using diffuse optical tomography. *Visual Computing for Industry, Biomed. Art* **2019**, *2*, 6. [CrossRef]
77. Mohammed, M.A.; Ghani, M.K.A.; Hamed, R.I.; Ibrahim, D.A.; Abdullah, M.K. Artificial neural networks for automatic segmentation and identification of nasopharyngeal carcinoma. *J. Comput. Sci.* **2017**, *21*, 263–274. [CrossRef]
78. Costa, F.F. Big data in biomedicine. *Drug Discov. Today* **2014**, *19*, 433–440. [CrossRef]
79. Landset, S.; Khoshgoftaar, T.M.; Richter, A.N.; Hasanin, T. A survey of open source tools for machine learning with big data in the Hadoop ecosystem. *J. Big Data* **2015**, *2*, 24. [CrossRef]
80. Shvachko, K.; Kuang, H.; Radia, S.; Chansler, R. The Hadoop Distributed File System. In Proceedings of the 2010 IEEE 26th Symposium on Mass Storage Systems and Technologies (MSST), Incline Village, NV, USA, 3–7 May 2010; pp. 1–10. [CrossRef]
81. Azeroual, O.; Fabre, R. Processing Big Data with Apache Hadoop in the Current Challenging Era of COVID-19. *Big Data Cogn. Comput.* **2021**, *5*, 12. [CrossRef]
82. Fu, J.; Sun, J.; Wang, K. SPARK—A Big Data Processing Platform for Machine Learning. In Proceedings of the 2016 International Conference on Industrial Informatics—Computing Technology, Intelligent Technology, Industrial Information Integration (ICIICII), Wuhan, China, 3–4 December 2016; pp. 48–51. [CrossRef]
83. Salloum, S.; Dautov, R.; Chen, X.; Peng, P.X.; Huang, J.Z. Big data analytics on Apache Spark. *Int. J. Data Sci. Anal.* **2016**, *1*, 145–164. [CrossRef]
84. Liu, W.; Li, Q.; Cai, Y.; Li, Y.; Li, X. A Prototype of Healthcare Big Data Processing System Based on Spark. In Proceedings of the 2015 8th International Conference on Biomedical Engineering and Informatics (BMEI), Shenyang, China, 14–16 October 2015; pp. 516–520. [CrossRef]
85. Ed-daoudy, A.; Maalmi, K. Application of Machine Learning Model on Streaming Health Data Event in Real-Time to Predict Health Status Using Spark. In Proceedings of the 2018 International Symposium on Advanced Electrical and Communication Technologies (ISAECT), Rabat, Morocco, 21–23 November 2018; pp. 1–4. [CrossRef]
86. Ed-Daoudy, A.; Maalmi, K. Real-Time Machine Learning for Early Detection of Heart Disease Using Big Data Approach. In Proceedings of the 2019 International Conference on Wireless Technologies, Embedded and Intelligent Systems (WITS), Fez, Morocco, 3–4 April 2019; pp. 1–5. [CrossRef]
87. Chandra, D.G. BASE analysis of NoSQL database. *Future Gener. Comput. Syst.* **2015**, *52*, 13–21. [CrossRef]
88. Williams, A.J.; Harland, L.; Groth, P.; Pettifer, S.; Chichester, C.; Willighagen, E.L.; Evelo, C.T.; Blomberg, N.; Ecker, G.; Goble, C.; et al. Open PHACTS: Semantic interoperability for drug discovery. *Drug Discov. Today* **2012**, *17*, 1188–1198. [CrossRef] [PubMed]
89. Khazaei, H.; Mench-Bressan, N.; McGregor, C.; Pugh, J.E. Health Informatics for Neonatal Intensive Care Units: An Analytical Modeling Perspective. *IEEE J. Transl. Eng. Health Med.* **2015**, *3*, 1–9. [CrossRef] [PubMed]
90. McGregor, C.; Inibhunu, C.; Glass, J.; Doyle, I.; Gates, A.; Madill, J.; Pugh, J.E. Health Analytics as a Service with Artemis Cloud: Service Availability. In Proceedings of the 2020 42nd Annual International Conference of the IEEE Engineering in Medicine & Biology Society (EMBC), Montreal, QC, Canada, 20–24 July 2020; pp. 5644–5648. [CrossRef]
91. Salvi, E.; Parimbelli, E.; Basadonne, A.; Viani, N.; Cavallini, A.; Micieli, G.; Quaglini, S.; Sacchi, L. Exploring IBM Watson to Extract Meaningful Information from the List of References of a Clinical Practice Guideline. In *Artificial Intelligence in Medicine*; Springer: Cham, Switzerland, 2017; pp. 193–197. [CrossRef]
92. Contractor, D.; Telang, A. (Eds.) *Applications of Cognitive Computing Systems and IBM Watson*; Springer: Singapore, 2017. [CrossRef]
93. Koutkias, V. From Data Silos to Standardized, Linked, and FAIR Data for Pharmacovigilance: Current Advances and Challenges with Observational Healthcare Data. *Drug Saf.* **2019**, *42*, 583–586. [CrossRef] [PubMed]

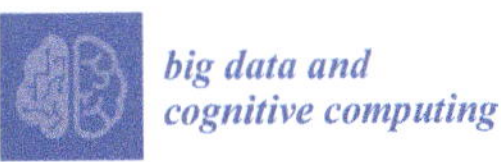
big data and cognitive computing

MDPI

Review

An Overview on the Challenges and Limitations Using Cloud Computing in Healthcare Corporations

Giuseppe Agapito [1,2,3,*] and Mario Cannataro [3,4]

1   Department of Law, Economics and Social Sciences, University "Magna Græcia" of Catanzaro, 88100 Catanzaro, Italy
2   "Cultura Romana del Diritto e Sistemi Giuridici Contemporanei" Research Center, University "Magna Græcia" of Catanzaro, 88100 Catanzaro, Italy
3   Data Analytics Research Center, University "Magna Græcia" of Catanzaro, 88100 Catanzaro, Italy; cannataro@unicz.it
4   Department of Medical and Surgical Sciences, University "Magna Græcia" of Catanzaro, 88100 Catanzaro, Italy
*   Correspondence: agapito@unicz.it

Abstract: Technological advances in high throughput platforms for biological systems enable the cost-efficient production of massive amounts of data, leading life science to the Big Data era. The availability of Big Data provides new opportunities and challenges for data analysis. Cloud Computing is ideal for digging with Big Data in omics sciences because it makes data analysis, sharing, access, and storage effective and able to scale when the amount of data increases. However, Cloud Computing presents several issues regarding the security and privacy of data that are particularly important when analyzing patients' data, such as in personalized medicine. The objective of the present study is to highlight the challenges, security issues, and impediments that restrict the widespread adoption of Cloud Computing in healthcare corporations.

Keywords: cloud computing; big data; omics data; healthcare; artificial intelligence; cryptography; IoT; edge computing

---

Citation: Agapito, G.; Cannataro, M. An Overview on the Challenges and Limitations Using Cloud Computing in Healthcare Corporations. *Big Data Cogn. Comput.* **2023**, *7*, 68. https://doi.org/10.3390/bdcc7020068

Academic Editor: Carson K. Leung

Received: 13 March 2023
Revised: 27 March 2023
Accepted: 29 March 2023
Published: 6 April 2023

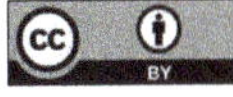

1. Introduction

The investigation of all living organisms and complex diseases, e.g., yeast, human, cancer, and Alzheimer's has highlighted the need for a new holistic vision to shed light on the multiple interactions among several biological players, such as genes, enzymes, and small molecules. In the reductionist approach [1], a single mutation or weakness is responsible for diseases and phenotype aberrancies. In contrast, the holistic approach [2] asserts that conditions and phenotype aberrancies are due to the intricate interactions network among several biological players.

The appearance of omics sciences [3] provides the approaches to consolidate the holistic idea mandatory for studying living organisms at all structural and functional levels, including humans. Omics includes the domains ending in -omics, such as proteomics, epigenomics, metabolomics, and microbiomics. In particular, the rapid advances in High-Throughput (HT) and Molecular Biology (MB) technologies make omics sciences a central part of medical research. The continuous technological advances in HT and MB have made it possible to comprehensively analyze a simple living organism's genome, e.g., a single bacteria, and a complex organism, e.g., humans, in a few hours or a few days [4,5]. The highest quality of HT and MB produces massive data per single experiment, transforming biology and genomics into data-driven sciences [6]. Only the practical analysis of this enormous amount of data will allow us to understand the complex aberrancies starting from the genome.

The transition of life sciences toward data-driven science provides researchers with new opportunities, making it possible to yield vast amounts of omics data in a cost-

---

and time-efficient manner. Simultaneously, acquiring, storing, distributing, analyzing, and interpreting these data is challenging [7]. The high data heterogeneity in terms of type and source requires technical improvements in many Information Technology (IT) domains, raising various privacy, security, storage, sharing, processing, and computing power issues. Hence, it is essential to develop specific algorithms and software tools for analyzing the different available types of omics data, such as protein sequences, single nucleotide polymorphisms (SNPs), and gene expressions, necessary for understanding the expression of genes and their regulation and the mutations in DNA underlying genetic diseases. A further contribution is the development of graphic interfaces that effectively display information from various data sources.

To meet these challenges, Cloud Computing and High-Performance Computing (HPC) architectures can significantly improve the speed of omics data investigation, analysis, reliability, and reproducibility.

Architectures based on multiprocessors, even multi-core, Graphics Processing Units (GPUs), and hybrids architectures, e.g., holding both GPUs and CPUs, make HPC architectures ideal for handling computations requiring significant amounts of computing power and memory. The strength of HPC systems is the extreme computational power obtained through parallel or distributed computing.

Parallel programming enables us to write code in order to take advantage of the multiple computational cores of modern CPUs. Parallel programming decomposes programs, e.g., the process, as several independent bunches, e.g., the threads allowing parallel and concurrent execution. Partitioning programs into smaller threads allows the exploitation of multiple cores within modern CPUs. Multiple cores on a single machine share memory. Hence, threads can be executed simultaneously using shared memory to synchronize and communicate with each other. A popular environment for threads is Java thread, while CUDA is a popular environment for exploiting the computational properties of Graphics Processing Units (GPU). Distributed computing uses network protocols such as TCP/IP, allowing applications to send and receive data to each other over the network by providing the services and protocols for exchanging data. Hence, a distributed application is built upon several layers. At the lower level, the network connects devices, allowing communication among them. At the higher level, services are defined on the network protocols. Finally, distributed applications run on top of these layers to perform tasks across the network. A popular library for distributed computing is Message Passing Interface (MPI) [8], which is available for many programming languages and architectures. Hence, parallel and distributed computing allows for solving complex problems in a short time by employing many computing resources simultaneously that would otherwise require a lot of time if performed sequentially.

Thus, programmers must explicitly develop parallel programs, e.g., in a global environment using a multi-threading paradigm or in a distributed environment through the Message-Passing Interface (MPI) standard [8], to exploit the computational power delivered from HPC systems. In addition, to ensure that HPC systems run at optimal performance, a suitable technical support service is required. All these constraints introduce additional expenses, e.g., purchase, maintenance, and development, making the HPC systems ideal for large IT research centers and limiting the spread in biological, medical, and genomics research centers. The limiting element for the significant employment of HPC is nowadays primarily computational. On the other hand, Cloud Computing [9,10] brings a new paradigm from the analogy with existing infrastructures, such as electricity or water. Consequently, the achievement of the results is guaranteed independently of where data or instruction sequences are stored or executed. When opening a tap or turning on a lamp, one does not wonder where the water or electricity comes from; the important thing is that these are made available. Similarly, when some commands or services need to be executed in the Cloud system, it does not matter who takes care of it; the overall system will have to deliver the correct results based on the user requests. Thus, Cloud Computing provides an on-demand system through the Internet. Therefore, it eliminates purchase, maintenance, and development costs, making high-performance computation available even for small research centers. Cloud Computing is available in three fundamental models, such as IaaS (Infrastructure as a Service), PaaS (Platform as a Service), and SaaS (Software as a Service).

Cloud Computing could be the ideal tool for dealing with many steps of the bioinformatics analysis pipeline, from pre-processing, selection, aggregation, and analysis, including exploration and visualization.

To take full advantage of the considerable benefits of Cloud Computing, healthcare corporations must face several management, technology, security, and legal issues that affect its rapid adoption in healthcare. For example, storing confidential health information in third-party remote data storage raises serious problems related to the patient's sensitive information because patient data could be lost or misused.

Thus, the present study aims to highlight the challenges, security issues, and impediments that limit the adoption of cloud computing in healthcare corporations.

The rest of the manuscript is arranged as follows: Section 2 describes the principal service and deployment models of Cloud Computing, highlighting the main difference between them. Section 3 introduces some well-known Cloud services suitable for handling Big omics Data. Section 4 describes challenges, security issues, and impediments that are limiting the spread of Cloud Computing in healthcare corporations. Section 5 discusses some of the possible challenges and issues to address underlying the low adoption of Cloud services in healthcare. Section 6 provides some guidelines to follow, when dealing with Cloud Computing in healthcare. Finally, Section 7 concludes the manuscript.

2. Cloud Computing

Cloud infrastructures comprise the front end and back end. The front end refers to the end users' devices (e.g., pc, tablets, or smartphones), an Internet connection, and a web browser or similar application indispensable to accessing the Cloud Computing environment. Two different types of users can benefit from the front end: (i) the user of the final Cloud service; (ii) the developer and owner of the provided Cloud service. Through the front end, the provider ensures the final users that data on its hosts are always available through Internet connections. Simultaneously, developers can always have access to enhance and maintain their services by interacting with the Cloud system through terminals-scripts, RESTfull services [11], and even using traditional browsers. The back end includes the data center resources providing security, storage capacity, and computing power necessary to keep all the Cloud ecosystems available to the users.

2.1. Service Models of Cloud Computing

Cloud Computing includes different standardized service models, among which are the following:

- Software as a Service (SaaS) [12] allows the use of the provider's applications running on remote architectures. The applications are obtainable through client applications, such as a web browser or an Application Program Interface (API). Users cannot control or manage the beneath Cloud infrastructure components such as network, servers, operating systems, storage, or individual application capabilities, excluding determinate user-specific application configuration settings.
- Platform as a Service (PaaS) [13] enables users to develop in the Cloud environment the users' applications created using libraries, services, and APIs compatible with the Cloud provider. Users cannot directly manage or control the infrastructure beneath the Cloud, including network, servers, operating systems, or storage, but retain the deployed applications and particular configuration settings for the application-hosting domain.
- Infrastructure as a Service (IaaS) [14] facilitates the user in provision processing, storage, networks, and other essential computing resources where the user can deploy and run the software, including operating systems and apps. Users cannot manage or

control the beneath-Cloud infrastructure, whereas having control of the operating systems, storage, deployed applications, and limited control on some select networking components, e.g., host firewalls or bridges.

Over the years, in addition to the essential service models, new Cloud service models have been added, including the following:

- Business Process as a Service (BPaaS) [15] exploits the Cloud to automate and drive down the costs of business processes carried out by organizations.
- Data as a Service (DaaS) [16] offers Cloud-based Big Data cleaning, filtering, and enrichment schemes to produce data sets suitable for predictive or prescriptive analyses.
- Connectivity as a Service (CaaS) [17] provides Voice-Over-IP (VOIP), video-conferencing, and Instant Messaging (IM) functions as Cloud-based subscription services for commercial institutions.
- Identity as a Service (IDaaS) [18] provides Cloud-based centralized authentication and Single-Sign-On (SSO) services on heterogeneous or federated Cloud schemes.

A critical aspect of each Cloud services model is the Multi-Tenancy (MT). MT is the Cloud platforms' power to satisfy multiple user requests concurrently, providing the highest separation between run time environment and data. MT is achieved by virtualizing the applications' run time environment and/or operating system, allowing users' applications to run on different Virtual Machines (VM). MT differs from multi-user operations, where multiple users share the same application. Still, the user applications and run time data, also known as user context, are only logically separated, e.g., held in different files or directories on the same physical storage.

2.2. Deployment Models of Cloud Computing

Deployment models have been developed alongside cloud service models to support users' business workloads. Today, business applications and processes rely on a complex ecosystem of hardware and services, each with its prerequisites in terms of privacy, availability, and scalability. Over the last decade, Cloud Computing has been embraced to improve business processes, and its models have been extended to meet the challenges in various scientific areas, including healthcare.

The Cloud Computing deployment models include the following:

- Public Cloud infrastructure is ideal for organizations needing quick access to computing resources without significant capital expenditure. Public Cloud infrastructure allows organizations to purchase virtualized computing services through the Internet. Since Public Cloud services are furnished as pay-per-use, no initial investments are required because new resources can be purchased when needed. Public Cloud services are ideal for healthcare organizations that cannot afford an investment in particular hardware and maintenance.
- Private Cloud infrastructure is intended for exclusive use by a single organization. The Private Cloud lets organizations complete control over how data are shared and stored, an optimal solution if security is the primary concern, e.g., in the healthcare domain, ensuring compliance with any ethical regulations and protecting the subject's sensitive data. Additionally, the Private Cloud provides on-demand data availability, guaranteeing trustworthiness and support for mission-critical tasks.
- Hybrid Cloud infrastructure combines Public and Private Cloud infrastructures by allowing data and applications to be moved between them. Cloud infrastructures are unique entities linked by standardized or proprietary technologies, enabling the portability of data and applications. Hence, Hybrid Cloud provides a unique integrated environment combining locally Private and Public Cloud services. Healthcare organizations using Hybrid Cloud could enhance the standard of security. In this regard, data and services that do not affect sensitive information can be available through the Public Cloud. In contrast, sensitive information held in the Private Cloud are under the institution's absolute control.

- Multicloud infrastructure handles several Cloud services by different providers, including organizations' Private Cloud resources and private computational assets, to accomplish various requirements and demands in a single heterogeneous Cloud environment. Multicloud gives more flexibility regarding service and computational capabilities, improving performance and increasing resource availability and redundancy, letting organizations and final users to use all available resources efficiently.
- Federated Cloud infrastructure is a heterogeneous Cloud environment connecting diverse providers through a partnership mechanism, e.g., a standard policy to share, access, and control infrastructure and services. Federated Cloud commonly combines multiple Private and Public Clouds. Federation members remain independent in resource sharing and access control, comprising federated identity management. Thus, the Federated Cloud increases reliability and, simultaneously, the scaling up of resources.
- Intercloud is a general model of Cloud infrastructures that incorporates heterogeneous Clouds from various providers and typically includes non-cloud resources. Intercloud models may use the Federated Cloud standard as the basis for creating or implementing more specific but customized control and management functions.

To sum up, the Public Cloud is suitable for use cases in which it is necessary to scale up quickly, execute short-term jobs, and mitigate the request for computational resources. The Private Cloud is ideal for use cases in which it is mandatory to protect sensitive information, including patents, meet data compliance requirements, ensuring high availability. The Federated Cloud infrastructure enables application scalability and workload optimization requirements through a federation paradigm between Public and Private Clouds. Hybrid Cloud is ideal for combining Public and Private Cloud services on-site in a unique integrated architecture. Multicloud is ideal for using multiple Cloud services, even from different providers. Multicloud can also incorporate physical and virtual infrastructures in a single heterogeneous Cloud environment. Intercloud is ideal for implementing more specific but customized common control and management functions for creating a virtual Private Cloud with restricted access based on federated access.

Table 1 shows the advantages and disadvantage of Deployment models.

Table 1. The table summarises the advantages and disadvantages of Cloud Deployment Models. In the table DM are the initials of Deployment Models; CP refers to Computational Power; S indicates the Security; AS introduces the Applications Scalability; AP denotes the Applications Portability; ToJ refers to Type of Job; HS refers to Heterogeneous Service; C refers to the Costs; EU indicates the Exclusive Use; T is the Trustness; sj, cj, and gj are the initials of short, critical, and general job, finally, the $\sqrt{}$ indicate feature availability, while $\times$ indicates absence of the feature.

DM	CP	S	AS	AP	ToJ	HS	C	EU	T
Public	$\sqrt{}$	$\times$	$\sqrt{}$	$\times$	sj	$\times$	$\times$	$\times$	$\times$
Private	$\sqrt{}$	$\sqrt{}$	$\sqrt{}$	$\times$	cj	$\times$	$\sqrt{}$	$\sqrt{}$	$\sqrt{}$
Federate	$\times$	$\sqrt{}$	$\sqrt{}$	$\times$	cj	$\sqrt{}$	$\sqrt{}$	$\sqrt{}$	$\sqrt{}$
Hybrid	$\times$	$\times$	$\times$	$\sqrt{}$	gj	$\sqrt{}$	$\sqrt{}$	$\times$	$\times$
Multicloud	$\sqrt{}$	$\times$	$\sqrt{}$	$\times$	gj	$\sqrt{}$	$\sqrt{}$	$\times$	$\times$
Intercloud	$\times$	$\sqrt{}$	$\times$	$\times$	gj	$\sqrt{}$	$\sqrt{}$	$\sqrt{}$	$\sqrt{}$

3. Background

Healthcare organizations generate a vast range of data and information. Thanks to the progress of HT omics technologies, there has been an exponential growth of omics data, e.g., gene expressions, sequences alignment, and protein sequences, rendering classical computational approaches ineffective for handling these massive amounts of heterogeneous data. Consequently, omics sciences turned into Big Data science. Big Data in health and medical areas need infrastructures to improve data storage and management. Data sharing and security are critical in health and medical care since researchers need easy and extensive access to data for scientific analysis and sharing results. Cloud Computing solutions for healthcare organizations can contribute to making data analysis, sharing, access, and storage effective through Cloud services able to scale when the amount of data increases. Thus, Cloud Computing services are a cost-effective solution for storing, accessing, analyzing, sharing, and protecting healthcare data and information.

The following is a list of well-known Cloud services models suitable for handling Big omics Data.

- Cloud BioLinux [19] provides a platform for developing bioinformatics infrastructures on the Cloud. Cloud BioLinux is a publicly accessible Virtual Machine (VM) to create on-demand frameworks for high-performance bioinformatics computing using Cloud architectures. Cloud BioLinux preconfigured command line and graphical software applications are available through the Amazon EC2 Cloud. Cloud BioLinux is distributed under the MIT Licence, including different Cloud BioLinux VMs, whereas source code and user guides are available at http://www.cloudbiolinux.org (accessed on 21 March 2023).
- Cloud4SNP [20] is a Cloud-based framework for the parallel preprocessing and statistical analysis of pharmacogenomics SNP DMET microarray data sets. Cloud4SNP extends the DMET-Analyzer [21] engine to be implemented as a Cloud Computing service through the Data Mining Cloud Framework [22]. Data Mining Cloud Framework is a software framework for creating and implementing knowledge discovery workflows on the Cloud [23]. Cloud4SNP performs massive statistical tests of SNPs relevance in case-control studies using the well-known Fisher test. Cloud4SNP exploits data parallelism and employs an optimized filtering technique to bypass the execution of ineffective Fisher tests by removing rows, e.g., probes with similar SNPs distributions.
- CloudBurst [24] is a parallel read-mapping algorithm optimized for mapping Next-Generation Sequence (NGS) data from several organisms, including homo sapiens, SNPs discovery, genotyping, and personal genomics. CloudBurst runs the short Read-Mapping Program (RMAP) linearly since running time decreases linearly with the number of reads mapped, reaching a linear speedup increasing the number of processors. These results are obtained by implementing Hadoop MapReduce [25] to parallelize execution using multiple computing nodes. In this way, CloudBurst improves performance by decreasing the running time to minutes for mapping millions of short reads to the human genome. CloudBurst is available as an open-source Java project for Amazon EC2 at https://sourceforge.net/projects/cloudburst-bio/ (accessed on 21 March 2023).
- CloudMan [26] is a Cloud manager that directs all of the steps required to create and control a complete data analysis environment on a Cloud infrastructure using a web browser. CloudMan provides an NGS analysis technique integrated with the Galaxy applications. CloudMan comes with a graphical interface to enable an easy access to Cloud Computing services. CloudMan is currently available for Amazon Web Services (AWS) Cloud infrastructure as part of the Galaxy Cloud [27] and CloudBioLinux [28].
- Crossbow [29] is a scalable, portable, and automatic Cloud service for identifying SNPs from high-coverage short-read resequencing data. Crossbow implements the MapReduce framework [25] distributed from Apache Hadoop. Alignment and variant calling in Crossbow are performed using the Bowtie [29] and SOAPsnp [30] software tools.
- Eoulsan [31] is a Cloud service implementing the Hadoop MapReduce approach devoted to HT sequencing RNA-seq data analysis. The Eoulsan differential analysis of transcript expression workflow comprises six steps: (i) quality control filtering; (ii) reads mapping; (iii) alignments filtering; (iv) transcript expression calculation. (v) normalization; (vi) detection of significant differential expression. Eoulsan is available as standalone, local cluster, or Cloud Computing on Amazon Elastic MapReduce (EMR).
- Eoulsan 2 [32] is the update of Eoulsan initially developed for analyzing RNA-seq data. Eoulsan 2 introduces the following updates to handling long-read RNA-seq and scRNA-seq data: (i) enhances the workflow manager; (ii) facilitates the development of new modules; (iii) expands its applications to long-read RNA-seq and scRNA-seq.

Eoulsan 2 is implemented in Java, available only for Linux systems, and distributed under the LGPL and CeCILL-C licenses at http://outils.genomique.biologie.ens.fr/eoulsan/ (accessed on 21 March 2023). The source code and sample workflows are available on GitHub https://github.com/GenomicParisCentre/eoulsan (accessed on 21 March 2023).

- HealtheDataLab [33] is a Cloud Computing platform for analyzing Electronic Medical Records (EMRs) data with computing capability for analyzing Big Data. HealtheData-Lab enables the building of statistical and machine learning models flexibly through the use of Amazon Web Services (AWS), allows for scalability and high-performance computing system, and complaints with the Health Insurance Portability and Accountability Act (HIPAA) standard. HealtheDataLab is available upon request made directly to Cerner Corporation.

- iMage Cloud [34] allows the analysis of medical images integrated with EMRs, enabling the sharing of images, EMRs, and merged images via the Internet. iMage uses Hybrid Cloud to deliver more convenient and secure services, allowing high-performance image processing and virtual applications to be delivered securely, conveniently, and efficiently. iMage provides a graphical user interface with which it is possible to share images after being combined with EMRs.

- PeakRanger [35] is a software package that resolves closely spaced peaks obtained from Chromatin Immunoprecipitation (ChIP) coupled with massively parallel short-read sequencing (seq) ChIP-seq datasets. PeakRanger provides high performance on extensive data sets by taking advantage of the MapReduce parallel environment. PeakRanger improves recognition of extremely closely-spaced peaks improving spatial accuracy in identifying the exact location of binding events and improving the run time by exploiting the parallel environment provided by a Cloud Computing architecture. PeakRanger is written in C++ and can be deployed on Linux, macOS, and Windows.

- STORMSeq (Scalable Tools for Open-source Read Mapping) [36] is a software pipeline for whole-genome and exome sequence data sets. STORMSeq is implemented as AWS Cloud service. STORMSeq presents an intuitive user interface for dealing with reading mapping and variant calling using genomic data.

- VAT (Variant Annotation Tool) [37] is a software package to annotate variants from multiple individual genomes at the transcript level and obtain descriptive statistics across genes and individuals. VAT visualizes different variants, integrating allele frequencies and genotype data, simplifying comparative analysis between distinct groups of individuals. VAT is implemented in C and PHP and it is available as a command-line tool or as a web application. Moreover, VAT can be run as a virtual machine in the AWS Cloud environment. VAT documentation and user guide are available at http://www.vat.gersteinlab.org (accessed on 21 March 2023).

4. Materials and Methods

This section aims to highlight some challenges, security issues, and impediments limiting the spread of the use of Cloud Computing in healthcare corporations. To identify some of the main relevant obstacles limiting the high adoption of Cloud methodologies in healthcare corporations, we searched the online knowledge database PubMed [38], to figure out from the available scientific literature suitable clues to identify possible advice that could help mitigate the current difficulties in the large use of Cloud Computing in healthcare corporations.

The first step regarded the keywords definition to use for selecting relevant manuscripts. The chosen keywords to implement the selection criteria of the manuscript are: cloud computing, healthcare, security, challenges, applications. Table 2 shows the produced queries obtained by combining the keywords and the selected range of publication years in which to search for manuscripts.

In the second step, we defined the inclusion criteria comprising the following: (i) the manuscripts available on PubMed from the 2009, up to the December 2022 meeting the selected keywords; (ii) all the types of abstracts, manuscripts, conference abstracts, reviews, and letters are eligible if they contain the chosen keywords in the title and are free full text.

Table 2. The table shows the defined queries to identify relevant manuscripts related to Cloud Computing in healthcare.

QueryID	Query	Publication Years Range
Q_1	cloud computing & healthcare	2009–2022
Q_2	cloud computing & healthcare & security	2009–2022
Q_3	cloud computing & healthcare & challenges	2009–2022
Q_4	cloud computing & healthcare & applications	2009–2022

Table 3 reports the number of identified manuscripts in PubMed that apply to the queries contained in Table 2. The results of the queries were analyzed using an in-house Python script, to parse and extract manuscripts' title keywords, computing for each keyword its frequency (excluding from the frequency terms counting articles, prepositions, adverbs etc). Finally, keyword frequency is used to produce the word cloud diagram shown in Figure 1.

Table 3. The table shows the total number of eligible PubMed manuscripts matching the defined queries.

QueryID	TotManuscripts	TotFreeFullText
Q_1	668	408
Q_2	237	151
Q_3	184	120
Q_4	273	186

Figure 1 presents the results of query Q_1 in the form of word cloud diagram.

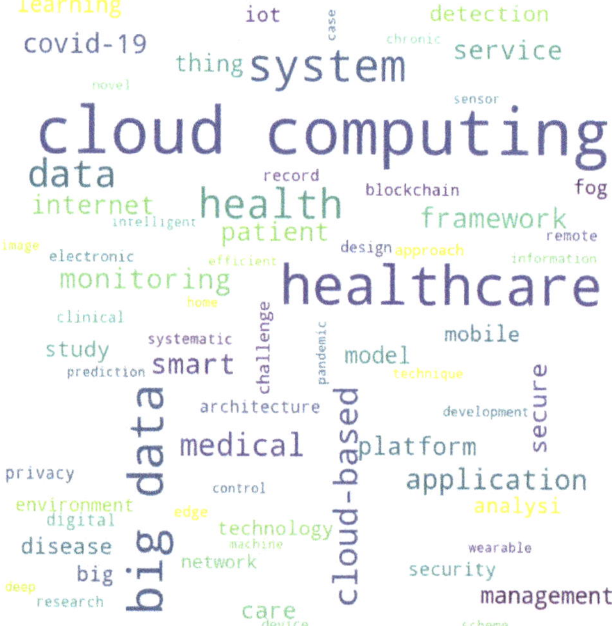

Figure 1. Figure shows the query Q_1 results as word cloud diagram.

Figure 2 shows the publication growth trend of manuscripts concerning the use of Cloud Computing in healthcare.

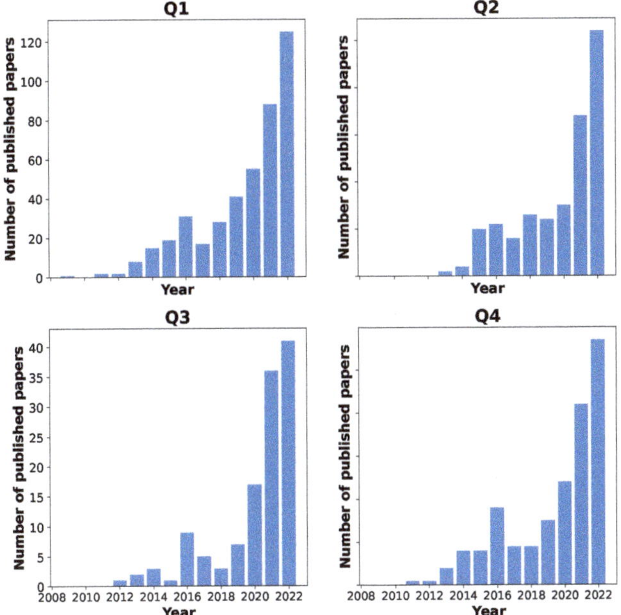

Figure 2. Figure shows the growth trend of Cloud Computing in healthcare starting from 2008 up to December 2022. Q_1 presents the growth per year of manuscripts dealing with cloud computing in healthcare. Q_2 shows the trends per year of the manuscripts focused on security issues in Cloud Computing especially within Cloud Computing in healthcare. Q_3 shows the growth of manuscripts focused on the challenges to be faced in Cloud Computing for healthcare. Finally, Q_4 provides an overview of the growth per year of Cloud application for healthcare.

To highlight the difficulties of adopting Cloud Computing in the healthcare sector, we will analyze the results obtained from the queries represented graphically using piecharts. Figure 3 shows the results of query Q_1.

Q_1 contains the following keywords cloud computing and healthcare, resulting in 67 keywords extracted (for readability reasons, the piechart visualize the first 30 keywords) from the titles of the scientific articles selected using the previously defined criteria concerning the use of Cloud Computing in Healthcare. Analyzing the frequency of keywords identified by query Q_1 shown in Figure 3, it is worth noting that many terms are related to healthcare, which could lead to misleading conclusions concerning the use of Cloud Computing in healthcare, considering that keywords such as security and privacy occupy the 35th and 38th position, respectively.

Query Q_2 adds the keyword security to query Q_1, extracting from scientific works compatible with the selection criteria 17 keywords. Adding the keyword security restricts the selection and search range of the query. In fact, from the result of Q_2 shown in Figure 4, it is possible to notice that the keywords related to security and privacy now leap respectively into 5th, 6th, and 8th position, highlighting the importance of the concepts of security and privacy in the various areas of use of the Cloud and, in particular, in the health sector.

Query Q_3, composed of keywords cloud computing, healthcare and challenges, locates 20 keywords, as shown in Figure 5.

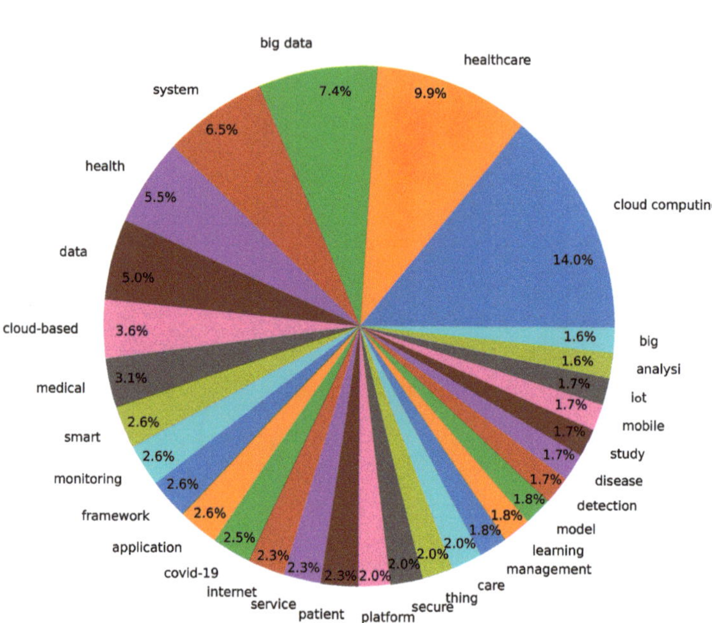

Figure 3. Figure shows the keyword frequency produced from query Q_1. To improve legibility, the percentage values have been truncated to the first value after the decimal point.

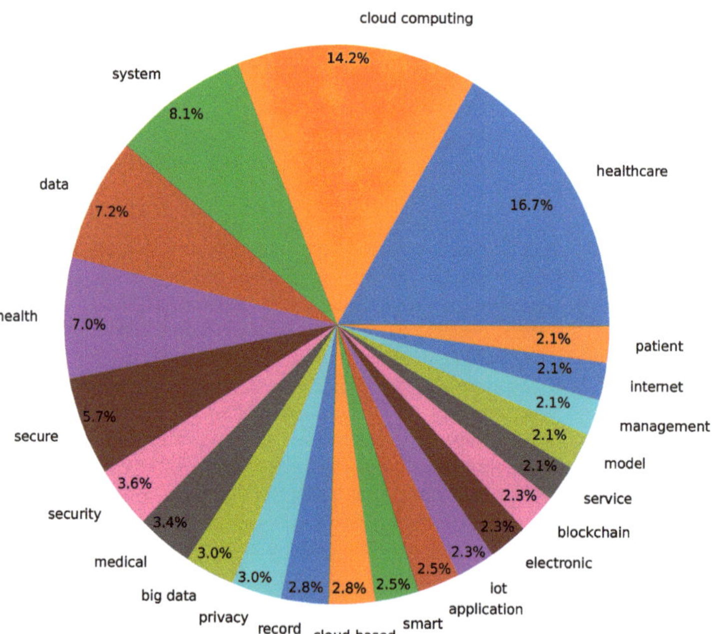

Figure 4. Figure shows the keyword frequency produced from query Q_2. To improve legibility, the percentage values have been truncated to the first value after the decimal point.

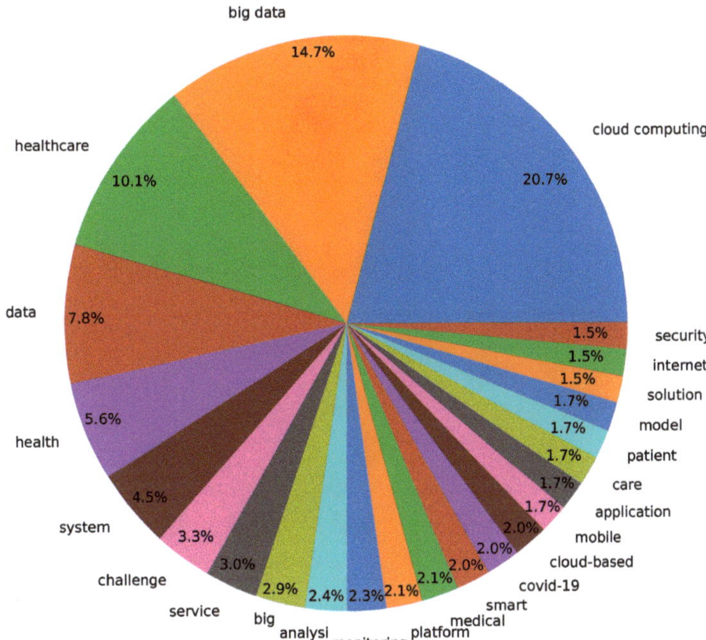

Figure 5. Figure shows the keyword frequency produced from query Q_3. To improve legibility, the percentage values have been truncated to the first value after the decimal point.

In particular, challenges occupies the 5th position, highlighting that the use of the Cloud in the healthcare sector must overcome various challenges, particularly related to the sensitive aspects of the data to be handled. Figure 6 displays the frequency of keywords extracted from query Q_4.

From the analysis of Figure 6 security occupies the 19th position, while privacy does not appear in the list of frequent keywords, introducing biases in the interpretation of the results, suggesting that the existing Cloud Computing applications are mainly aimed at sectors other than healthcare, as less stringent privacy requirements regulate them. In light of these conclusions, decisions regarding the relevant scientific papers to be analyzed were made using the intersection of the results produced by the four queries as a selection criterion.

To limit the manuscripts investigation, we computed the intersection among the results obtained from the four queries performed in PubMed. Figure 7 shows the intersection among the manuscripts' keywords retrieved from each query). The manuscripts intersection was computed using Venny 2.0 [39] a web application used to draw Venn diagrams.

Analysing Figure 7 it is wort noting that the intersection among the four queries contains 27 manuscripts. According to the eligibility criteria, 21 manuscripts have been excluded since they are not explicitly related to Cloud Computing. Finally, only the 6 manuscripts meeting the eligibility criteria have been assessed.

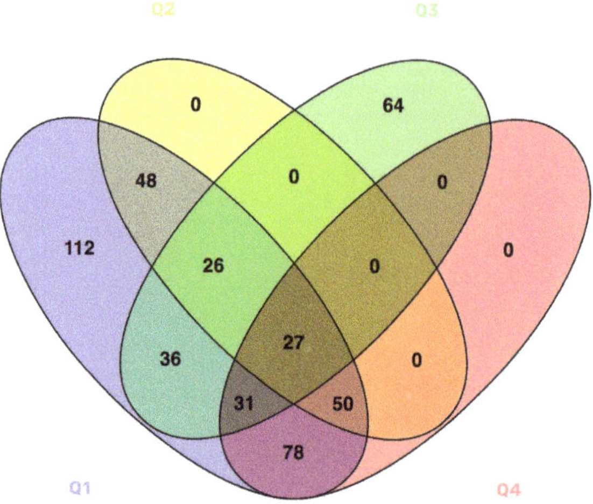

Figure 6. Figure shows the keywords' frequency produced from query Q_4. To improve legibility, the percentage values have been truncated to the first value after the decimal point.

Figure 7. Figure shows the intersection among the manuscripts' keywords retrieved from each query.

5. Discussion

Although Cloud Computing is a consolidated technology in computational and storage resources, with the explicit goals of reducing operating costs and improving results in many scientific domains, Cloud Computing is slowly gathering steam in healthcare despite those premises. This impasse may be due to the critical challenges to face, such as encryption, user identification, storage, access, etc.

Patient clinical information is now collected in Electronic Medical Records (EMRs), even known as Electronic Health Records (EHRs). Using Cloud tools to analyze and share

EMRs data can improve the performance of healthy corporations. Cloud services lowered the cost of care, improved outcomes, and increased customer/patient loyalty and satisfaction while yielding growth and profitability. At the same time, EMRs data must be stored and handled according to well-defined privacy and security rules [40]. Cloud environments must face several challenges in data handling, notably the native heterogeneity of healthcare data and the need to harmonize data sets from different healthcare organizations. Cloud storage is the ideal solution for storing data from different healthcare organizations. It can spur multi center data analysis, data summarization, integration, and harmonization, contributing to new knowledge, improving clinical trials, and developing new drugs. The need for suitable integration and harmonization functions hamper the collaboration between healthcare institutions. Traditional harmonization and integration methods are ineffective with healthcare data. In [41], authors present HarmonicSS, a PaaS Cloud Computing model encouraging collaboration among multiple organizations, providing several data harmonization functions based on semantic data models to identify concepts automatically without a human supervisor. In addition, HarmonicSS provides trustworthy AI models based on the Cloud Federated environment, allowing secure, legal, and ethical uploads compliant with HL7 standards ideal for the healthcare domain. The ubiquity of EMRs in recent years through Cloud Computing could lead to the wide use of artificial intelligence (AI) [42] to analyze these vast amounts of data. AI tools are unhurriedly supplanting humans in many application domains, such as deciding who should get a loan, hiring new workers, and supporting doctors in clinical reporting, decisions, and treatments design. The use of AI in fields where data-driven algorithmic decision-making may affect human life, e.g., healthcare, raises concerns regarding their reliability [43]. Indeed, since AI is a data-driven decision-making tool, using unbalanced, poor, or misleading data sets can increase the probability that these tools could be biased. Improving AI reliability can increase its adoption in healthcare environments. Thus, the challenge is establishing an end-to-end Cloud Computing service able to increase the reliability of AI tools. A potential Cloud Computing service includes the following steps: data acquisition, preprocessing, and AI model training. A possible strategy for increasing end-to-end reliability consists of the following: data labeling, which allows one to figure out the quality of data for the application; results aggregation to simplify the quality assessment; and finally, detection of unbalanced groups, which enables one to obtain more accurate and expressive knowledge models. Hence, the combination of Cloud Computing and reliable AI tools provides Cloud services that can help to increase the adoption of Cloud Computing services in healthcare organizations.

EMR data storage in Cloud repositories throws security problems, such as protecting patients' personal information [44]. Cloud providers can protect EMR-sensitive information by employing noncryptographic techniques such as anonymization and splitting [45]. Data anonymization [46] is a privacy technique to protect a user's personal information, hiding sensitive information that could reveal the identity. Data anonymization can be accomplished by applying various methods, such as removing or hiding identifiers or attributes. The primary intent of data anonymization is to obscure the person's identity in any way. Data splitting divides sensitive data into smaller chunks, distributing those smaller units to distinct storage locations to protect it from unauthorized access. In this manner, data anonymization and splitting protect patients' sensitive information without compromising Cloud Computing performance since data retrieval is accomplished without further computations such as decryption. Noncryptographic techniques provide a basic security level for Cloud environments because intruders can obtain access to complete sensitive information in case of a breach.

Thus, using cryptography [47] can improve Cloud environment security. Cryptography is a fundamental and widely used approach for hiding and securing classified information. Cryptography transforms the raw data into ciphertext using encryption algorithms to protect data during network transfer and storage. Today, cryptography is employed to pursue different targets, such as data confidentiality and integrity. Due to the increased data violations in the last few years, some Cloud service providers are moving toward cryptographic techniques to attain more safety. In [48], Hassan et al. discuss the relevance of synthesizing, classifying, and identifying different data protection methodologies. Although cryptography increases the security and trust of Cloud environments, it negatively affects Cloud environments' performance. Users want to retrieve their data stored in a Cloud database. Searching for encrypted data is a crucial element of cryptography because every user who stores sensitive data in a local or Cloud database wants to retrieve it. Data retrieving is completed by searching sensitive data through queries. Consequently, the procedure of retrieving data is complicated, since it is not possible to carry out computation on encrypted data without ever decrypting the content.

Cryptography approaches [49,50] are classified into Asymmetric and Symmetric. Asymmetric cryptography [51], also known as a public key, is a technique that uses a couple of keys to encrypt and decrypt information. A key in the pair is public that, as the name implies, can be distributed without affecting security. At the same time, the second key in the pair is private and known exclusively to the owner. In this approach, anyone can use the public key to encrypt messages, but only the paired private key can decrypt those encrypted messages. Public keys are usually stored in digital certificates, which allows them to be easily and securely shared. Private keys are not shared and must be held by users in suitable software systems or hardware, such as USB tokens. Symmetric cryptography [52], also known as a secret key, is a technique that uses a single key for encryption and decryption purposes. In symmetric cryptography, the secret key is private and a secure channel is required to distribute it. This requirement has proved challenging to maintain, representing the main weaknesses of this cryptographic schema. Hence, the key length can mitigate this weakness. In fact, the longer the key, the more secure the communication will be. For instance, to force a key of 128-bit with the computing power of current computers would take millions of years, a sufficient time to guarantee a secure outcome of communications. In asymmetric cryptography, on the other hand, public keys can be distributed on a (possibly) insecure channel, while private keys are generated locally without requiring to be transmitted. This public distribution allows for encrypted and authenticated communications between parties who have not previously met or exchanged information. To summarize, given their different nature, the two types of encryptions are used in purely different fields. Symmetric encryption is used to encrypt files and data when it is necessary to transfer large blocks of information, as well as during data transmission in HTTPS. In contrast, asymmetric cryptography is used in encryption and authentication procedures such as digital signatures. In this regard, healthcare corporations can use symmetric cryptography to achieve more security when sharing data through the network and choose asymmetric cryptography to provide secure authentication procedures to limit access to the stored sensitive information exclusively to the legitimate owner.

Blockchain technology is well known and used in cryptocurrency, safety, and trust management, making it suitable even for Cloud Computing services in healthcare. In [53], Rahmani et al. discussed the issues related to security breaches that occurred in Cloud platforms. Trust handling is critical for delivering secure and trustworthy service to users. The traditional trust-handling protocols in Cloud Computing are centralized, resulting in single-point failure. Hence, Rahmani et al. propose as a solution the use of Blockchain in Cloud domains, e.g., healthcare, that requires trust and trustworthiness in several aspects. An essential feature of Blockchain is the decentralization of the trust model that produces a trust Cloud environment. In [54], Ismail et al. present the limitations of a healthcare system based on either Cloud or Blockchain, highlighting the importance of implementing an integrated Blockchain-Cloud (BcC) system for further improve the Blockchain decentralization and, consequently, the Cloud environment trust.

The Internet of things (IoT) is a paradigm that allows different objects, e.g., intelligent entities and sensors, to communicate with each other on the Internet network. The IoT provides several benefits in many domains, from home to private and public corporations and government institutions. The IoT provides endless opportunities to connect homes, wearable devices, smart cities, and how patients interact with healthcare corporations. Smart devices, sensors, and wearables, even called smart-objects, are changing how personal care is delivered. Sensors like wearable trackers, e.g., smartwatches and bands, enable automatic self-monitoring and controlling health conditions such as hypertension and blood pressure. Patients can monitor their health status and, if necessary, communicate with their medical doctors to receive expert care directions, improving the quality of their medical care. In [55], the authors provide a picture of how IoT device use changes health care delivery. Thus, despite the above benefits, many issues must be considered, especially data security and privacy, because sensitive patient and hospital information are exchanged over the Internet.

In [56], Kibiwott et al. argue that if the IoT data are far from the owner's physical domain, privacy and security cannot be ensured. In this regard, Kibiwott et al. propose adopting attribute-based signcryption (ABSC) to mitigate security issues and protect sensitive data. ABSC cryptographic properties include fine-grained access control, authentication, confidentiality, and data owner privacy.

To bypass exchanging sensitive information over the network and preventing in this way to face data security and privacy issues, it is possible to use Edge Computing. Edge Computing is a novel programming model aiming to keep the computing step as near to the data source as possible, enabled by the availability of novel devices such as NVIDIA Jetson [57,58]. Moreover, the computation close to the data source guarantees a faster response with low latency, one of the essential requirements in decision-making or mission-critical processes. In [59], the authors present E-ALPHA (Edge-based Assisted Living Platform for Home cAre), which supports both Edge and Cloud Computing paradigms to design innovative Ambient Assisted Living (AAL) services in scenarios of different scales. E-ALPHA flexibly combines Edge and Cloud, assisting users in the preliminary assessment. In particular, it helps to determine the desired performance of the service. Next, it assists users in configuring applications or platforms for real deployment. IoT devices are continuously increasing in many domains, such as scientific, corporate, and domestic, presenting new challenges in the real-time elaboration of these vast amounts of different types of data produced. For these reasons, many initiatives investigating the deployment of architecture-based Edge Computing services and their impact on performance and cost are arising [60]. Moreover, Edge Computing, Machine Learning and Data Mining can put forward the analysis of IoT data based on Edge Computing, Machine Learning, and Deep Learning [61]. In [57], the authors present an approach based on Machine Learning and Edge Computing to diagnose early-stage cancer, allowing efficient and fast analysis without compromising the privacy of sensitive information. In [62] authors proposed EdgeMiningSim, a methodology aimed at IoT domain experts, for creating descriptive or predictive models to take actions in the IoT field.

In [63], Bertuccio et al. describe ReportFlow as an application to transfer sensitive data over the Public Cloud, speeding and simplifying the medical report process of EEGs. ReportFlow exploits the Role-Based Access Control (RBAC) to limit system access only to authorized users. ReportFlow deals with all cryptographic activities, managing certificates and checking their validity using OpenSSL, an open-source general-purpose cryptography library. Public keys and other information are held in specific folders on the Cloud. ReportFlow encrypts the data through a Triple Data Encryption Symmetric Algorithm (Triple DES or 3DES). Finally, Mehrtak et al. in [64] investigated several manuscripts to highlight the importance of accurately determining security challenges and their proper solutions that are fundamental for both Cloud Computing providers and corporations using Cloud services.

To summarize, the slow adoption of Cloud solutions in healthcare organizations could be related to the types of data produced by healthcare organizations. Healthcare data contain sensitive and confidential information about patients, requiring special handling. Thus, it is mandatory to develop special protocols and methods able to protect healthcare data that will be transferred through unsecured channels, i.e., through the internet network, up to the storage, analysis, retrieving etc.

6. Tips to Effectively Use Cloud Computing in Healthcare

This section provides some tips to facilitate the choice of the ideal Cloud Computing provider and how an user can deal with Cloud Computing to meet all the law requirements for healthcare corporations. Customers should choose a Cloud service holding stringent HIPAA and HITECH Act security requirements. Meet HIPAA and HITECH Act security requirements allow to limitate the common vulnerabilities that lead to breaches in security, implementing natively security protocols such as data encryption, multi-factor authentication, intrusion detection, and prevention. In this scenario, Cloud services will be more secure against data breaches, tampering, loss, and damage than on-premise data centers. Consumers would put data in the Cloud storage to create a central point of sharing, intending to promote interoperability. Interoperability can be achieved only if the Cloud provider supplies access to all services to constrained authenticated and authorized entities. Restricted data access with authentication and qualification reduces inappropriate and forbidden data changes. In this manner, data remain intact, secure, and adequately protected. Further consideration should regard the data transfer from local to Cloud repositories. Before uploading sensitive data, users must protect data using cryptography approaches like the HL7 standard and a secure channel like the https. In this way, data remain safe and adequately protected even during the transfer. Before uploading, data summarization, aggregation, and harmonization, in conjunction with encryption, promote secure data analysis, even using advanced AI tools. In this manner, it is possible to prevent AI tools from misusing sensitive information that can harm privacy by introducing biases in the outcomes, contributing to increasing AI reliability. Finally, before choosing a Cloud Computing provider, one must identify the geographic position of Cloud facilities since the security principles depend on the laws of the State and the corresponding legal jurisdiction where it will be held. For programmers, Cloud platforms provide a much faster and more secure method of developing and deploying collaborative, customized, and analytical workflows for dealing with heterogeneous data. In addition, Cloud platforms provide all the software tools, libraries, and APIs to design and develop robust services concerning security threats because the Cloud infrastructure has already been certified. Moreover, the Cloud also reduces the costs associated with maintaining existing infrastructure. In this manner, the internal IT resources can be concentrated on specific tasks rather than handling or maintaining data center hardware.

7. Conclusions

In this paper, we highlighted the importance of identifying Cloud security issues essential to defend patient privacy, complying with healthcare laws and ensuring that only authorized persons can access patients' sensitive data. Thus, the spread use of Cloud in healthcare could be enhanced by providing trusted Cloud architectures and services where the privacy and security of all data types is explicitly ensured, rendering information misuse impossible.

Author Contributions: Conceptualization, G.A.; methodology, G.A.; investigation, G.A.; writing, review and editing, G.A. and M.C. All authors have read and agreed to the published version of the manuscript.

Funding: This work has been partially funded by the Data Analytics Research Center, and the "Cultura Romana del Diritto e Sistemi Giuridici Contemporanei" Research Center, Catanzaro, Italy.

Institutional Review Board Statement: Not applicable.

Informed Consent Statement: Not applicable.

Data Availability Statement: Not applicable.

Conflicts of Interest: The authors declare no conflict of interest.

Abbreviations

The following abbreviations are used in this manuscript:

MC	Molecular Biology
HT	High-throughput
AWS	Amazon Web Services
BPaaS	Business Process as a Service
CaaS	Connectivity as a Service
ChIP	Chromatin immunoprecipitation
ChiPseq	Short read sequencing
DaaS	Data as a Service
DNA	DeoxyriboNucleic Acid
EMR	Elastic MapReduce
EMR	Hectronic medical record
GPU	raphics processing units
HIPAA	Health Insurance Portability and Accountability Act
HPC	High-Performance Computing
IaaS	Infrastructure as a Service
IDaaS	Identity as a Service
IT	Information Technology
MPI	Message-Passing Interface
NGS	Next-Generation Sequence
PaaS	Platform as a Service
RMAP	short read-mapping program
RNA-seq	RNA sequence
SaaS	Software as a Service
scRNA-seq	Single-cell RNA-sequence
SNP	Single Nucleotide Polymorphism
STORMSeq	Scalable Tools for Open-source Read Mapping
VAT	Variant Annotation Tool
VM	Virtual machines

References

1. Ahn, A.C.; Tewari, M.; Poon, C.S.; Phillips, R.S. The limits of reductionism in medicine: Could systems biology offer an alternative? *PLoS Med.* **2006**, *3*, e208. [CrossRef] [PubMed]
2. Loscalzo, J.; Barabasi, A.L. Systems biology and the future of medicine. *Wiley Interdiscip. Rev. Syst. Biol. Med.* **2011**, *3*, 619–627. [CrossRef] [PubMed]
3. Vailati-Riboni, M.; Palombo, V.; Loor, J.J. What are omics sciences? In *Periparturient Diseases of Dairy Cows*; Springer: Berlin/Heidelberg, Germany, 2017; pp. 1–7.
4. Mardis, E.R. Next-generation DNA sequencing methods. *Annu. Rev. Genom. Hum. Genet.* **2008**, *9*, 387–402. [CrossRef] [PubMed]
5. Shendure, J.; Balasubramanian, S.; Church, G.M.; Gilbert, W.; Rogers, J.; Schloss, J.A.; Waterston, R.H. DNA sequencing at 40: Past, present and future. *Nature* **2017**, *550*, 345–353. [CrossRef]
6. D'Adamo, G.L.; Widdop, J.T.; Giles, E.M. The future is now? Clinical and translational aspects of "Omics" technologies. *Immunol. Cell Biol.* **2021**, *99*, 168–176. [CrossRef]
7. Schneider, M.V.; Orchard, S. Omics technologies, data and bioinformatics principles. *Bioinform. Omics Data* **2011**, *719*, 3–30.
8. Clarke, L.; Glendinning, I.; Hempel, R. The MPI message passing interface standard. In *Programming Environments for Massively Parallel Distributed Systems*; Springer: Berlin/Heidelberg, Germany, 1994; pp. 213–218.
9. Kim, W. Cloud computing: Today and tomorrow. *J. Object Technol.* **2009**, *8*, 65–72. [CrossRef]
10. Dillon, T.; Wu, C.; Chang, E. Cloud computing: Issues and challenges. In Proceedings of the 2010 24th IEEE International Conference on Advanced Information Networking and Applications, Perth, WA, Australia, 20–23 April 2010; pp. 27–33.
11. Pautasso, C.; Wilde, E. RESTful web services: Principles, patterns, emerging technologies. In Proceedings of the 19th International Conference on World Wide Web, Raleigh, NC, USA, 26–30 April 2010; pp. 1359–1360.
12. Cusumano, M. Cloud computing and SaaS as new computing platforms. *Commun. ACM* **2010**, *53*, 27–29. [CrossRef]
13. Pahl, C. Containerization and the paas cloud. *IEEE Cloud Comput.* **2015**, *2*, 24–31. [CrossRef]
14. Bhardwaj, S.; Jain, L.; Jain, S. Cloud computing: A study of infrastructure as a service (IAAS). *Int. J. Eng. Inf. Technol.* **2010**, *2*, 60–63.
15. Woitsch, R.; Utz, W. Business process as a service (BPaaS). In Proceedings of the Conference on e-Business, e-Services and e-Society, Delft, The Netherlands, 13–15 October 2015; pp. 435–440.

16. Rajesh, S.; Swapna, S.; Reddy, P.S. Data as a service (daas) in cloud computing. *Glob. J. Comput. Sci. Technol.* **2012**, *12*, 25–29.

17. Ni, Y.; Xing, C.L.; Zhang, K. Connectivity as a service: Outsourcing Enterprise connectivity over cloud computing environment. In Proceedings of the 2011 International Conference on Computer and Management (CAMAN), Wuhan, China, 19–21 May 2011; pp. 1–7.

18. Ducatel, G. Identity as a service: A cloud based common capability. In Proceedings of the 2015 IEEE Conference on Communications and Network Security (CNS), Florence, Italy, 28–30 September 2015; pp. 675–679.

19. Krampis, K.; Booth, T.; Chapman, B.; Tiwari, B.; Bicak, M.; Field, D.; Nelson, K.E. Cloud BioLinux: Pre-configured and on-demand bioinformatics computing for the genomics community. *BMC Bioinform.* **2012**, *13*, 42. [CrossRef]

20. Agapito, G.; Cannataro, M.; Guzzi, P.H.; Marozzo, F.; Talia, D.; Trunfio, P. Cloud4SNP: Distributed analysis of SNP microarray data on the cloud. In Proceedings of the International Conference on Bioinformatics, Computational Biology and Biomedical Informatics, Washington, DC, USA, 22–25 September 2013; pp. 468–475.

21. Guzzi, P.H.; Agapito, G.; Di Martino, M.T.; Arbitrio, M.; Tassone, P.; Tagliaferri, P.; Cannataro, M. DMET-analyzer: Automatic analysis of Affymetrix DMET data. *BMC Bioinform.* **2012**, *13*, 258. [CrossRef]

22. Marozzo, F.; Talia, D.; Trunfio, P. A Cloud Framework for Big Data Analytics Workflows on Azure. In *Proceedings of the Post-Proceedings of the High Performance Computing Workshop 2012*; Catlett, C., Gentzsch, W., Grandinetti, L., Joubert, G., Vazquez-Poletti, J.L., Eds.; IOS Press: Cetraro, Italy, 2013; Volume 23, pp. 182–191, ISBN 978-1-61499-321-6.

23. Marozzo, F.; Talia, D.; Trunfio, P. Using clouds for scalable knowledge discovery applications. In Proceedings of the European Conference on Parallel Processing, Aachen, Germany, 26–30 August 2013; pp. 220–227.

24. Schatz, M.C. CloudBurst: Highly sensitive read mapping with MapReduce. *Bioinformatics* **2009**, *25*, 1363–1369. [CrossRef]

25. Dean, J.; Ghemawat, S. MapReduce: Simplified data processing on large clusters. *Commun. ACM* **2008**, *51*, 107–113. [CrossRef]

26. Afgan, E.; Chapman, B.; Taylor, J. CloudMan as a platform for tool, data, and analysis distribution. *BMC Bioinform.* **2012**, *13*, 315. [CrossRef]

27. Afgan, E.; Lonie, A.; Taylor, J.; Goonasekera, N. CloudLaunch: Discover and deploy cloud applications. *Future Gener. Comput. Syst.* **2019**, *94*, 802–810. [CrossRef]

28. Afgan, E.; Baker, D.; Coraor, N.; Chapman, B.; Nekrutenko, A.; Taylor, J. Galaxy CloudMan: Delivering cloud compute clusters. In Proceedings of the BMC Bioinformatics, Boston, MA, USA, 9–10 July 2010; Volume 11, pp. 1–6.

29. Langmead, B.; Schatz, M.; Lin, J.; Pop, M.; Salzberg, S. Searching for snps with cloud computing. *Genome Biol.* **2009**, *10*, R134. [CrossRef]

30. Li, R.; Li, Y.; Fang, X.; Yang, H.; Wang, J.; Kristiansen, K.; Wang, J. SNP detection for massively parallel whole-genome resequencing. *Genome Res.* **2009**, *19*, 1124–1132. [CrossRef]

31. Jourdren, L.; Bernard, M.; Dillies, M.A.; Le Crom, S. Eoulsan: A cloud computing-based framework facilitating high throughput sequencing analyses. *Bioinformatics* **2012**, *28*, 1542–1543. [CrossRef]

32. Lehmann, N.; Perrin, S.; Wallon, C.; Bauquet, X.; Deshaies, V.; Firmo, C.; Du, R.; Berthelier, C.; Hernandez, C.; Michaud, C.; et al. Eoulsan 2: An efficient workflow manager for reproducible bulk, long-read and single-cell transcriptomics analyses. *bioRxiv* **2021**. [CrossRef]

33. Ehwerhemuepha, L.; Gasperino, G.; Bischoff, N.; Taraman, S.; Chang, A.; Feaster, W. HealtheDataLab—A cloud computing solution for data science and advanced analytics in healthcare with application to predicting multi-center pediatric readmissions. *BMC Med. Informatics Decis. Mak.* **2020**, *20*, 115. [CrossRef] [PubMed]

34. Liu, L.; Chen, W.; Nie, M.; Zhang, F.; Wang, Y.; He, A.; Wang, X.; Yan, G. iMAGE cloud: Medical image processing as a service for regional healthcare in a hybrid cloud environment. *Environ. Health Prev. Med.* **2016**, *21*, 563–571. [CrossRef] [PubMed]

35. Feng, X.; Grossman, R.; Stein, L. PeakRanger: A cloud-enabled peak caller for ChIP-seq data. *BMC Bioinform.* **2011**, *12*, 139. [CrossRef]

36. Karczewski, K.J.; Fernald, G.H.; Martin, A.R.; Snyder, M.; Tatonetti, N.P.; Dudley, J.T. STORMSeq: An open-source, user-friendly pipeline for processing personal genomics data in the cloud. *PloS ONE* **2014**, *9*, e84860. [CrossRef]

37. Habegger, L.; Balasubramanian, S.; Chen, D.Z.; Khurana, E.; Sboner, A.; Harmanci, A.; Rozowsky, J.; Clarke, D.; Snyder, M.; Gerstein, M. VAT: A computational framework to functionally annotate variants in personal genomes within a cloud-computing environment. *Bioinformatics* **2012**, *28*, 2267–2269. [CrossRef]

38. Roberts, R.J. PubMed Central: The GenBank of the published literature. *Proc. Natl. Acad. Sci. USA* **2001**, *98*, 381–382. [CrossRef]

39. Oliveros, J.C. VENNY. An Interactive Tool for Comparing Lists with Venn Diagrams. 2007. Available online: http://bioinfogp.cnb.csic.es/tools/venny/index.html (accessed on 15 March 2023).

40. Calabrese, B.; Cannataro, M. Cloud computing in healthcare and biomedicine. *Scalable Comput. Pract. Exp.* **2015**, *16*, 1–18. [CrossRef]

41. Pezoulas, V.C.; Goules, A.; Kalatzis, F.; Chatzis, L.; Kourou, K.D.; Venetsanopoulou, A.; Exarchos, T.P.; Gandolfo, S.; Votis, K.; Zampeli, E.; et al. Addressing the clinical unmet needs in primary Sjögren's Syndrome through the sharing, harmonization and federated analysis of 21 European cohorts. *Comput. Struct. Biotechnol. J.* **2022**, *20*, 471–484. [CrossRef]

42. Bukowski, M.; Farkas, R.; Beyan, O.; Moll, L.; Hahn, H.; Kiessling, F.; Schmitz-Rode, T. Implementation of eHealth and AI integrated diagnostics with multidisciplinary digitized data: Are we ready from an international perspective? *Eur. Radiol.* **2020**, *30*, 5510–5524. [CrossRef]

43. Shneiderman, B. Human-centered artificial intelligence: Reliable, safe & trustworthy. *Int. J. Hum. Comput. Interact.* **2020**, *36*, 495–504.

44. Wu, Z.; Xuan, S.; Xie, J.; Lin, C.; Lu, C. How to ensure the confidentiality of electronic medical records on the cloud: A technical perspective. *Comput. Biol. Med.* **2022**, *147*, 105726. [CrossRef]
45. Gkoulalas-Divanis, A.; Loukides, G. *Anonymization of Electronic Medical Records to Support Clinical Analysis*; Springer: Berlin/Heidelberg, Germany, 2012.
46. Majeed, A.; Lee, S. Anonymization techniques for privacy preserving data publishing: A comprehensive survey. *IEEE Access* **2020**, *9*, 8512–8545. [CrossRef]
47. Ayoub, F.; Singh, K. Cryptographic techniques and network security. In *Proceedings of the IEE Proceedings F-Communications, Radar and Signal Processing*; IEEE: Piscataway, NJ, USA, 1984; Volume 7, pp. 684–694.
48. Hassan, J.; Shehzad, D.; Habib, U.; Aftab, M.U.; Ahmad, M.; Kuleev, R.; Mazzara, M. The Rise of Cloud Computing: Data Protection, Privacy, and Open Research Challenges—A Systematic Literature Review (SLR). *Comput. Intell. Neurosci.* **2022**, *2022*, 8303504. [CrossRef]
49. Forouzan, B.A.; Mukhopadhyay, D. *Cryptography and Network Security*; Mc Graw Hill Education Private Limited: New York, NY, USA, 2015; Volume 12.
50. Abood, O.G.; Guirguis, S.K. A survey on cryptography algorithms. *Int. J. Sci. Res. Publ.* **2018**, *8*, 495–516. [CrossRef]
51. Gordon, A.D.; Jeffrey, A. Types and effects for asymmetric cryptographic protocols. *J. Comput. Secur.* **2004**, *12*, 435–483. [CrossRef]
52. Biryukov, A.; Perrin, L. State of the art in lightweight symmetric cryptography. *Cryptol. ePrint Arch.* **2017**. Available online: https://eprint.iacr.org/2017/511 (accessed on 15 March 2023)
53. Rahmani, M.K.I.; Shuaib, M.; Alam, S.; Siddiqui, S.T.; Ahmad, S.; Bhatia, S.; Mashat, A. Blockchain-Based Trust Management Framework for Cloud Computing-Based Internet of Medical Things (IoMT): A Systematic Review. *Comput. Intell. Neurosci.* **2022**, *2022*, 9766844. [CrossRef]
54. Ismail, L.; Materwala, H.; Hennebelle, A. A scoping review of integrated blockchain-cloud (BcC) architecture for healthcare: Applications, challenges and solutions. *Sensors* **2021**, *21*, 3753. [CrossRef]
55. Metcalf, D.; Milliard, S.T.; Gomez, M.; Schwartz, M. Wearables and the Internet of Things for Health: Wearable, Interconnected Devices Promise More Efficient and Comprehensive Health Care. *IEEE Pulse* **2016**, *7*, 35–39. [CrossRef]
56. Kibiwott, K.P.; Zhao, Y.; Kogo, J.; Zhang, F. Verifiable fully outsourced attribute-based signcryption system for IoT eHealth big data in cloud computing. *Math. Biosci. Eng.* **2019**, *16*, 3561–3594. [CrossRef]
57. Barillaro, L.; Agapito, G.; Cannataro, M. Edge-based Deep Learning in Medicine: Classification of ECG signals. In Proceedings of the 2022 IEEE International Conference on Bioinformatics and Biomedicine (BIBM), Las Vegas, NV, USA, 6–8 December 2022; pp. 2169–2174.
58. Crespo-Cepeda, R.; Agapito, G.; Vazquez-Poletti, J.L.; Cannataro, M. Challenges and Opportunities of Amazon Serverless Lambda Services in Bioinformatics. In Proceedings of the 10th ACM International Conference on Bioinformatics, Computational Biology and Health Informatics, Niagara Falls, NY, USA, 7–10 September 2019; pp. 663–668. [CrossRef]
59. Aloi, G.; Fortino, G.; Gravina, R.; Pace, P.; Savaglio, C. Simulation-driven platform for Edge-based AAL systems. *IEEE J. Sel. Areas Commun.* **2020**, *39*, 446–462. [CrossRef]
60. Casadei, R.; Fortino, G.; Pianini, D.; Placuzzi, A.; Savaglio, C.; Viroli, M. A methodology and simulation-based toolchain for estimating deployment performance of smart collective services at the edge. *IEEE Internet Things J.* **2022**, *9*, 20136–20148. [CrossRef]
61. Barillaro, L.; Agapito, G.; Cannataro, M. Scalable Deep Learning for Healthcare: Methods and Applications. In Proceedings of the 13th ACM International Conference on Bioinformatics, Computational Biology and Health Informatics, Northbrook, IL, USA, 7–10 August 2022. [CrossRef]
62. Savaglio, C.; Fortino, G. A simulation-driven methodology for IoT data mining based on edge computing. *ACM Trans. Internet Technol. (TOIT)* **2021**, *21*, 1–22. [CrossRef]
63. Bertuccio, S.; Tardiolo, G.; Giambò, F.M.; Giuffrè, G.; Muratore, R.; Settimo, C.; Raffa, A.; Rigano, S.; Bramanti, A.; Muscarà, N.; et al. ReportFlow: An application for EEG visualization and reporting using cloud platform. *BMC Med. Inform. Decis. Mak.* **2021**, *21*, 7. [CrossRef] [PubMed]
64. Mehrtak, M.; SeyedAlinaghi, S.; MohsseniPour, M.; Noori, T.; Karimi, A.; Shamsabadi, A.; Heydari, M.; Barzegary, A.; Mirzapour, P.; Soleymanzadeh, M.; et al. Security challenges and solutions using healthcare cloud computing. *J. Med. Life* **2021**, *14*, 448. [CrossRef]

MDPI
St. Alban-Anlage 66
4052 Basel
Switzerland
Tel. +41 61 683 77 34
Fax +41 61 302 89 18
www.mdpi.com

Big Data and Cognitive Computing Editorial Office
E-mail: bdcc@mdpi.com
www.mdpi.com/journal/bdcc

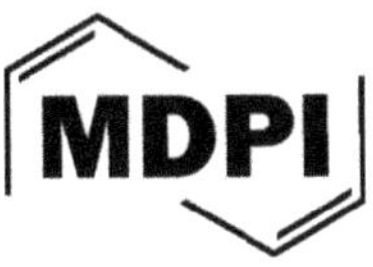